AF652484

# SOCIAL WORK PRACTICES IN HEALTH AND MEDICAL PROFESSION

# SOCIAL WORK PRACTICES IN HEALTH AND MEDICAL PROFESSION

by
**Dr. I. Sundar**
Reader in Economics
Directorate of Distance Education
Annamalai University
Tamil Nadu, India

**SARUP BOOK PUBLISHERS PVT. LTD.**
NEW DELHI - 110002

*Published by*
**SARUP BOOK PUBLISHERS PVT. LTD.**
4740/23, Ansari Road
Darya Ganj, New Delhi-110002
Tel. : 23281029, 23244664, 41010989
Fax : 011-23277098
E-mail : sarupandsonsin@hotmail.com.
Website: www.sarupbooks.com

*Social Work Practices in Health and Medical Profession*

© *Editor*
1st Published 2009
ISBN-978-81-7625-982-8

Printed in India
Published by Prabhat Kumar Sharma
for Sarup Book Publishers Pvt. Ltd.
Laser Typesetting at Chitra Computers and
Printed at Mehra Offset Printers, Delhi

# Preface

Social work provides persons, families, or vulnerable populations with the psychosocial support needed to cope with chronic acute, or terminal illnesses, such as Alzheimer's, cancer, or AIDS. Services include advising family care givers, providing patient education and counseling, and making necessary referrals for other social services.

Social work prepares individuals for the professional practice of social welfare administration and counseling, and that focus on the study of organized means of providing basic support services for vulnerable individuals and groups. It Includes instruction in social welfare policy; case work planning; social counseling and intervention strategies; administrative procedures and regulations; and specific applications in areas such as child welfare and family services, probation, employment services, and disability counseling.

Clinical or Medical Social Work prepares individuals for the specialized professional practice of social work, in collaboration with other health care professionals, in hospitals and other health care facilities and organizations. It includes instruction in social work, psychiatric case work, clinical interviewing techniques, therapeutic intervention strategies, patient testing and evaluation, patient and family counseling, social rehabilitation, patient care planning, record-keeping, and support services liaison. This book is organized in 13 chapters. The first chapter deals with Origin and Development of Social Work. This chapter discusses modern social work, the development of social work, types of professional intervention, concept of medical social work,

work settings, advanced education and training, future outlook and typical tasks. The second chapter discusses public health. It covers topics such as history of Public Health, the dawn of history to the fall of Rome, the dark ages and the medieval period, the renaissance and the plague centuries, the enlightenment and sanitary reform, medical sociology, bacteriology, colonialism and public health, the early twentieth century and evaluation of public health programs. The third chapter narrates about Interdisciplinary Approach to Health and Medicine. It analyses application of social theories in analyzing the phenomena of health and medicine, opportunities of development of medical sociology, sociology in public health, sociological concepts in public health and sociology and evaluation in public health. The fourth chapter is Medical Social Theory. It analyses medical ideology, professional social control, the traditional format of the medical encounter and critical theory of medical discourse. The fifth chapter discusses Social Workers in Public Health. It covers topics such as Social Work Guiding Principles, Case Management, Continuity of Care, Health Care Settings, Health Planning and Public Health Model. The sixth chapter deals with Hospital Social Work. It explains the professional skills, personal characteristics and hospital work plan. The seventh chapter makes a detailed discussion on Clinical Social Work. In this chapter we see Goals of the Standards, Clinical Social Work, Psychotherapy, Therapy and Hospitalization Risk Assessment. The eighth chapter explains Genetics and Medical Social Work Practice. The ninth chapter discusses about Community Health. The tenth chapter deals with Community Health Workers and this chapter discusses factors that affect community and population health and three tools of community health practice. The eleventh chapter is Social Epidemiology. It discusses current theoretical trends in social epidemiology, psychosocial theory, social production of disease or political economy of health, ecosocial theory and related multilevel dynamic perspectives, two types of theory for the practice of epidemiology and theory matters. Twelfth chapter is

Bioethics in Medical profession and last chapter explain Clinical Ethics.

I express my sincere gratitude to our revered Vice Chancellor Dr. M. Ramanathan and S.B. Nageshwara Rao, Director, Directorate of Distance Education of Annamalai University who have been the source of constant inspiration. I express my sincere gratitude to Dr. N. Malathi, Professor and Head, Department of Economics, Dr. D. Namasivayam, Professor and Economics Wing Head, Directorate of Distance Education, Annamalai University for their constant encouragement.

It is with heart and soul that I thank to Shri. Prabhat Kumar Sharma, Proprietor Sarup Book Publishers Pvt. Ltd., New Delhi for evincing keen interest in publishing this book.

**Dr. I. Sundar**

# Contents

# Contents

# 1

# Origin and Development of Social Work

Social work in health care helps people who are dealing with a medical problem to function within their situation. The who specializes in health care works with clients and their families to provide services necessary to make their lives easier for the duration of the client's illness, and to help them deal with the consequences directly related to that illness?

The profession of social work is dedicated to a set of core values. These values include social justice, service, dignity and worth of the person, importance of human relationships, integrity, and competence, and they form the foundation of social work. Social workers in the medical field provide a wide variety of services to clients who are going through a short-term medical crisis, suffering from facing a life-threatening disease, or in need of long-term care or rehabilitation.

The main concern of the social worker is to assist the client and the client's family in coping with their health care situation. Clients are faced with many problems when they have an accident, contract a sudden and debilitating illness, or are diagnosed with a chronic or life-threatening disease. Social workers help them assess these problems, identify their immediate and long-term needs, and find to supply the needs.

If the social worker is working in a hospital, these duties may include setting up home health care services after the client's discharge, arranging for meals to be delivered to the client's home, and setting appointments for follow-up care. The worker may also make arrangements for transportation to doctor's appointments and community social service agencies, and for long-term care within another facility. Organized work intended to advance the social conditions of a community, and especially of the disadvantaged, by providing psychological counseling, guidance, and assistance, especially in the form of social services.

In the public health arena, social workers are a valuable resource for the development of treatment plans for patients, for locating supportive resources, and in facilitating referrals. Under the auspices of government and non-government public health organizations and institutions, social workers often provide behavioural and social assessments along with mental health assessment, treatment, and short-term or ongoing case management. Social workers may also work in the community as planners or community organizers capable of engaging groups of people, neighbourhoods, or entire communities to address social problems such as drug abuse or teen pregnancy. Social work is a distinct profession, requiring college training, and a masters degree is often a necessity.

Any of various professional activities or methods concerned with providing social services such as investigatory and treatment services or material aid to disadvantaged, distressed, or vulnerable persons or groups. The field originated in the charity organizations in Europe and the U.S. in the late 19th century. The training of volunteer workers by these organizations led directly to the founding of the first schools of social work and indirectly to increased government responsibility for the welfare of the disadvantaged. Social service providers may serve the needs of children and families, the poor or homeless, immigrants, veterans, the mentally ill, the handicapped, victims of rape or domestic violence, and persons dependent on alcohol or drugs.

The profession of social work emerged in the early twentieth century as charitable organizations began employing trained workers rather than relying on volunteers. Pioneers developed two competing approaches for addressing social problems. Early social workers took that as a challenge and mobilized workers to produce professional literature, organizations, and a code of ethics.

The profession of social work responds to wider historical changes, shifting its focus from environmental reform to individual change, as the nation's social climate fluctuates. For example, social workers aimed to radically change institutions and rejected the traditional establishment during the Progressive Era of the 1900s, the depression of the 1930s, and the social unrest of the 1960s. However, in more conservative times, such as the 1920s, 1950s and 1980s, the profession attended to direct service and individual change. In the 1920s, social workers debated whether the profession would include caseworkers across a broad range of fields or limit membership to professional elite with high educational standards. The latter position won, and social workers were required to complete masters-level training.

Entry-level social workers are trained as generalists and are expected to provide service to a broad range of clients, maintain a wide scope of knowledge, and practice a great diversity of skills. Advanced practitioners with graduate-level training may specialize in areas such as clinical, medical, or school social work, as well as planning and development, aging, mental health, or corrections. In the late 1960s and 1970s, states began establishing licensing requirements to legally regulate practice. While all states require some form of licensure, current trends are moving toward "declassification": downgrading requirements for social work in order to employ persons with neither a license nor a degree to do case management and other functions traditionally reserved for social workers.

## Modern Social Work

Modern social work employs three methods of assistance: case work, group work, and community organization. Case work is the method by which individual persons and families are assisted. The person in need of case work may be physically, mentally, or socially handicapped. Among those regarded as socially handicapped are: the unemployed, the homeless, members of broken families, alcoholics, drug addicts, and neglected or problem children. To determine the cause of maladjustment, the social worker must understand individual psychology as well as the sociology of the community. Physicians, psychiatrists, and other specialists may be required to help diagnose the difficulty.

Social group work is exemplified by the social settlement, the supervised playground and gymnasium, and the classroom, where handicrafts may be learned. The community may be called upon to provide the buildings and grounds for such activities; often the services of volunteers and of public groups are utilized; in recent years people living in poverty areas have been employed to work in and direct poverty projects in their own communities. Through community organization the welfare work of single agencies as well as of whole communities is directed, cooperation between public and private agencies is secured, and funds are raised and administered. The funds required by private agencies are often pooled in a community chest, from which each agency receives a share. Community welfare councils are organized to map programs of rehabilitation, to eliminate duplication of services, and to discover and meet overlooked needs.

## The Development of Social Work

Social work emerged as a profession out of the early efforts of churches and philanthropic groups to relieve the effects of poverty, to bring the comforts of religion to the poor, to promote temperance and encourage thrift, to care for children, the sick, and the aged, and to correct the delinquent. Orphanages and homes for the elderly were typical results of these activities. The word *charity* best describes the early activities, which were aimed at the piecemeal alleviation of particular maladjustments. In such charitable work the principal criterion in determining aid to families was worthiness, while the emphasis in later social work was on restoring individuals to normal life both for their own sake and for the sake of the community.

The first attempts to solve the problem of poverty in a modern scientific way was made by P. G. F. Le Play, who in the 1850s made a detailed study of the budgets of hundreds of French workers' families. Forty years later Charles Booth investigated wages and prices, working conditions, housing and health, standards of living, and leisure activities among the poor of London and revealed the extreme poverty of a third of the population. Booth's social survey became a method for determining the extent of social maladjustment, and through surveys in other cities in Europe and the United States a vast number of facts were accumulated, and methods were developed that provided the basis for modern social work.

Social work is a social science involving the application of social theory and research methods to study and improve the lives of people, groups, and societies. It incorporates and uses other social sciences as a means to improve the human condition and positively change society's response to chronic problems. Social work is a profession committed to the pursuit of social justice, to the enhancement of the quality of life, and to the development of the full potential of each individual, group and community in the society. It seeks to simultaneously address and resolve social issues at every level of society and economic status, but especially among the poor and sick. Social workers are concerned with social problems, their causes, their solutions and their human impacts. They work with individuals, families, groups, organizations and communities.

Social work and human history go together. Social work was always in human societies although it began to be a defined pursuit and profession in the 19th century. This definition was in response to societal problems that resulted from the Industrial Revolution and an increased interest in applying scientific theory to various aspects of study. Eventually an increasing number of educational institutions began to offer social work programmes. The settlement movement's emphasis on advocacy and case work became part of social work practice. During the 20th century, the profession began to rely more on research and evidence-based practice as it attempted to improve its professionalism. Today social workers are employed in a myriad of pursuits and settings. Professional social workers are generally considered those who hold a professional degree in social work and often also have a license or are professionally registered. Social workers have organized themselves into local, national, and international professional bodies to further the aims of the profession.

Social work has its roots in the struggle of society to deal with poverty and the resultant problems. Therefore, social work is intricately linked with the idea of charity work; but must be understood in broader terms. The concept of charity goes back to ancient times, and the practice of providing for the poor has roots in all major world religions. Social Work Education begins in a systematised manner in universities, but is also an ongoing process that occurs though research and in the workplace.

The International Federation of Social Workers states, of social work today, social work bases its methodology on a systematic body of evidence-based knowledge derived from research and practice evaluation, including local and indigenous knowledge specific to its context. It recognizes the complexity of interactions between human beings and their environment, and the capacity of people both to be affected by and to alter the multiple influences upon them including bio-psychosocial factors. The social work profession draws on theories of human development and behaviour and social systems to analyse complex situations and to facilitate individual, organizational, social and cultural changes.

The current state of social work professional development is characterized by two realities. There is a great deal of traditional social and psychological research both qualitative and quantitative being carried out primarily by university-based researchers and by researchers based in institutes, foundations, or social service agencies. Meanwhile, many social work practitioners continue to look to their own experience for knowledge. This is a continuation of the debate that has persisted since the outset of the profession in the first decade of the twentieth century. One reason for the gap between information obtained through practice, as opposed to through research, is that practitioners deal with situations that are unique and idiosyncratic, while research concentrates on similarities. The combining of these two types of knowledge is often imperfect. A hopeful development for bridging this gap is the compilation, in many practice fields, of collections of "best practices" which attempt to distill research findings and the experience of respected practitioners into effective practice techniques. Although social work has roots in the informatics revolution, an important contemporary development in the profession is overcoming suspicion of technology and taking advantage of the potential of information technology to empower clients.

Professional social workers have a strong tradition of working for social justice and of refusing to recreate unequal social structures The main tasks of professional social workers can include a variety of services such as case management linking clients with agencies and programs that will meet their psychosocial needs, medical social work, counseling psychotherapy, human services management, social welfare policy analysis, community organizing, advocacy, teaching in schools of social work, and social science research, Professional social workers work in a variety of non-profit, for-profit, or public social service settings, including: grassroots advocacy organizations, hospitals, hospices, community health agencies, schools, faith-based organizations, employee assistance, philanthropy, and even the military. Some social workers work as psychotherapists, counselors, or mental health practitioners, often working in collaboration with psychiatrists, psychologists, or other medical professionals. Social workers may also work independently as private practice psychotherapists in the United States and are able to bill most third party payers such as insurance companies. Additionally, some social workers focus their efforts on social policy or conduct academic research into the practice or ethics of social work. The emphasis has varied among these task areas by historical era and country. Some of these areas have been the subject of controversy as to whether they are properly part of social work's mission.

A variety of settings employ social workers, including governmental departments especially in the areas of child and family welfare, mental health, correctional services, and education departments, hospitals, non-government welfare agencies and private practice — working independently as counselors, family therapists or researchers.

## Types of Professional Intervention

There are three general categories or levels of intervention. The first is "Macro" social work which involves society or communities as a whole. This type of social work practice would include policy forming and advocacy on a national or international scale. The second level of intervention is described as "Mezzo" social work practice. This level would involve work with agencies, small organizations, and other small groups. This practice would include policymaking within a social work agency or developing programs for a particular neighborhood. The final level is the "Micro" level that involves service to individuals and families.

There are a wide variety of activities that can be considered social work and professional social workers are employed in many different types of environments. In general, social workers employed in clinical or direct practice work on a micro level. Social workers who serve in community practice are occupied in the mezzo or macro levels of social work.

## Concept of Medical Social Work

Social work research addresses psychosocial problems, preventive interventions, treatment of acute and chronic conditions, and community, organizational, policy and administrative issues. Covering the lifespan, social work research may address clinical, services and policy issues. It benefits consumers, practitioners, policymakers, educators, and the general public by: Examining prevention and intervention strategies for health and mental health, child welfare, aging, substance abuse, community development, managed care, housing, economic self-sufficiency, family well-being, etc.; Studying the strengths, needs, and inter-relationships of individuals, families, groups, neighborhoods, and social institutions; and providing evidence for improved service delivery and public policies.

Recent contributions from social work research include studies that address:

- Psychosocial assessment and intervention strategies for persons at risk of and living with cancer

- Access to mental health services for youths in urban and rural settings
- Depression among elders in long-term care and home health care settings
- HIV/AIDS prevention and intervention in urban communities
- School-based violence prevention efforts targeted to youths
- Risk factors associated with poverty and mental illness
- Community-based child maltreatment prevention models
- Resilience factors for diverse groups experiencing trauma
- Co-occurring disorders of substance abuse and mental illness
- Assessment and interventions for individuals dealing with the multiple risk factors associated with poverty and domestic violence

**Work Settings**

Duties of the social worker vary with the health care setting. Medical social workers may work in a hospital, hospice, assisted living center, nursing home, physical rehabilitation center, clinic, home health care agency, or drug rehabilitation or mental health center. Social workers may work in the health care facility or make home visits to work with their clients. They often work with other agencies and have to travel short distances for meetings with the agency members. Social workers confer with other agency workers or with health care team members to assess client needs and to make plans for the client's care.

Hours of work vary for the social worker, depending upon the facility or agency within which he is employed.

Usually the work hours are between 8 a.m. and 5 p.m. Monday through Friday, but the worker may be required to work hours as needed for emergencies. In larger urban areas or rural areas, the social worker may also be required to work during evening hours and on weekends to better serve the clients.

## Advanced Education and Training

Social education work qualifies the social worker to make clinical assessments, choose an area of specialization, manage large caseloads, and supervise social workers with lesser degrees.

## Future Outlook

Social work is a growing profession. The occupational outlook is optimistic. There are several reasons why the field of social work in health care continues to grow: the aging population of "baby boomers" advanced medical treatment longer life expectancy growth of home health care due to growing trend of early release of patients from hospitals replacement of workers seeking career change stress and burnout among social workers causing them to leave profession and increase in population of people living with AIDS

**Medical Social Work** is a sub-discipline of social work, also known as Hospital social work. Medical social workers typically work in a hospital, skilled nursing facility or hospice, have a graduate degree in the field, and work with patients and their families in need of psychosocial help. Medical social workers assess the psychosocial functioning of patients and families and intervene as necessary. Interventions may include connecting patients and families to necessary resources and supports in the community; providing psychotherapy, supportive counseling, or grief counseling; or helping a patient to expand and strengthen their network of social supports. Medical social workers typically work on an interdisciplinary team with professionals of other disciplines such as medicine, nursing, physical, occupational, speech and recreational therapy, etc.

The medical social worker has a critical role in the area of discharge planning. It is the medical social worker's responsibility to ensure that the services the patient requires are in place in order to facilitate a timely discharge and prevent delays in discharge that can cost the hospital thousands of per day.

Other skills required of the medical social worker is an ability to work cooperatively with other health care staff as part of a multidisciplinary treatment team, good analytical and assessment skills, an ability to communicate clearly with both patients and staff, an ability to quickly engage the patient in a therapeutic relationship, an ability to process almost an never-ending flow of paperwork, and a willingness to advocate for the patient, especially in situations where the medical social worker has identified a problem that may compromise the discharge and put the patient at risk in the community. For example, the medical doctor reports that a frail elderly patient is medically cleared for discharge and plans to discharge the patient home with home care services. However, after assessing the patient's psychosocial needs, the medical social worker determines that the patient does not have the requisite ability to direct a home care worker and recommends that the discharge be deferred pending further assessment of this problem. In such a case, it is the medical social worker's ethical duty to inform the medical doctor that the discharge may place the patient at risk and advocate for another, more appropriate discharge even if it means that the patient's discharge has to be postponed. It is precisely in such cases that the medical social worker proves his or her worth — by placing the needs of the patient above all other considerations.

Advocate for clients or patients to resolve crises. Collaborate with other professionals to evaluate patients' medical or physical condition and to assess client needs. Refer patient, client, or family to community resources to assist in recovery from mental or physical illness and to provide access to services such as financial assistance, legal aid, housing, job placement or education. Counsel clients and patients in individual and group sessions to help them overcome dependencies, recover from illness, and adjust to life. Utilize consultation data and social work experience to plan and coordinate client or patient care and rehabilitation, following through to ensure service efficacy. Plan discharge from care facility to home or other care facility. Organize support groups or counsel family members to assist them in understanding, dealing with, and supporting the client or patient. Modify treatment plans to comply with changes in clients' status. Monitor, evaluate, and record client progress according to measurable goals described in treatment and care plan and Identify environmental impediments to client or patient progress through interviews and review of patient records.

**Typical Tasks**

Interviews clinic patients and parents to obtain social data relating to problems of the patients; prepares case histories of patients receiving treatment; participates in staff conferences with other members of the clinic staff to interpret information collected and to specify the possible effect of social factors in the patient's personality and adjustment problems; recommends admission, discharge, or referral of patients or clients to other agencies or treatment units; executes social treatment phase of total treatment program as determined by diagnostic staff; confers periodically with patients or other members of the household to interpret the bearing of social factors on the patient's mental and emotional condition; determines casework services appropriate for families presenting personal adjustment problems; explains the objectives and principles of psychiatric or medical social work to teachers, social workers, civic groups, and the public through talks and round-table discussions; prepares interpretive reports of the social adjustment problems and progress of cases referred to the clinic when requested by relatives, physicians, and referring agencies.

## Typical Tasks

Receive casework referrals from medical and nursing staff, other agencies, relatives and friends of the patient, or the patient Interviews patient, patient's associates, friends and/or relatives to secure relevant social information, and to determine the effect of the illness upon the patient and the patient's family. Attempts to instill feelings of personal significance in the patient, and works with emotional problems, which may hinder acceptance of medical care. Participate as a member of a multidisciplinary treatment team, in ward rounds and therapy conferences to develop problem understanding and effective treatment plans. These plans include consideration of patient, family, and community resources counsels with patient and family relating to hospitalization, discharge and/or rehabilitation. Provides professional guidance and consultation to lower level staff and may assign, review, and coordinate the work of lower level staff.

## Required Knowledge, Skills and Abilities

Knowledge of the principles and techniques of psychiatric or medical social worker including casework methods and techniques knowledge of the functions of social service agencies; Knowledge of the fundamental types and problems of mental retardation and abnormal behavior; Ability to plan and execute casework services; Ability to develop social service resources in a community; Ability to work effectively with other professional disciplines and Ability to establish and maintain effective relationships with professional associations, civic groups and the general public.

As medical social workers often have large caseloads and have to meet tight deadlines to arrange for necessary services, medical social work is a highly demanding job and as a result the turnover rate is high. In addition, medical social worker often confront highly complex cases involving patients with multiple psychosocial issues, all of which requiring intervention and leading to delays in discharge. For instance, in a major urban acute care medical center, it is not uncommon for the medical social worker to assess patients who are simultaneously homeless, without health insurance coverage, have multiple chronic medical and psychiatric conditions, are unemployed, have just been released from incarceration, and have substance abuse problems, all of which, separately and together, can impede timely discharge. Sometimes situations as mundane as the patient needing carfare or shoes can lead to delays in discharge, especially if these needs are not identified early. This is why a complete and timely assessment of the patient's psychosocial needs is critical. Other skills required of the medical social worker is an ability to work cooperatively with other health care staff as part of a multidisciplinary treatment team, good analytical and assessment skills, an ability to communicate clearly with both patients and staff, an ability to quickly engage the patient in a therapeutic relationship, an ability to process almost an neverending flow of paperwork, and a willingness to advocate for the patient, especially in situations where the medical social worker has identified a problem that may compromise the discharge and put the patient at risk in the community. For example, the medical doctor reports that a frail elderly patient is medically cleared for discharge and plans to discharge the patient home with home care services. However, after assessing the patient's psychosocial needs, the medical social worker determines that the patient does not have the requisite ability to direct a home care worker and recommends that the discharge be deferred pending further assessment of this problem. In such a case, it is the medical social worker's ethical duty to inform the medical doctor that the discharge may place the patient at risk and advocate for another, more appropriate discharge even if it means that the patient's discharge has to be postponed. It is precisely in such cases that the medical social worker proves his or her worth — by placing the needs of the patient above all other considerations.

## Definition

Under general supervision, performs the most complex medical social work in coordination with a program of medical care; may act in a lead capacity; and performs related work as required.

## Distinguishing Characteristics

The medical social work classification series is primarily oriented to assisting patients and their families cope with personal and social problems arising as a result of illness and medical care. Positions in this classification may be utilized in the Medical Center or the Health Department.

Medical Social Worker III is the third level classification in this series. This classification differs from Medical Social Worker II in that Medical Social Worker III is utilized to perform the most complex assignments and may act in a lead capacity. In addition, the Medical Social Worker III requires a current California license as a Licensed Clinical Social Worker

Medical Social Worker I is the first level of the Medical Social Worker series. This class is distinguished from the next higher class of Medical Social Worker II primarily by the amount of direction and assistance they receive in their work. Incumbents who meet the minimum qualification for Medical Social Worker II are eligible to be considered for promotion on a merit basis subject to recommendation of the Department Head and approval of the Director of Personnel.

## Essential Functions

### *Dependent upon assignment*

Functions at a highly skilled level in such areas as counseling, medical social work, protective services, family services, community organization and research interviews and counsels patients and relatives in order to determine appropriateness of services, to determine extent of social and emotional problems, and to plan for patient's illness and related problems evaluates problems and makes treatment plans; provides casework and group work treatment for patients Interprets diagnoses and prognoses to patients and their families to insure best adjustment to treatment and/or medical condition counsels patients on rehabilitation and employment programs performs assessments and provides information for use in diagnosis and treatment and participates in research projects, mental health educational programs, treatment intervention and assists in discharge transition

Observes effects of current policies and informs supervisor of gaps in the program participates in conferences, meetings and committees cooperates with other agencies to insure adequate resources to assist in the patient's maximum level of functioning and adjustment evaluates patient's community behavior and assists in determining need for further treatment arranges for follow-up care prepares case records, reports, and correspondence develops the cultural competency program in the internal medicine department develops professional interviewing skills for residents of the internal medicine department and dependent upon area of practice or department assignments, demonstrates clinical knowledge and skill in the care of the newborn, infant, toddler, child, adolescent, adult and geriatric patient ranging up to 100+ years of age.

Knowledge of the principles, procedures, techniques, trends and literature of social work; knowledge of social, emotional, behavioral, and economic implications of illness, disease, incapacitation, and disfigurement; knowledge of modern hospital organization and functions; knowledge of general laws relating to health and welfare; ability to evaluate information and form logical and sound conclusions; ability to prepare reports and case records; ability to maintain effective and cooperative relationships with professional personnel, patients and community agencies; ability to interview and obtain accurate personal and psychosocial data for records.

# 2

# Public Health

## History of Public Health

Public health was defined by the American public health leader, Charles-Edward A. Winslow, in 1920 as, "the science and art of preventing disease, prolonging life, and promoting physical health and efficiency through organized community efforts for the sanitation of the environment, the control of community infections, the education of the individual in principles of personal hygiene, the organization of medical and nursing service for the early diagnosis and preventive treatment of disease, and the development of the social machinery which will ensure to every individual in the community a standard of living adequate for the maintenance of health." Although a modern nosologist would add *mental* to *physical* aspects of health, Winslow's definition has not been superseded. It provided the basis for the World Health Organization's definition of health: "A state of complete physical, mental, and social well-being and not merely the absence of disease or infirmity" (1948).

## The Dawn of History to the fall of Rome

Elements of Winslow's concept of public health can be found in the earliest evidence of communal living. Paleopathology, the study of fossils and other artifacts, reveals that early *Homo sapiens*, who were hunter-gatherers, suffered from essentially the same diseases that afflict people today.

In remote parts of the world—in the Amazon, Indonesia, Australia, and Africa—isolated communities exist that anthropologists believe follow lifestyles typical of prehistoric populations. These peoples share the belief that diseases are caused by malevolent supernatural forces. To diagnose, treat, and, in some cases, prevent the spread of these malevolent forces, all primitive societies have created a class of "shamans"—persons specially trained to intervene on the spiritual and physical level. Thus, the most primitive societies provide an "organized" approach to the recognition and management of disease.

The social structure of the earliest primitive villages was probably not very different from that of the earlier hunter—gatherer tribes, and physical amenities were, no doubt, similarly unchanged. However, the establishment of cities brought about major developments. Archaeologists have found that all the great cities of antiquity in Asia, Europe, Africa, and South America had municipal water supplies and sewerage systems. The culmination of ancient sanitary engineering was accomplished in Rome, where aqueducts supplied the city with water in amounts comparable to many modern municipal systems and sewers and drains carried away the wastewater. Part of the great central drain of ancient Rome, the *Cloaca Maxima*, still serves as part of the sewerage of the modern city.

It was the exigencies of urban living, not considerations of health and disease that necessitated sanitary engineering. Supernatural explanations of disease did not evoke or require an environmental origin for disease. However, in the fifth and fourth centuries B.C.E., in Greece, an empirical explanation of disease was proposed by the physician Hippocrates and his followers who described diseases in objective terms, and rejected supernatural causes. In his book *On Airs, Waters, Places*, the relations of disease to physical, social, and behavioral settings are presented for the first time. This book served as a guide for decisions regarding the location of urban sites in the Greco-Roman world, and may be considered the first rational guide to the establishment of a science-based public health.

## The Dark Ages and the Medieval Period

During the Dark Ages (about 500–1000 C.E.), Western Europe experienced a period of social and political disintegration. Large cities disappeared, replaced by small villages surrounding the castles of feudal chiefs. The only unifying force was Christianity, and it was in the monasteries that the learning and culture of the Greco-Roman world was preserved. Furthermore, in many of these institutions, piped water supplies, sanitary sewers, privies, bathing facilities, and heating and ventilation were provided. In addition, some monasteries constructed hospices to shelter travelers and sick persons, though the medical care provided in them was primitive at best. In Eastern Europe and Asia Minor, however, feudalism did not exist, and medicine advanced and became centered in major secular hospitals established in Byzantium, Baghdad, and Cairo.

The most important disease of the period was leprosy, manifested by a continent-wide epidemic beginning in the sixth century and lasting through the fifteenth. Lepers were excluded from communities and segregated. Elaborate rules and regulations were set up to diagnose the disease and isolate cases. Leper houses (leprosaria) were established, and it is estimated that by the end of the twelfth century there were 19,000 such houses throughout Europe. Isolation of cases of leprosy in medieval times represents the earliest application of a public health practice still in use.

By about 1000 C.E., the stagnation in the West gave way to change. Feudal fieldoms were being consolidated into nation states, cities and towns were growing, education was beginning to be secularized, and the Crusades were bringing increased interaction between the Islamic East and the Christian West. As these changes occurred, the responsibility for communal functions was transferred from the feudal lords and ecclesiastic authorities to lay councils presided over by a hierarchy of hereditary or appointed officials. Public health activities, such as overseeing the water supply and sewerage, street cleaning, and supervision of the markets, fell under the jurisdiction of the councils.

The establishment, in Salerno, Italy, of the first organized medical school was indicative of the changes occurring in Western Europe. This institution, founded in the eleventh or twelfth century, was particularly remarkable for two reasons: It was a lay organization, independent of the church, and it welcomed students of any race or creed. Its faculty included women, who apparently dealt with obstetric issues, and the renowned peripatetic scholar, Constantine the African (1020–87), who translated many important Arabic works into Latin. Its most prominent literary product was the *Regimen Sanitatis Salernitanum*, a lengthy poem, prescribing healthy habits from birth to old age. Drawing on the whole corpus of Greco-Roman and Arabian medical writings the *Regimen* emphasized personal hygiene, diet, exercise, and temperance. It was the first "health guide" for the masses.

## The Renaissance and the Plague Centuries

It was during the Renaissance, a period of great commercial, scientific, cultural, and political development, that the bubonic plague, or "Black Death," swept over Europe and the Near East killing an estimated one-fourth to one-third of the population between 1347 and 1351. For the following two-and-a-half centuries, periodic epidemics of plague decimated these populations.

There were other epidemics as well. In the sixteenth century two new diseases, syphilis and the "English sweat," an ill-defined condition, possibly a form of influenza, were widespread in Europe. The ever-present smallpox was transported to the Americas, where it decimated the native populations. These catastrophic events precipitated the three most important contributions to public health of the Renaissance: the organization of boards of health, the promulgation of a theory of contagion, and the introduction of health statistics.

With the recurrence of plague epidemics, it finally became apparent in the cities of Northern Italy that the *ad hoc* arrangements of the city councils were inadequate to deal with these episodes. By the middle of the fifteenth century, the major cities of the region had established permanent boards of health that were responsible for determining the existence of plague, establishing quarantine, issuing health passes, arranging for the burial of plague victims and the fumigation of their residences, and the management of *lazarettos* (houses and institutions of quarantine). The boards maintained close relations with the local physicians who provided medical care and prophylactic advice. As time passed, the boards expanded their purview to the control of markets, sewage systems, water supplies, cemeteries, and the cleanliness of streets; and they took jurisdiction over the professional activities of physicians and surgeons, the preparation and sale of drugs, and the activities of beggars and prostitutes. With the disappearance of plague at the end of the seventeenth century, the boards of health of Northern Italy withered away. Nevertheless, they provided a model for nineteenth-century organization of public health activities.

Although vague theories of the contagious nature of certain diseases had existed since ancient times, it was the Italian physician and scholar, Girolamo Fracastoro who had written an epochal description of syphilis, giving the disease its name, who, in 1546, published *On Contagions and the Cure of Contagious Diseases*. Fracastoro proposed that many diseases are caused by transmissible, self-propagating, disease-specific agents called "germs", viz; seminaria which propagate themselves in tissues of the infected host and cause disease by setting up chemical processes. Most importantly, Fracastoro proposed that germs are spread by direct contact person to person, by contact with fomites, viz; inanimate objects, and by distant transmission.

By early in the fifteenth century, the Italian boards of health instituted a system of death registration, first for contagious diseases and subsequently for all diseases. The resulting bills of mortality have provided continuous data on mortality in Italy from the Renaissance to the present. In seventeenth-century London, analysis of bills of mortality by John Graunt in his epochal treatise *Natural and Political Observations Made upon the Bills of Mortality* (1662) laid the basis for the modern use of statistics for the planning and evaluation of public health activities.

## The Enlightenment and Sanitary Reform

The Enlightenment the period from 1750 until the mid–nineteenth century was characterized by unprecedented industrial, social, and political developments, and the resulting societal impacts were immense, culminating in the Industrial Revolution. It was in Germany that the first major contribution of the period to public health occurred. Between 1779 and 1816, Johann Peter Frank, a leading clinician, medical educator, and hospital administrator, published a six-volume treatise, *System of a Complete Medical Policy*, in which he proposed a sweeping scheme of governmental regulations and programs to protect the population against disease and to promote health. His proposals covered the entire life span from birth to death. The actions that he advocated ranged from measures of personal hygiene and medical care to environmental regulation and social engineering.

Meanwhile, in England, Jeremy Bentham (1748–1832) was enunciating a similar humanitarian social philosophy and consequent political reform. In *Introduction to the Principles of Morals and Legislation* (1789), Bentham argued, among other ideas, that society should be organized for the greatest benefit for the greatest number, viz; Utilitarianism. In his *Constitutional Code* (1830), Bentham proposed radical new legislation dealing with such issues as prison reform, the establishment of a ministry of health, birth control, and a variety of sanitary measures.

Implementing these concepts in the mid–nineteenth century fell to Bentham's disciples, particularly Edwin Chadwick. Chadwick had been secretary of England's Poor Law Commission, established in 1834 to effectuate the New Poor Law, and was aware of the pervading interaction of disease and poverty. Thus, when the Commission undertook a special study in 1839 of the prevalence and causation of preventable diseases, particularly of the working poor, Chadwick took the lead. The resulting publication, *General Report on the Sanitary Condition of the Labouring Population of Great Britain* (1842), is considered one of the most important documents of modern public health.

Chadwick documented the status of housing of the working population, the lack of sewerage and adequate supplies of water, the unhygienic circumstances of places of work, the life expectancy of various social classes, the economic impact of unsanitary conditions, and the evidence for the beneficial health effects of preventive measures. As a result, sewerage, potable and plentiful water supplies, refuse disposal, proper ventilation of residences and places of work, supervision of public works by qualified professionals, and legislative authorization of measures to obtain these results were put forward.

Chadwick's report was widely circulated and carefully considered. In the United States, it stimulated a similar survey based on more sophisticated survey methods and with more comprehensive recommendations. The *Report of a General Plan for the Promotion of Public and Personal Health* (1850), authored by the organizer and first president of the American Statistical Association, Lemuel Shattuck, put forward fifty recommendations many still worthy of implementation but not yet realized and a model state public health law. Although both of these reports impacted national and local legislation, their more enduring effect was to define the purview and establish the organizational framework of the field of public health in the late nineteenth and early twentieth centuries.

## Medical Sociology

Some have argued that medical sociology should be thought of as a loosely connected network of disparate subgroups rather than as a single discipline. Many medical sociologists tend to argue against certain axioms in the biomedical model of health and illness. They reject the reductivist approach of biomedicine, which claims that health and disease are natural phenomena that exist in the individual body rather than in the interaction of the individual and the social world; they reject the doctrine of specific etiology, the vision that disease can be induced by introducing a single specific factor into a healthy animal; and they reject biomedicine's claim to scientific neutrality. Like sociology in general, subgroups within medical sociology vary according to dichotomies such as human agency *versus* social structure, conflict *versus* consensus, and idealism *versus* realism. Subgroups also vary according to subject matter, thus the sociology of medicine can be distinguished from the sociology of health and illness, the sociology of healers, and the sociology of the health care system. Medical sociologists also distinguish between the sociology of health, the study of health, illness, and health care to further sociological theory; and sociology in health, the use of sociological insights to complement biomedicine's objectives and priorities. There are four often interrelated areas of research in medical sociology: the social production of health and illness, the social construction of health and illness, postmodern perspectives on health and illness, and the study of the health care system and its constituent parts.

Research in the social production of health and illness tends to explore variations in biomedical indicators of health such as self-reported health status and morbidity or mortality statistics. Social epidemiology shows that the distribution of disease is related to the structure of social inequalities i.e., to occupational class, socioeconomic status, gender, marital status, age, ethnicity, area of residence, housing, family structure, and employment status, although it does little to explain these microlevel relationships.

The political economy perspective incorporates a broader political and economic framework, arguing that relations of domination within patriarchal capitalism create conditions of deprivation within which some people must struggle to maintain health. It claims that there is a contradiction between the pursuit of health and the pursuit of profit. It notes the large differentials in health found among social classes, sometimes pointing to unhealthy work environments of the lower classes as an explanation, and also notes the strong relationship found among Western countries between aggregate health and degree of income inequality. This perspective has been criticized, however for failing to recognize the substantial health gains that have accompanied capitalist development and for proposing a scenario with little opportunity for intervention or change.

Social relations such as social support for individuals and social capital or social cohesion for communities have been investigated as determinants of the health of individuals and communities. There is also strong empirical support for the importance of lifestyle practices and behaviors embedded in social environments and cultural contexts. On a global scale, some authors argue that capitalist imperialism influences the presence and distribution of illness in developing nations, through the transfer of modern medicine, industry, and technology from the West, which is motivated in part by profit-driven pharmaceutical companies, for example. Finally, some authors investigate the role of Western medicine in creating as well as preventing illness. They argue that improvements in health have come mainly from nonmedical factors, and that medicine reproduces the legitimacy of the dominant social order by serving as a means of social control.

Social construction research views illness behaviors and the experience of health and illness as social states. Interactionist theory argues that people bestow meaning on their interactions with others—that selves are emergent and socially constructed. An early sociological contribution was the distinction between disease an objective state, illness the subjective experience of disorder, and sickness the social state associated with being ill. Talcott Parsons's sick role, a social role with certain rights and obligations for those so labeled, shows the power of medicine to define illness and shows that illness is a form of social deviance. Subsequent work has introduced core sociological concepts such as deviance, labeling, career, medicalization, socialization, self, and identity to the field. Interactionist approaches have been criticized for neglecting the hard realities of power and politics and for their cognitivist bias, sharply separating the mind and body.

Postmodernist thought rejects binary oppositions, instead focusing on a shifting reality with multiple truths. Foucauldian social constructionism of claims that diseases are fabrications of powerful discourses wherein individuals explore the boundaries of their self-identity, engaging in the endless task of self-transformation. Others argue that the body is a liquid commodity, an object of circulating capital, in a new world of hyper reality filled with new forms of technology. The sociology of the body stresses the re-entrance of the physical body within sociological discourse, exploring how socially structured physiology affects social behavior and *vice versa*. These perspectives are criticized for their lack of an ethic, extreme relativism and abstraction, and lack of attention to the greater political context.

Some micro-level concerns when studying the health care system are entry into and experience with the health care system and patient-practitioner relationships, which have shifted focus from the provider's interest in compliance to a power-based perspective. Some argue that medicalization providers defining needs impinges on patient autonomy and acts as a form of social control directing deviance into controllable channels. Others explore the behaviors of providers, the management of uncertainty in practice, and implicit theories of professional knowledge. A prevailing theme at the meso-level, the interactional region between the face-to-face encounter and the wider social structure, is medical dominance, the power of medicine to define matters in its own interests, applied to the study of professions, occupations, hospitals, and medical schools, for example. Some have studied the adoption of a cloak of competence in the socialization of medical students. Community involvement in planning and decision-making—the democratization of medical care—received attention in the late 1990s. Finally, some macro-level concerns are the role of multinational pharmaceutical companies in shaping the nature of health care and the reasons for and historical development of health insurance.

Social welfare is very much related to the better health or morbidity indicators of the society, thus medical sociology is one of the fundamental developing areas of the science of public health. Phenomena of urbanization, industrialization, and globalization in all over the world are about to change not only the developing direction of medicine itself, but the attitude of the society towards the disease, its curing, or the activity of institutions, ensuring health care as well. Medical sociology becomes the new "glasses" for public health specialists, where the view looking through them seems wider, and the opportunities of tackling the health care problems for instance, doctor patient interactions are higher.

## Bacteriology

With the discoveries of pathogenic bacteria by Louis Pasteur in France and Robert Koch in Germany in the late 1870s and early 1880s, the science of microbiology was born. Consequent developments in immunology and parasitology provided epidemiologists and other public health workers with the tools to study and understand epidemic phenomena. Sanitation could become science-based and the development of vaccines promised the prevention of many infectious diseases. A new era of rational public health was established.

## Colonialism and Public Health

From the sixteenth through the nineteenth century, European countries had competitively colonized most of the tropical world. The contagious diseases they brought with them frequently ravaged indigenous populations. Conversely, the prevalent diseases of colonized areas threatened the invaders. Colonial sanitation and medical care was originally designed to serve the interests of the colonists. However, after the establishment of biomedical science, there was enhanced incentive to control the major tropical diseases that were interfering with the economic development of the colonies e.g., malaria and yellow fever. In India, in 1897, Ronald Ross identified the mosquito vector of malaria, leading to the partial control of the world's most prevalent endemic disease and vastly increasing the agricultural output and, incidentally, the population of the subcontinent. In Cuba, in 1900, Walter Reed and his colleagues identified the mosquito vector of yellow fever. Subsequently, William C. Gorgas, by extensive application of larvicide, eradicated the disease from Cuba and controlled it, along with malaria, in Panama. This action permitted the construction of the canal that had previously been abandoned because of the devastating impact of these diseases.

When these colonies gained independence, mostly during the twentieth century, much of the public health infrastructures put in place by the colonial powers were transferred intact to the new nations. The ability to effectively utilize these resources has varied considerably, contributing to the development of international public health organizations.

## The Early Twentieth Century

Although the Sanitary movement of the nineteenth century and the development of bacteriology substantially lowered death rates from enteric diseases, other serious health problems still existed. One was the appalling and ubiquitous rate of infant mortality. First in Europe, then in Britain and in the United States, maternal and child health programs were initiated with an emphasis on nutrition, medical care, and, eventually, health inspection in schools. Muckraking journalists exposed disgraceful conditions in the food processing industry, leading to the imposition of widespread governmental regulation. High rates of occupational diseases and industrial injuries led to programs for industrial hygiene and occupational health. Mental health was identified as a public health issue, and specific nutritional deficiencies were recognized as risk factors for a spectrum of diseases. Furthermore, pioneering studies of pellagra, a vitamin-deficiency disease, by Joseph Goldberger and Edgar Sydenstricker, revealed the complex environmental, social, and biological interactions responsible for the occurrence and distribution of such diseases.

The growing scope and complexity of public health concerns led to the establishment of academic programs to expand research and train relevant technical personnel. At the University of London, a school of Tropical Medicine was established in 1905 and, in the United States, a School for Health Officers was created jointly by Harvard University and the Massachusetts Institute of Technology in 1913.

The first school of public health in the United States was established in 1916 at Johns Hopkins University with a grant of $ 267,000 from the Rockefeller Foundation. Subsequently, the Foundation supported the establishment of schools of public health at Harvard, the University of Michigan, the University of London, and in several other locations around the world.

By midcentury, the basic activities of public health had been widely recognized in the industrialized world. These components were: communicable diseases control, environmental sanitation, maternal and child health services, health education, occupational and industrial hygiene, nutrition, and, in most developed countries, the provision of medical care. In the United States, only medical care for the indigent, the aged, and for certain diseases e.g., tuberculosis were considered within the purview of public health.

An important role has also been played by the philanthropic foundations and voluntary health organizations. For example, the Rockefeller Foundation provided the impetus and financial resources to initiate public health professional education and the Milbank Fund pioneered the establishment of local health departments in New York State by carrying out demonstration projects around the state. Other important foundations include the Julius Rosenwald Fund, the Russell Sage Foundation, and the Twentieth Century Fund.

Voluntary health agencies evolved in the late nineteenth and early twentieth centuries in Europe and North America, growing out of the failure of public health organizations to fully apply knowledge created by the new biomedical sciences, and by the continuing deplorable condition of the urban poor. Organizations like the Pennsylvania Society for the Prevention of Tuberculosis which evolved into the American Lung Association took on the task of public education, case counseling, financial aid, and advocacy for relevant legislative action, while organizations like the Henry Street Settlement in New York City and Hull House in Chicago provided social and medical services in slum neighborhoods. By the mid–twentieth century there were more than 20,000 voluntary health agencies in the United States alone.

### The Late Twentieth Century

In the last half of the twentieth century, public health continued to expand its established roles. However, new forces were at work to further broaden its purview. Among these were the aging of the populations in industrialized regions, recognition of the importance of behavioral factors in determining the health of populations, exacerbation of social inequalities in health, increasing violence at the domestic level as well as at the civil and international level, and globalization.

As infant and child mortality declined in the industrialized countries, life expectancy and the proportions of the elderly in populations increased. Consequently, diseases such as heart disease and cancer became more important. After World War II, epidemiological research concentrated on identifying risk factors for these and other chronic diseases. A prominent role for behavioral factors was readily demonstrated. Particularly, cigarette smoking was identified as a major etiological factor for heart disease and for several cancers, particularly lung cancer. Other behavioral factors, such as diet, exercise, and obesity, were found to be causally associated with several other diseases. Ameliorating adverse behavioral risk factors has become a major function of public health agencies.

Since the mid–nineteenth century, the relationship between socioeconomic status and health has been widely recognized. However, in the late twentieth century epidemiological research has pointed out additional differences in health status between gender, ethnic, and occupational groups. Such inequalities appear to be increasing and are being recognized as a major challenge for modern public health.

Domestic violence, gang warfare, ethnic conflicts and genocide, and civil wars and wars between nations have resulted in substantial mortality and a vast disruption of societies. In some countries, including the United States, homicide has become a major cause of death among those under twenty years of age. Around the world, many millions of displaced persons live in enormous refugee camps with minimum medical and public health facilities. Clearly, the health effects of war and violence demand to be addressed.

Increased globalization and technological advances have resulted in worldwide economic, political, and social interdependence. However, recognition of the interdependence of regions and nations with respect to health and disease was institutionalized in 1902, when the Pan American Health Organization was established to coordinate communicable disease surveillance and quarantine in the western hemisphere. By the end of the century, the major global public health problems included the manifold consequences of atmospheric warming; pollution of the oceans and fresh waters of the world and the depletion of fisheries; the rapid growth of the world's population; the emergence of new infectious diseases, including HIV/AIDS (human immunodeficiency virus/acquired immunodeficiency syndrome); and the increased production and use of addictive drugs. These are daunting challenges for the World Health Organization and other international agencies.

Nevertheless, in 1977, public health registered its greatest historical feat. In that year, the eradication of one of the human species' most dreaded and lethal diseases, smallpox, was completed. The last case occurred in 1977 in the East African nation of Somalia and the eradication was certified by a Commission of the World Health Organization in 1979.

**Evaluation of Public Health Programs**

Public health programs are essential to protect and enhance the health of the population and are, by definition, publicly funded. It is, therefore essential that they be evaluated. The benefits of public health programs often extend well beyond the immediate target population—reductions in communicable diseases or environmental hazards may benefit the whole world. Different disciplines approach evaluation in different ways.

Epidemiologists distinguish between an intervention's efficacy its ability to work under ideal circumstances, its effectiveness results obtained under real-world circumstances, and its efficiency results obtained relative to the resources expended. An intervention cannot be effective unless it is efficacious. Randomized studies are the gold standard for studies of efficacy, since they ensure that study groups are comparable in the long run. They thereby help to ensure that the results are due to the intervention. But they are more feasible for single interventions directed at individuals than for complex programs directed at groups, so their potential for evaluating public health programs is limited. Community trials, in which groups are the unit of randomization, are difficult and expensive. Quasi-experimental approaches try to obtain the advantages of randomization through careful selection of comparison groups often multiple groups and sophisticated statistical analysis.

Administrative sciences tend to assume that a program's efficacy has been demonstrated and concentrate on other dimensions of evaluation. Using the World Health Organization's 1991 *Health Programme Evaluation* as a basis, J. E. Veney and A. D. Kaluzny (1991) recommend that five aspects of a health program be evaluated: its relevance to the needs of the population and to social priorities, progress implementation, efficiency in terms outcomes achieved in relation to resources expended, effectiveness in terms of extent to which predetermined objectives are met, and impact long-term outcomes. Approaches for measuring these dimensions include monitoring, case studies, and various epidemiologic designs.

Economists compare a particular program to a possible alternative. Costs are expressed in monetary units and should be marginal cost of producing the last unit of output rather than average across all units of output. Outcomes may be assumed to be identical and, therefore not measured in terms of cost-minimization analysis or expressed in natural units like cases prevented in terms of cost-effectiveness monetary units cost-benefit, or universal units like quality-adjusted life years costutility.

Public health managers often use logic models for evaluating public health programs, setting out the program's expected operation in matrix format and showing the activities, target groups, and short-and long-term outcomes for each component. Much more highly developed is the Precede-Proceed framework of L. W. Green and M. W. Kreuter, a nine-step process for the design of a health-promotion program social, epidemiologic, behavioral/environmental, educational/organization, and administrative/policy diagnoses and its evaluation such as implementation and process, impact, and outcome evaluation. All these approaches force program developers to think through a program systematically, and they show program evaluators what to measure. By sampling the program process at various stages evaluators can distinguish between an implementation failure potentially good idea that was never properly tested and a program failure (a bad idea). Governments often produce standards against which local public health programs can be tested. The National Public Health Performance Standards Program is the standard being developed in the United States.

### Practice of Public Health

The phrase "practice of public health" which will be used interchangeably with the term "public health practice" fails to evoke a single compelling image, even for public health professionals who have spent years working in the field. Unlike medicine, or law, or even engineering, both those who contribute to and those who benefit from public health practice's efforts poorly understand what it is and how it works? Here we discuss the key aspects of public health practice by addressing the following basic questions:

- What is public health practice?
- Where did it come from?
- What does it do?
- How is it organized and structured?
- What challenges does it face in the twenty-first century?

### What is Public Health Practice?

One approach to describing public health practice is to compare it to some similar activity that most people understand and appreciate. Medical practice appears to fit this bill. The major functions of medical practice are to diagnose diseases and other conditions, develop a treatment plan for those health problems, and see that the treatment regimen achieves its therapeutic goals.

Public health practice has remarkably similar functions that focus on populations rather than individual patients. Public health functions involve identifying health problems and the factors that cause them, developing a strategy to address these problems, and seeing that these strategies are implemented in a way that works. In this light, public health practice is the development and application of preventive strategies and interventions in order to promote and protect the health of populations. Public health practitioners serve the health needs of populations in very much the same ways that physicians tend to the health needs of individual patients. Medical practice focuses primarily on diseases, injuries, and other conditions while public health practice focuses at the community level on factors that contribute to higher rates of these same health problems.

The practice of public health involves both individual and collective efforts. Many different professions and disciplines contribute to public health practice, including public health nurses, nutritionists, health educators, environmental health specialists, and physicians, just to name a few. But public health practice also includes the collective efforts of public health professionals acting in concert with others, often community partners, to identify and address health problems affecting defined populations.

The need for these different disciplines and skills indicates the complexity of the factors contributing to health and disease. Various bacteria and viruses cause many infectious diseases. But other factors can cause or contribute to the development of health problems. For example, the use of tobacco and alcohol contributes to heart disease, cancer, and injuries. Behavioral choices can place an individual at risk of certain infectious diseases sexually transmitted diseases, chronic diseases emphysema, injuries drug overdoses, and other conditions. There are also aspects of the physical environment that affect health in terms of contaminated air, water, or food. The social environment can also determine health risks, viz, low income and education levels, overcrowding, and personal safety. Other social factors related to the use of health and medical services, such as travel distance, the number of providers, and even the availability of day-care services, also influence health. With so many elements affecting health, there is no one body of scientific knowledge that guides public health practice. Instead there are many. These include epidemiology, statistics, environmental sciences, management, biological sciences, and the behavioral sciences such as anthropology, sociology, psychology, and more. Political science, economics, and law are also involved in modern public health practice. Public health is grounded in many different sciences and supported by a variety of other disciplines.

Many people think of public health practice as only those activities performed by governmental public health agencies. Public health practice certainly includes, but is not limited to, the activities of federal, state, and local health agencies such as the federal centers for Disease Control, state health departments, and local public health departments. But many other individuals, organizations, institutions, and collaborations contribute to public health practice—and these efforts take place in private and voluntary, as well as in public, settings. For example, hospitals and businesses are often involved in communitywide health fairs and heart and lung associations continuously promote healthy lifestyles.

With so many different participants, the practice of public health can appear to be fragmented and chaotic. But, ideally, public health practice is strategic and purposeful; it is organized perhaps most effectively at the community level and it is both interdisciplinary and multidisciplinary. In sum, the practice of public health embodies what a community or society does collectively in order to ensure conditions in which people can be healthy. The skills and competencies necessary for public health practice are both individual and collective.

## Where did Public Health Practice come from

Many different forces have shaped modern public health practice. These include diseases and other health threats, history, science, social values, and the role of government. Health threats have always challenged human populations; nearly all of the diseases that have wreaked havoc on society over the centuries are still with us today, including tuberculosis, cholera, malaria, yellow fever, and plague. While some diseases have disappeared due to intensive prevention and control initiatives smallpox is a good example, there is little expectation that all diseases and illnesses can be avoided. The infectious diseases of the past have been joined by dozens of other conditions, most recently by AIDS and by a host of chronic disease risks and environmental threats. The identification of and responses to these threats, over-time and across the globe, especially responses that represent collective decisions and actions have evolved into what we know as public health practice?

In past centuries, health risks and threats were addressed in a variety of ways. For much of recorded history, diseases were accepted as phenomena beyond human control. Acceptance and avoidance were major strategies as recently as the nineteenth century. For example, when cholera appeared in cities or neighborhoods in Europe and the United States as recently as the mid-nineteenth century, residents if not immediately infected could accept the risk or choose to move away until the risk subsided.

While diseases and the microorganisms that cause them have cohabited with humankind for all of history, their spread was greatly aided by industrialism, nationalism, and mercantilism in recent centuries. Industrialism brought previously agrarian societies into urban centers where the population density and unsanitary living and working conditions fostered the spread of many diseases. Nationalism and mercantilism fostered travel and trade across the globe and provided increased opportunities for diseases to be carried from one densely populated area to another. European societies that had centuries of experience with many diseases—and had developed an ecological balance with those diseases through changes in their collective immunological status—brought diseases never before seen to Native-American populations in North and South America. Small wonder that relatively tiny armies of European explorers easily conquered civilizations with much larger populations, encouraging the belief that they were indeed supernatural figures and that the diseases they brought with them were beyond human control.

It was the spread of epidemic diseases largely through seaport towns and cities that prompted the first U.S. public health responses. Boards of distinguished citizens, the first local boards of health, were appointed in cities like Philadelphia, New York, and Chicago to provide the credibility and support necessary to pursue the restrictive policies of quarantining ships and their crews, or placing notices or placards to warn citizens to avoid locations where diseases had occurred. But until the latter part of the nineteenth century, little was known about the causes and pathways of these epidemics. The work of pioneering scientists in the latter half of the nineteenth century, such as Louis Pasteur in France and Robert Koch in Germany, opened the way to the identification of specific microorganisms and eventually to the development of specific approaches to battle those germs and break the chain of transmission.

These scientific advances established that many health threats could be addressed through communitywide interventions, such as those that would ensure clean water supplies and sanitary disposal of human waste and sewage. Public health laboratories were developed to assist in diagnosing new cases so that prevention and control activities could be put in place to avoid further spread. Immunizations were developed from these scientific advances and provided to susceptible populations through massive vaccination programs. Because these efforts required both citizen support and public resources, local governments became increasingly involved in public health responses. State governments became active at a slightly later stage, primarily because infectious disease risks did not respect municipal boundaries.

The increasing involvement and expectations for governmental participation in public health responses represents an important facet of public health practice. The U.S. system of government divides duties and responsibilities between the federal government and the states. There are no specific powers related to protecting or promoting the health of its citizens identified for the national government in the U.S. constitution. As a result, the basic responsibility for health and public health resides with the states and, as established by those states, with local governments. The federal role in health has nonetheless grown, especially over the twentieth century, as a result of its ability to pursue health goals as a power implied though not explicitly stated by the Constitution to promote the general welfare. With immense resources available through the federal income tax and with the ability to influence the activities of state and local governments by offering financial resources for specific programs and services through "grant in aid" mechanisms, the federal government emerged as an important player in the health field. Later its role as a major purchaser of health services through massive national programs such as Medicare and Medicaid brought the federal government even greater power and influence in the health sector. Today it maintains a substantial role in health and public health.

The extensive social and economic chaos accompanying the Great Depression in the 1930s raised public expectations that government would involve itself in protecting the health and welfare of all-U.S. citizens. Prior to this time, most Americans didn't want government to have powers over their lives and welfare. Government's role as an important force in public health arose out of other needs as well. Only government can implement and enforce some of the policies and interventions necessary to battle health risks—ensuring safe public water supplies and effective municipal sewage disposal programs, for example, or investigating contacts of persons diagnosed with infectious diseases. To the extent that public resources are utilized for these ends, governmental forums are the appropriate places for these decisions. This is but one of the unique features of public health practice, its link with government. But there are several others that have come to distinguish public heath from other forms of health practice.

The public nature of public health practice means it must depend on social values and popular support for both its ends and its means. This makes public health practice inherently political in that different values and perspectives exist in various communities as to what needs to be done about important public policy problems. These sentiments and viewpoints change over-time and, as a result, the problems to be addressed by public health practice have changed over-time as well. For example, infectious diseases were major concerns through the middle of the twentieth century. Chronic diseases became a major focus after the middle of the twentieth century, as did problems and gaps in the health system. Mental health and substance abuse issues became priorities in the 1970s and 1980s, while the 1990s saw violence emerge as a new problem for the public health practice agenda. The ever-changing agenda of public health practice reflects the dynamic nature of its two most influential forces: science and social values. While public health practice is grounded in science, what we choose to do with that scientific knowledge is determined by social values?

One of the most unique features of public health practice is its basis in social justice. Social justice seeks to distribute the benefits of science and technology equally among all segments of society. In the case of health benefits, this would mean eliminating disparities in mortality, disease incidence, disability, and the like. With the considerable differences in health status and outcomes between African Americans and European Americans, for example, or between rich and poor, it is clear that not all parts of the U.S. population share health benefits equally. These social links help explain why public health practitioners share an uncommon bond: the commitment to improve the health status of others.

## What Does Public Health do Today

The complete description for public health practice has yet to be written. The simplest and most straightforward depiction of what public health practice is all about today is best illustrated in the mission, vision, and functions outlined in the "Public Health in America" statement. This one-page document was developed to become the hymnal from which all public health practitioners would sing in the twenty-first century.

The statement articulates a vision i.e., healthy people in healthy communities, a mission promoting physical and mental health and preventing disease, injury, and disability and statements of what public health practice does and how it accomplishes those ends. Six broad commitments characterize what public health does. Public health:

Prevents epidemics and the spread of disease, protects against environmental hazards, Prevents injuries. Promotes and encourages healthy behaviors. Responds to disasters and assists communities in recovery and assures the quality and accessibility of health services. How public health practice accomplishes these objectives and serves its mission is characterized by ten essential public health services that seek to:

Monitor health status to identify community health problems. Diagnose and investigate health problems and health hazards in the community. Inform, educate, and empower people about health issues. Mobilize community partnerships to identify and solve health problems. Develop policies and plans that support individual and community health efforts. Enforce laws and regulations that protect health and ensure safety. Link people to needed personal health services and assure the provision of health care when otherwise unavailable. Assure a competent public and personal health care work force. Evaluate effectiveness, accessibility, and quality of personal and population-based health services and provide research for new insights and innovative solutions to health problems.

These statements establish a high standard for performance. But by many different measures of performance, it appears that public health practice has not fully achieved these standards. Signs of sub-optimal performance include continuing high rates of morbidity, mortality, and disability for many conditions; huge disparities among various segments of the population; and persistently unequal access to health services. Improvement in these areas requires a well organized and effectively functioning system of public health practice.

### How is Public Health Practice Organized and Structured?

The final decades of the twentieth century witnessed a series of examinations and initiatives that changed the face of public health practice. These began with a landmark report issued by the prestigious Institute of Medicine in 1988 entitled *The Future of Public Health*. This report examined the state of public health practice in the 1980s and concluded that the public health system was in a state of "disarray" and that it required a major reengineering effort.

The report proposed that governmental public health organize around three broad functions: assessment, policy development, and assurance. Basically these translate into identifying what should be done assessment, what will be done on policy development, and achieving those ends assurance. Identifying what should be done comes from a comprehensive and broadly participatory assessment of needs and assets and involves both science and values. Determining what will be done recognizes that not all needs can be met, and that some needs are more important than others. Achieving agreed—upon ends involves evidence-based decisions about what works and what doesn't in a particular setting and about who needs to be involved in community interventions?

Some needs are identified by scientific means, such as data showing higher death rates from cardiovascular disease in a community or from reports of an increasing number of AIDS cases. However, other needs are identified by the willingness of people and organizations to mobilize over problems and issues that are important to them and their communities. In some instances, problems are identified for which there may not be convincing data. Yet these problems can be given as high or even higher priority than those advanced by the so called experts. For example, a community may decide that leaf burning is a more important public health problem than childhood lead poisoning even when the number of reported cases of elevated blood lead levels is much greater than illnesses that are linked to leaf burning.

## What Challenges Does Public Health Practice Face in the Year 2001 and Beyond

Public health practice faces many challenges. There are scores of continuing health problems such as cancer and injuries, emerging health problems such as AIDS and violence, and re-emerging ones such as tuberculosis, and a slew of new issues on the public health practice agenda. While health status has never been better as measured by life expectancy and infant mortality, the gains have not been shared equally by all segments of the population. These widening differences reflect the increasing gap between the "haves" and the "havenots" and the widespread prevalence of negative social determinants of health among sub-populations in the developing counties and entire societies across the globe. Despite the most expensive and effective medical services in the world, health status gains have not kept pace with immense investments. These unacceptable realities challenge public health practitioners' core values of realizing public health's dream of social justice and creating a health system organized around health. To meet the challenges, public health practice will have to relearn the lessons of its past and move to expand its circle to include new sectors of society at every level of government—namely, more community partners and stakeholders and a more involved citizenry.

In sum, further improvements in health status that eliminate disparities in outcomes remains the greatest challenge to the practice of public health. A continuing commitment to realize the dream of social justice in health will, in all probability, continue to drive public health practice in the twenty-first century.

## Anthropology in Public Health

Public health is often described as having the population or community as its patient, in contrast to the individual-level focus of clinical medicine. This focus on community creates a natural foundation for partnership between public health and anthropology, which takes as its primary focus the study of people in groups, and especially in local communities. Anthropology has four major subfields: cultural anthropology, physical or biological anthropology, archeology, and linguistics. Crosscutting the subfields are several subdisciplinary foci that have much to contribute to the achievement of public health objectives. The most important for public health is *medical anthropology*, a field that first emerged as a coherent subdiscipline in the 1950s and has rapidly grown to become one of the largest areas of research and practice within anthropology. The richness of this subdiscipline is apparent in the range of theoretical perspectives encompassed by it.

Anthropology has also made important methodological contributions to public health, especially with regard to the use of ethnography for the systematic collection of field data; qualitative methods for the collection and analysis of descriptive, interpretative, and formative data; and the integration of qualitative and quantitative approaches. The ability to translate scientific knowledge into effective practice at the community level is a third area where anthropological approaches have much to offer public health.

**Theoretical Contributions**

As with anthropology and public health, the basic unit of study in ecology is the population. The *medical-ecological* approach links biomedicine with biological and cultural anthropology, resulting in important contributions to understanding health and disease as dynamic, adaptive, population-based processes. The ecological model builds on three key assumptions:

There are no single causes of disease; rather, disease is ultimately due to a chain of factors related to ecosystem imbalances. Health and disease are part of a set of physical, biological, and cultural subsystems that continually affect one another and the ecological model provides a framework for the study of health in an environmental context, but it does not specify what factors maintain health within any given local system?

*Critical medical anthropology* raises important questions about the impact of global political and economic structures and processes on health and disease. It expands the context within which medical anthropology operates and brings it closer to the perspective of public health practice by explicitly seeking to contribute to the creation of global health systems that "serve the people." Critical medical anthropology focuses on health care systems and how they function at multiple levels, including the individual level of patient experience, the *microlevel* of physician-patient relationships, the *intermediate* level of local health care systems, particularly hospitals and clinics, and the *macrosocial* level of global political-economic systems. At each of these levels, the goal is to understand how existing social relations structure the relationships among the participants in the systems. In particular, critical medical anthropologists study the way health care is embedded within dominant relations such as those of class, race, and gender.

The individual level of patient experience has been the focus of *interpretative anthropology* approaches. A. Kleinman (1997) introduced the cultural interpretative model to provide a means of balancing the externalized, objective view of disease with the subjective experience of illness. M. Lock and N. Scheper-Hughes (1990), in turn, developed the concept of "sufferer experience" as an important dimension to the study of health. They developed a metaphorical framework of "the three bodies" to facilitate understanding of the multiple layers of health and illness. The *individual body* constitutes the layer of lived experience, with an explicit rejection of Cartesian mind-body dualism. The *social body* encompasses the way in which the individual body becomes a kind of canvas upon which nature, society, and culture is represented. The *body politic* refers to "the regulation, surveillance, and control of bodies individual and collective in reproduction and sexuality, work, leisure, and sickness". Sickness, in this framework, is understood as a "form of communication" among all three levels, a kind of individual-level expression of social truths and social contradictions. It then follows that, in order to effectively treat the individual expression of sickness, the role of social and political factors in generating sickness must also be considered.

The microlevel of physician-patient relationships and the intermediate level of local health care systems have been the focus of *clinical anthropology*. M. Konner (1993) provides a global overview of the many political and economic factors that impact the way doctors are trained and socialized, as well as how they shape the way medical care is enacted in clinics and hospitals. P. Farmer (1999) examines inequalities in the distribution and outcome of infectious diseases such as tuberculosis, AIDS acquired immunodeficiency syndrome, Ebola, and malaria, as well as social responses such as quarantine and accusations of sorcery that often are associated with infectious diseases. His particular concern is with the emergence of disease from socially produced phenomena such as poverty and political upheaval, which he describes as the "biological reflections of social fault lines". Farmer also critiqued simplistic models of disease causality that fail to incorporate dynamic, systematic global factors and, therefore, slight the need for preventive models that target the social determinants of health.

In a similar mode, M. Singer (1994) proposed a synthesis of two key concepts from the ecological model—that health and disease are ultimately due to a chain of factors, and that they are part of a set of interacting subsystems—with the broader global perspective of critical medical anthropology to describe and explain the dynamics of the AIDS pandemic. Singer coined the term "syndemic" to describe the synergistic interaction of social factors, especially local and global inequities, with the epidemiological risk factors for HIV TB, hepatitis, and substance abuse. The syndemic model provides an important intermediate model that frames the investigation of community-level outcomes in terms of individual behavior, local processes, and higher level processes. This model raises difficult questions, and it challenges public health to address the root causes of health disparities. By introducing a multilevel, dynamic epidemiological perspective, it points toward the need to develop and evaluate systems—and community-level interventions that target linked processes.

## Methodological Contributions

The application of anthropological methods to public health problems has been another important area of contribution. The use of systematic, descriptive, and qualitative methods has proven effective in identifying context-specific factors that contribute to health and disease outcomes. Another important methodological contribution is the use of triangulation, or the systematic application of multiple methods in order to reduce bias in situations where controlled comparison is not feasible. For example, anthropologists typically use natural observation of behavior along with self-report data and descriptions of normative expectations to obtain highly accurate descriptions of events and social relationships.

The development of rapid assessment techniques, variously called rapid appraisal, rapid assessment, and rapid rural appraisal, is a prime example of anthropological contributions to the public health methodological toolkit. As described by J. Beebe (1995) this is a multidisciplinary team-based approach designed to generate reasonably valid, reliable, and qualitative results within a short-time frame. Rapid assessments can provide the contextual information needed to design in-depth community-level and community-based public health research and to guide decisions about implementing programs in local settings.

J. A. Trostle and J. Sommerfeld (1996) describe a number of mutual methodological benefits to be gained from combining anthropological and epidemiological approaches, including:

Anthropological knowledge of cross-cultural variability can be used to improve the development and measurement of epidemiologic variables. Research results can be communicated more effectively to policymakers and to a public audience when both anthropological and epidemiological descriptions are employed. Conceptual and experimental work can be undertaken to determine the best measures of complex cultural and behavioral variables and ethnographic and epidemiological information can be used to design health surveillance systems that return data to communities in more comprehensible forms, creating new meanings for the "popular epidemiology."

The authors also provide a useful overview of the way anthropologists and epidemiologists have approached key social and cultural concepts relevant to the study of health and disease, including culture change and stress; social stratification; risk vulnerability; behavior; and illness constructs. They also review a number of areas of mutual methodological interest. They propose the label of "cultural epidemiology" to describe "cross-cultural analyses of the distribution and determinants of disease and illness and with unpacking variables e.g., race, class, religion, time to illustrate and specify their theoretical context and meaning".

## Translating Knowledge into Action

Anthropological theory and methods have much to offer public health in the area of translating public health knowledge into effective action. Contributions range from basic issues of cultural sensitivity to enhance the acceptability and effectiveness of proven practices in clinic settings to the development of policy for the provision of complex treatment regimens for emerging epidemics under conditions of inequity in access to health care. As such, anthropologists are asking questions about the root causes of public health's toughest problems. These problems are not often amenable to study using controlled clinical trials or cross-sectional survey designs. Rather, they are dynamic, systems-level problems that require fieldbased observation and the use of multiple methods that are both qualitative and quantitative.

## Social Assessment in Health Promotion Planning

Within the context of health promotion, social assessment refers to a process in which objective and subjective information are used to identify high-priority problems, or assets, that affect the common good. Ideally, this process will use a variety of social, economic, and quality-of-life indicators, including the perceptions and concerns of representatives from the area or community being assessed.

There are strong connections between major health problems e.g., violence, chronic disease, teen pregnancy and their social determinants e.g., cultural differences, variability in levels of income, social support, housing, and education. While these factors tend to cluster within neighborhoods or communities, they vary considerably between communities. Any social assessment should be designed to take these realities into account. Armed with the information generated from a social assessment, planners will be in a better position to tailor interventions to meet the unique needs of a given community.

## Multiple Indicators

There are different ways of knowing, and different interpretations of reality. An epidemiologist, an anthropologist, a health educator, and a layperson are all likely to view a given problem through different lenses. More importantly, each is quite likely to detect a glimpse of reality that the others may miss. The social assessment process will be productive to the extent that: (1) it serves as a first step in a planning process, (2) it reflects a spirit of inclusion, (3) time is dedicated to allow all stakeholders to discuss and interpret information gained in the process, and (4) those discussions are carried out in an atmosphere of mutual respect and trust.

The literature describing methods and instruments to assess quality-of-life and social indicators is extensive and growing. Included among the objective and subjective indicators that may be used as a part of social assessment include perceptions of quality of life; sense of community; perceived functional capacity; employment rates; differences in levels of income; access to transportation and transportation services; alcohol-related auto crashes; housing density; crime; trust or distrust in government; air and water quality; access to health, mental health, and social services; and education.

A wide range of methods have been used to collect data for social assessments. These include, but are not limited to, interviewing those who have a stake in the outcomes of a relevant program or project, community town meetings, focus groups, community polls and surveys, archival research, reviews of income, housing status, access to health services and other relevant social indicators, and synthetic estimates from national data interpolated to the local level. As a means to save limited resources, some planners retrieve existing information, whenever possible, rather than generate new data.

### Assets

As implied in the definition, a social assessment in health promotion should involve an accounting of community and individual assets as well as identification of problems or concerns. John McKnight and John Kretzmann describe a process of community asset mapping, wherein relevant skills and capacities of individuals, as well as other assets that may exist in a given community, are documented. These assets are classified into three tiers of primary, secondary, and potential building blocks. Primary building blocks are those that exist and are controlled within a given community e.g., a local health agency, or a local teacher; they are also the assets that are most accessible. Secondary building blocks are those that exist within a community but are controlled from outside the community e.g., a health clinic which is a satellite of a regional or corporate medical system. Potential building blocks are those located and controlled outside of the community e.g., federal grant programs or national campaigns. An analysis of this kind will help planners keep a realistic perspective on the comparative difficulty of accessing the assets they have identified.

Another example of using positive indicators is found in Peter Benson's work on the developmental assets that influence children and adolescents. Benson describes forty developmental assets, which are classified equally into two categories: (1) internal assets related to the personal qualities of children (e.g., self-esteem, achievement motivation) and (2) external assets (e.g., family and adult support, safety, programs and services). Analysis of developmental assets reveals a consistent pattern where, among youth, developmental assets are inversely related to high-risk health behaviors— the more developmental assets children have, the less likely they are to engage in behavior that puts them at health risk. High levels of developmental assets are associated with success in school and valuing diversity.

## Respect

Lawrence Green and others have made the point that health is an instrumental value, that is, a value that facilitates the striving for, or attainment of, higher order, or ultimate values. For example, a company may value a commitment to physical fitness and nutrition to the extent that it influences employee performance and satisfaction. The implication is that health has value to the extent that it either supports or enables higher order values, which may include social benefits, overall quality of life, the capacity to function, or even an organization's bottom line. This point is relevant to social assessment because information gleaned from the process can be used to illustrate how the effective application of health-promotion programs contributes to the improvement of social benefits beyond improvements in health.

In a study designed to improve the immunization rates among children 0 to 2 years of age and born to low-income mothers in an urban setting, researchers found that marked increases in immunization coverage were attributable to tailored messages created from assessments that took into account the family characteristics, social and environmental conditions, and selected cultural factors unique to the participants. Irrespective of the methods, indicators, or instruments used in the social assessment process, a commitment to engaging the people of a community in identifying and assessing their own perceived problems and aspirations is essential. Not only does such a commitment assure that a critical view of reality will not be left out of the health-promotion program planning process, it signals a tangible sign of respect toward the members of a community.

## Health Risk Appraisal

A health risk appraisal (HRA) is a computer-based health-promotion tool, consisting of a questionnaire, a formula for estimating health risks (e.g., premature death), an advice database, and a means to generate reports. Its roots lie in efforts to guide physicians in promoting health as well as treating illness. HRAs are widely used in worksite wellness programs and community-based health programs as well as health care settings.

Typical aims are to assess health risks and lifestyle choices; to motivate individuals to adopt or maintain beneficial lifestyle practices; to guide health-promotion activities of health plans, employers, and health agencies; and to create a database profile of the population appraised. A key element of any HRA is personalized feedback to identify areas of excess health risk and recommend actions.

## Public Health Nursing

Public health nursing is a specialized form of registered nursing that combines nursing and public health principles. According to the American Public Health Association, the primary focus of public health nursing is improving the health of the community as a whole rather than just that of an individual or family. Public health nursing is sometimes called a type of community health nursing. Some experts use the terms "public health nursing" and "community health nursing" interchangeably.

## History

Public health nursing traces its roots to England where, in 1859, Florence Nightingale assisted in organizing district public health nursing. Each nurse was assigned a specific geographic area of London and was responsible for the health of the people living in that neighborhood. This type of organization finds its echo today in many public health departments, where public health nurses organize their work by groups of census tracts called districts and the nurse is known as the district public health nurse.

In the United States, modern public health nursing was defined by pioneering nurse Lillian Wald in the late 1800s. She established the Henry Street Settlement in New York City, where nurses lived in the neighborhoods where they worked. In the beginning, public health nursing was primarily concerned with taking care of the sick poor in their homes. Lillian Wald came to the realization that sickness found in the home had its origin in larger societal problems. She set about directing nursing efforts toward employment, sanitation, recreation, and education. It was Lillian Wald who coined the term "public health nurse." Hospital-based schools of nursing which granted nursing diplomas provided the educational preparation for nurses at this time.

In the early part of the twentieth century, Visiting Nurses Associations were formed to continue the tradition of providing care for the sick in their homes, which eventually became known as home health nursing. Public health nursing began to be practiced in both voluntary agencies such as the American Red Cross, and governmental agencies, such as local county and city health departments. Serving the needs of the poor remained a key aspect of public health nursing. In the mid twentieth century, care shifted from the home to the clinic, where nurses worked in well baby and immunization clinics for the uninsured and were active in controlling communicable diseases such as tuberculosis.

In the latter part of the twentieth century, nursing education began to move out of hospital based programs and into community colleges and universities. Educational preparation for public health nurses varies widely in the United States with some jurisdictions requiring a bachelor's degree in nursing and others accepting a hospital diploma or associate degree from a community college. A bachelor's degree in nursing is considered a minimum requirement for public health nursing practice by many nursing professionals and professional nursing organizations. A bachelor's degree in nursing is thought to provide the background in social science and public health science such as epidemiology and environmental health that a public health nurse needs. Increasingly, public health nurses are enrolling in advanced degree programs in public health, community health nursing, and other public health specialties.

## The Role of the Public Health Nurse

Ideally, the work of public health nurses is defined as "primary prevention," which means preventing disease, injury, disability and premature death. Public health nurses work as a team with other public health professionals such as environmental health specialists, health educators, epidemiologists, public health physicians, and nutritionists. As members of this team, they work with local communities to assess and prioritize the major health problems and work on a plan to alleviate or eliminate these problems and the conditions that contribute to their development.

Public health nurses are able to assist individuals and families to take action to improve their health status. Often this takes the form of teaching about healthy lifestyle choices in the home, in the workplace, and in community settings. Public health nurses assist people in applying improved health behavior choices to their everyday lives. Examples of personal behaviors that can contribute to health problems are tobacco use, improper diet, lack of physical exercise, unsafe sexual practices, and driving while intoxicated.

Public health nurses also recognize that the community and environment in which people live can affect their ability to make healthy lifestyle choices and can affect whether or not such choices exist at all. Thus, public health nurses may spend a significant portion of their time on ensuring healthy living conditions in the neighborhoods where they work and on improving the health status of the entire community, not just that of individuals. Examples of community issues on which the public health nurse may work are reducing tobacco sales to minors, fluoridation of drinking water, identifying and reducing workplace hazards, immunization of all children against communicable diseases, and reducing the risk of drowning through community education, pool safety, and construction regulation.

Public health nurses are found in a variety of settings, including schools and the workplace. Public health nurses who assist workers at the job site are called occupational health nurses. Some nurses work in local government health departments as general practice nurses in neighborhoods. In some health departments, the community intervention role of public health nurses is not well established and their work is confined to home visits and clinic work. Their primary role is that of case manager and they have a varied caseload of individuals and families whom they assist with illness-oriented concerns, such as communicable diseases and health problems of mothers and children. Sometimes, these case manager public health nurses specialize in one area, such as follow up of cases of lead poisoning or sudden infant death syndrome. Much of the funding for public health work has been fragmented, coming to local government jurisdictions from state and federal sources for a specific problem or intervention only. As a consequence, public health nursing in many settings has become more specialized and even more concentrated on caring for individuals and families, usually in the home.

Many public health nursing experts feel that this emphasis on caring for people with a disease or condition has hindered public health nurses from being full participants in public health and has diverted public health nursing away from its prevention role. Some in public health nursing would even argue that, as a result, the practice of public health nursing has lost its way and needs to refocus on the true mission of public health: to look at the health problems of a community as a whole and work with the community in alleviating those problems. They would argue that there is the mistaken perception of public health nurses as providers of personal care only. The challenge for public health nurses in the future is to apply the nursing process such as assessment, diagnosis, planning, implementation, and evaluation of interventions to improve health, not just of individuals, but also with larger segments of the population in partnership with the community.

## Participation in Community Health Planning

The health of a community depends on many factors, including the health protection and promotion activities of local government agencies e.g., public health, transportation, public works, parks and recreation, not-for-profit agencies e.g., Red Cross, American Cancer Society, YMCA/YWCA and private sector organizations e.g., plastic recycling firms. Because the determinants of health lie, to a great extent, outside the health sector including socioeconomic, cultural, and working conditions), involving citizens in making decisions on issues that affect their health has long been supported by public health. Theory and practice in community health suggests that planning is best done by those individuals who will be the recipients of, or will be affected by, the resulting programs, policies, or services. Efforts to get people to change their lifestyle behaviors, their worksites e.g., to implement a no smoking policy, or their schools e.g., to adopt a healthier lunch menu, will be most successful if those asked to make such changes are included in the planning process. In addition to engendering positive program outcomes, participation is also thought to: Empower individual participants by increasing their knowledge and skill levels, their feelings of control and competence to make a difference, and their sense of self-worth and dignity. Nurture local planning skills and abilities. Build community capacity to tackle future health issues and foster the overall health of the community by strengthening citizens' trust in each other and their connectedness to the community.

Opportunities for citizens to participate in health planning has often been hindered or blocked, however, by resistance from the state and from the professions, precluding citizens from making decisions and shaping policy about their own lives. Participation can be, and often is, tokenistic or consultative rather than meaningful. While it remains an attractive concept, it is one that has been realized only in a limited sense.

Community participation is often narrowly defined as simply asking community members about their health needs. Opinions are often confined to prepackaged formulas, and delegating the actual planning, implementation, and evaluation of programs is left to professional practitioners. While needs assessments and pretesting programs are crucial components of planning, participation needs to go beyond responding to surveys or opinion polls, with people actively involved in defining the issues and in all subsequent phases of the process.

It is often difficult to attract participants that reflect the diversity of a community. The participation process itself can discriminate against those in the community who are not well-educated, well-spoken, or well-off. Committee meetings and public forums can be inconvenient, inaccessible, and intimidating to all but the few who possess the requisite professional experience and educational and discretionary resources to attend. In addition to meetings being convenient and welcoming, citizens must be able to see some reflection of themselves in the participatory endeavor in order to trust the process and become involved. In the absence of broad-based participation, particularly when economy of time and problems of scale restrict participation by all, experiential participation may be a step toward achieving better representation of diverse perspectives.

Experiential participation abandons the "meeting mindset." Participation takes place in schools, worksites, churches, street corners, and coffee houses, and engages citizens in a planning process that reflects their life experiences. It also demands acknowledging and respecting the diverse and non-traditional contributions and strengths of different groups of citizens. Meaningful participation may constitute sharing experiences as recipients of services, providing input about the delivery and quality of health programs, as well as chairing meetings, interpreting statistics, and penning community health plans. A final challenge lies in maintaining the momentum of and interest in, participatory initiatives when much of the work relies on lay volunteers with busy lives.

# 3

# Interdisciplinary Approach to Health and Medicine

Sociology is the scientific study of groups, organizations, institutions, relationships, and interpersonal behavior. The field of medical sociology brings an eclectic approach to the study of health behavior, professional work roles, and medical institutions. Medical sociologist is trained to appraise how cultures, institutions, and organizations are influencing individual beliefs, behaviors and patterns of social interaction and ultimately affect the physical and mental health of individuals, groups, and organizations. Medical sociologists are especially well suited to understand practitioner—patient relationships in health care system, which is the complex of technical, organizational, economical, and ethical approaches. This multidimentional perspective, coupled with knowledge about how groups and organizations are functioning, allows medical sociologist to facilitate communication among the various clinicians, researchers, administrators, and patients in health care delivery settings. Medical sociologists hold teaching positions not only in sociology departments but also in public health, medical, and nursing schools. In addition, they are employed as researchers and research directors in public and private health agencies and in health-related industries, such as insurance, pharmaceutical, and hospital management companies.

In general, sociology tends to focus on basic research, for which practical applications are not always obvious.

In contrast, medical sociology has an applied focus which takes researchers into health service settings for on-site data collection and intervention. Medical sociologists utilize applied sociology methods, such as needs assessment and social impact assessment. In addition, medical sociology lends itself to formulating and testing case management options in health care settings using evaluation research methods.

The meaning of medical sociology appeared in the USA, in the second half of the 19th century, and the development of urbanization, industry, and other social issues had a significant impact on it. The term "medical sociology" was used for the first time in the paper of Ch. McIntire called "The importance of studies of medical sociology" and published in 1894.

Thus, R. Strauss in 1957, analyzing the meaning of medical sociology was paying more attention to the main terms – sociology in medicine and sociology of medicine. The mentioned two could be supposed as two different approaches in medical sociology. The meaning of sociology in medicine in some scientific literature found as sociology of health and disease reflects more applied approach of medical sociology and is understandable as the application of sociological of social sciences methods in analyzing the exact, different problems of medicine and health such as treatment of diseases and prevention, resource allocation, etc. (1). Thus sociology in medicine is understandable as applied social researches, the main object of which is not the social, but medical-based problems or phenomena (2). In the case of medical sociology sometimes called as sociology of health care institutions, medicine itself is supposed as social institution, pretty the same as, for instance, family, religion, education, economics, politics, and so far (3). So, the studies of social nature, which are being proceeded in investigating medicine from the social point of view, give the opportunity to develop certain providences about the social interactions, social networks, social organizations, etc., which are influencing the social problems of medicine and health.

J. Siegrist tried to delineate the disciplinary structure of medical sociology in terms of five important areas of knowledge:

Sociology of healthy lifestyles (prevention); Sociology of patients' careers (rehabilitation); Sociology of client–professional interaction (diagnosis, therapy); Sociological (social epidemiological) studies of causes of health and disease and Sociology of health care systems.

It is argued that intensified exchange according to these areas between the academic disciplines of medical sociology and social medicine is needed to generate a significant impact on future training and research both in medicine and in public health.

## Application of Social Theories in Analyzing the Phenomena of Health and Medicine

### *Structural functionalism*

Structural functionalism looks at the role the sick person plays in society. The focus is on how being ill is given a specific form in human societies so that the social system's stability and cohesion can be maintained. Talcott Parsons is often considered the father of Medical Sociology because of his description of the "Sick Role." This describes the difference between the role of a sick person as opposed to the "Social Role" of a healthy person. He defines the sick role as defining the motivation of the patient. Curiously enough, T. Parsons makes no mention of the role of the doctor or other medical institutions. The sick role comprises four aspects: exemption from normal social role responsibilities, the privilege of not being held responsible for being sick, the desire to get better, and the obligation to find proper help and follow that advice. A pivotal event occurred in 1951 that oriented medical sociology towards theoretical concerns and initiated the establishment of its academic credentials.

This was the publication of T. Parsons' long-anticipated book "The Social System," which established the author at the time as the dominant figure in American sociology. Anything T. Parsons published attracted great attention because he was supposed to be charting a course for all of sociology. T. Parsons was interested in the different roles of professionals in capitalistic and socialist societies and decided to include physicians and their relationship with their clients/patients in his analysis, because this topic was an area of long-standing interest and one in which he felt he had familiarity.

T. Parsons' concept of the sick role is a clear and straightforward statement of four basic propositions outlining the normative pattern of physician utilization by the sick and their respective social roles. T. Parsons not only constructed the first theoretical concept directly applicable to medical sociology, but by utilizing the work of E. Durkheim and M. Weber, he did so within the parameters of classical sociological theory. His formulation was recognized as "a penetrating and apt analysis of sickness from a distinctly sociological point of view," which indeed it was. T. Parsons also influenced the study of professions by using the medical profession as the model for professions based on expertise and a service orientation.

E. Durkheim's only work that had a direct application to medical sociology was his theory of suicide in which the act of taking one's life was determined by the individual's ties to his or her community or society. This is seen in his typology of three major types of suicide: 1) egoistic (social detachment); 2) anomic (state of normlessness); and 3) altruistic a normative demand for suicide. The merit of his concept is that it shows the capability of the larger society to create stressful situations where people are forced to respond to conditions not of their own choice. Thus, E.

Durkheim helps us to not only understand the social facets of suicide, but to recognize that macro-level social events like economic recessions can affect health in a variety of ways through stress and that the effects of stress can be mitigated through social support. Structural functionalism, with its emphasis on value consensus, social order, stability, and functional processes at the macro-level of society, had a short lived period as the leading theoretical paradigm in medical sociology.

## Conflict Theory

Conflict theory is concerned with the relationship between health and illness and capitalist social organization. The focus is on how the definition and treatment of health and illness are influenced by the nature of economic activity in a capitalist society. Conflict theory is based on the assumption that society is composed of various groups struggling for advantage that inequality is a basic feature of social life, and conflict is the major cause of social change. C. Marx's perspective in conflict theory is seen in the rejection of the view expressed by structural functionalism that society is held together by shared norms and values. Conflict theory claims that true consensus does not exist; rather, society's norms and values are those of the dominant elite and imposed by them on the less privileged to maintain their advantaged position. Since all social systems contain such inequality, conflict inevitably results, and conflict, in turn, is responsible for social change. Whereas, the Marxian-oriented features of conflict theory have emphasized class struggle, other theorists have moved toward emphasizing conflicts that occur between interest groups and the unequal distribution of political power. According to B. Turner, modern societies are the best understood as having a conflict between the principles of democratic politics emphasizing equality and universal rights and the organization of their economic systems involving the production, exchange, and consumption of goods and services, about which there is considerable inequality. Therefore, while people have political equality, they lack social equality. This unresolved contradiction is relatively permanent and remains a major source of conflict. Ideologies of fairness are constantly challenged by the realities of inequalities, and they influence governments to try to resolve the situation through politics and welfare benefits.

This situation represents one of conflict theory's most important assets for medical sociology; namely, the capacity to explain the politics associated with health reform. Conflict theory allows us to chart the maneuvers of various entities, like the medical profession, insurance companies, drug companies, the business community, and the public, as they struggle to acquire, protect, or expand their interests against existing government regulations and programs and those under consideration. Other conflict approaches are connected more directly to classical Marxism by relying on class struggle to explain health policy outcomes and the disadvantages of the lower and working classes in capitalist medical systems where the emphasis is on profit. While a major focus of conflict theory in medical sociology is on the role of competing interests in health care delivery and policy, other interests concern the sources of illness and disability in work environments, working-class health, differences in health lifestyles, and capitalist ideologies supportive of physician–patient interaction. However, there are inherent limitations in the use of conflict theory in medical sociology. While some health situations are affected by conflict-related conditions, others are not. People may maintain their health or become sick, and these outcomes can have little or nothing to do with conflict, politics, interest-group competition, class struggles, and the like.

The greatest potential of conflict theory for medical sociology thus lies in its non-Marxist aspects, as interest-group competition in welfare states proves more relevant for health concerns than class struggle.

## Symbolic Interaction

How we interact in the society? What is the way we understand each other? What determines the success of our social interaction? Symbolic interaction is one of the social theories, which is attempting to answer to the questions above. This is theory of modern sociology and social psychology, which analyzes the social interactions and appeals on their symbolic content. The sense of symbolic interaction is based on the look at the interaction among people as continuous dialog, where the participants are observing each other and thinking about each other's intentions and react on them differently. Social meanings are being created and changed during this dialog. Human behavior is social and based on the communication. Individuals are responding both to the behavior of others and to the other's intentions.

Symbolic interactionism is concerned with examining the interaction among the different role players in the health and illness drama. The focus is on how illness and the subjective experience of being sick are constructed through the doctor–patient exchange. The argument is here that illness is a social accomplishment among actors rather than just a matter of physiological malfunction.

J. Elinson raises somewhat rhetorical questions about the value of medical care and medical sociology. Behind them is a serious concern with the type and scope of medicalization in modern society as well as its sociological criticism. This raises the issue of whether the various theoretical images of medicine and the patient which sociology provides are able to account for the effect of the social environment upon morbidity and mortality as shown, for instance, by the Alameda County Study. Three theoretically distinct approaches are discussed in detail, structural functionalism, symbolic interactionism and conflict theory. These characterize medical sociology over the last 30 years.

The theory of symbolic interactionism is widely used in the investigations of population health. Traditionally, symbolic interactionism has been viewed as one perspective underpinning qualitative research, but it is also the basis for quantitative studies. Rooted in social psychology, symbolic interactionism has a rich intellectual heritage that spans more than a century. Underlying symbolic interactionism is the major assumption that individuals act on the basis of the meaning that things have for them. Symbolic interactionism can serve as a theoretical perspective for conceptually clear and soundly implemented multiple method research that will expand the understanding of human health behavior.

## Feminist Theory

Feminist theory explores the gendered nature of the definition of illness and treatment of patients. Its main concern is the way in which medical treatment involves male control over women's bodies and identities. Feminist theory in medical sociology also has poststructural roots, especially in regard to social constructionist accounts of the female body and its regulation by a male-dominated society. Social and cultural assumptions are held to influence our perceptions of the body, including the use of the male body as the standard for medical training, the assignment of less socially desirable physical and emotional traits to women, and the ways in which women's illnesses are socially constructed. Other feminist theory is grounded in conflict theory or symbolic interaction and deals with the sexist treatment of women patients by male doctors and the less than equal status of female physicians in professional settings and hierarchies. There is, however, no unified perspective among feminist theorists other than a "woman-centered" perspective that examines the various facets of women's health and seeks an end to sexist orientations in health and illness and society at large. Regardless of its widespread influence on many facets of contemporary theory in medical sociology, post structuralism has its critics.

Some argue that post structuralism has been overtaken and surpassed by postmodern theory or, at best, cannot be easily distinguished from postmodernism. Others suggest that the perspective does not take limits on power into account, nor explain relations between macro-level power structures other than dwell on their mechanisms for reproduction; moreover, there is a disregard of agency in post structural concepts, especially those of M. Foucault.

Oppression based on gender exists in all aspects of women's lives and transcends contemporary cultures, economic systems, and even health care services. Radical feminism provides an alternative philosophic framework of health care that is based on a women centered viewpoint, with the experiences of women as its unifying philosophy. Midwifery is a means to apply this new philosophic approach to the health care of women. A partnership between midwifery and feminist philosophy will allow women's voices to be heard, while guiding research in women's health care in new directions and illuminating new approaches to current health problems. The new millennium provides an opportunity to explore an alternative framework and philosophy that will change the current paradigm of women's health care.

By its very nature, the field of medical sociology has considerable potential for incorporating a consideration of gender in its research. After approximately a generation of the women's movement, women's studies, and the study of gender in sociology, now is an appropriate time to assess the impact of feminism on the mainstream of the field. Such an assessment is distinct from a feminist critique of medical sociology, with its implication that the field has many shortcomings, and also from a review of the growing sociological study of women's health and their role in providing as well as receiving care. The purpose to examine a representative research in mainstream medical sociology for evidence of the extent and nature of feminism's influence is necessary. Overall, one may argue that by the 1990s mainstream medical sociology has been significantly affected by feminism, but that this effect is qualified in important ways.

**Post Structuralism**

Post structuralism concentrates on the dominant medical discourse, which has constructed definitions of normality health and deviance sickness. This discourse provides subjects in modern societies with the vocabulary through which their medical needs and remedies are defined. The source and beneficiary of this discourse is the medical profession. Post structuralism theorists also argue that medical discourse plays an important role in the management of individual bodies what M. Foucault called "anatomopolitics" and bodies *en masse* bio-politics. Medicine is not just about medicine as it is conventionally understood, but also about wider structures of power and control. The leading representative of post structuralism is M. Foucault, who focused on the relationship between knowledge and power. M. Foucault provided social histories of the manner in which knowledge produced expertise that was used by professions and institutions, including medicine, to shape social behavior. Knowledge and power were depicted as being so closely connected that an extension of one meant a simultaneous expansion of the other. In fact, M. Foucault often used the term "knowledge/power" to express this unity. The knowledge/power link is not only repressive, but also productive and enabling, as it is a decisive basis upon which people are allocated to positions in society. A major contribution of M. Foucault to medical sociology is his analysis of the social functions of the medical profession, including the use of medical knowledge as a means of social control and regulation, as he studied madness, clinics, and sexuality. M. Foucault found two distinct trends emerging in the history of medical practice: "medicine of the species" the classification, diagnosis, and treatment of disease and "medicine of social spaces" the prevention of disease. The former defined the human body as an object of study subject to medical intervention and control, while the latter made the public's health subject to medical and civil regulation. The surveillance of human sexuality by the state, church, and medicine subjected the most intimate bodily activities to institutional discourse and monitoring. Thus, bodies themselves came under the jurisdiction of experts on behalf of society.

Another area of investigation is the social construction of bodies, illness, and emotions. In medical sociology, the social constructionist approach is closely tied to M. Foucault and analyzes the body as a product of power and knowledge. It focuses on examining the manner in which people shape, decorate, present, manage, and socially evaluate the body.

## Opportunities of Development of Medical Sociology

In paradigmatic – basically directions of social theories– attitude contemporary medical sociology is rather differentiated and in some aspects fragmented. From the other hand, investigations, especially sociological, are usually deeper integrated in sociopolitical, socio economical, and socio cultural environment of certain social structure. Medical sociology should combine two things, which are far from each other: inherited conservative tradition of quantitative methods and more often interdisciplinary qualitative principals of social health coming from the Western world of science. The processes of international integration of science raise very important questions: what is the perspective of medical sociology in integrating in the wider and more dynamic context of directions of biomedical researches or different directions of public health researches? Should medical sociology remain as only passive watcher of processes running around? It is obvious that to answer to this question it would be necessary to evaluate the heritage of traditions of conservative quantitative researches and modern opportunities of development of qualitative researches. Any tradition creates certain pyramidical and hierarchical structures, which have the independent power as dominating norms and further support the existing and institutionalized meaning of science. Thus, the problems of differentiation of medical sociology are related not only to the possible administrative changes, but to the real relations of power and questions of institutionalization as well. The last mentioned are important because the definitions of medical sociology are substantially changing today – medical sociology is acquiring the peculiarities of multiparadigmatic academic activity. All this allows forming different, sometimes even alternative theoretical and empirical strategies of researches, which in overall orient towards the wider interpretation of the directions of contemporary medical sociology. While discussing the theories of medical sociology and proportion of methodology and methods, it is crucial to understand that social theories, which are based on the certain theoretical paradigm, are not the final consequence of academic investigations or approximately set collection of truth which covers the direct historical perspective. The latter attitude pays an important role for methodology, which helps to understand that social theoretical paradigms as systems of reading and the choice of certain methods of researches are not set once for ever. Medical sociology and its branch, sociology of health and medicine, are not only the sciences of accumulative nature as, for instance, nature sciences but the science of critical thinking and interpretational nature as well. One of the main aims of medical sociology is to understand, evaluate, and forecast the social problems of health in different levels of the analysis of society for instance, levels of community, regional, societal, and global levels, which come from their general source – experience. It is vital to combine aspects of experience and thinking. Theoretical activity is also both observing and taking part in analytical interpretational researches. That is why it is important for medical sociology to participate in investigating intellectual, ethical, or political health problems of society. It is important to note that strategy mentioned promotes critical evaluation of methodological problems of researches, especially too much pretentious tradition of positivism, which was dominating during the 20th century and is still dominating in contemporary medical sociology. Thus, the question whether we should think about the training of professionals of medical sociology. Recent graduate of high medical school is very much familiar about the cells, human organs, biochemical structures, and so on, but seeing the offered list of subjects to study, there is a doubt whether graduate is aware enough about at least core peculiarities, interactions and relations of individual, as social being and society, as the system, whether graduate is able to analyze these questions in certain level? Besides, it is vital today to reorient medical thinking in the direction of sociologization within the society and medicine itself; it is important to develop not only researches of medical sociology but theory as well and construct certain terminology using the Western standards and experience. It is the time to think about the establishment of the association and specialized scientific journal of medical sociology i.e., sociology of health, which would stimulate the development of medical sociology and would help to tackle the retardation of it from the Western part of the world related to the past experience and events. Thus, it is logically to think that in the present and in the future, it would be purposive to work systematically in developing the studies and researches of medical sociology. The attempts of looking for the reasons and explanations of medical phenomena not only using demographical approaches but socio-cultural contexts as well show that medical sociology has very good opportunities to develop and reflect the strivings to explore the winnings and achievements of public health science more effectively and oriented towards the improvement of human well-being in every country.

## Disability: Usage in Medical Sociology

Medical sociologists generally work with the lay or commonsense meaning of 'disability', or with 'official' re-workings of the lay view. In Anglophone cultures, disability refers to 'limited activity' – not being able 'to do things', and a 'disabled person' is someone who has a medically certifiable 'condition' that prevents him or her carrying out the full range of age-related activities considered normal. This understanding of disability is deeprooted and pervasive, and is reflected in the UK's Disability Discrimination Acts of 1995 and 2005 (DDA). To paraphrase the DDA: a person 'has a disability' if he or she has a physical or mental impairment that has a substantial and long-term adverse effect on his or her ability to carry out normal day-to-day activities.

The commonsense perspective assumes that an injury to the body – through illness, accident or 'developmental abnormalities' in gestation – is the cause of disability, of 'being disabled' and of 'disablement'. For any individual, the degree of her disablement, or the extent of his 'disabilities', depends on the severity and nature of the condition involved. Collectively, reference is made to 'people with disabilities'. Medical and rehabilitative services are believed to possess the scientific expertise required to identify with precision the failings of the body that 'cause disability', and to offer the best hope for corrective solutions.

In the main, medical sociologists' interests lie not in contesting or examining the meaning of the concept 'disability' *per se*, but in exploring the social dimensions and consequences of disability and its causes – at societal and individual levels. The prevalence of disability rises with age: because impairment increases with age so too does disability or disablement. It also follows that disability is a universal phenomenon: 'The existence of impairment and disability are as old as the human body and early societies; they are a human constant'. Medical sociologists have long recognised that disabled people are also subject to degrees of social discrimination and disadvantage, and some have made these *additional* limitations the subject for research

## Disability and Disablism: Usage in Disability Studies

In the 1970s, disability activists in the UK challenged the commonsense meaning of disability and its *individualising* essence and consequences. The best-known outcome of this struggle to redefine what being disabled means is 'the social model of disability', formulated by Michael Oliver in 1983. In his words:

> In the broadest sense, the social model of disability is about nothing more complicated than a clear focus on the economic, environmental and cultural barriers encountered by people who are viewed by others as having some form of impairment – whether physical, mental or intellectual. The barriers disabled people encounter include inaccessible education systems, working environments, inadequate disability benefits, discriminatory health and social support services, inaccessible transport, houses and public buildings and amenities, and the devaluing of disabled people through negative images in the media – films, television, and newspapers.

This shifts the focus to the imposition of limits on activity *from the outside*. As we shall see, writers and researchers in disability studies have worked to substantiate and elaborate *social* definitions and interpretations of disability eversince.

*Disablism*, a term introduced by Paul Abberley (1987), refers to the social beliefs and actions that oppress/exclude/disadvantage people with impairments. It is a term that is used widely in disability studies – one that belongs to the social oppression paradigm. Its meaning is easily grasped because its sister concepts – racism, sexism and ageism–are so familiar and well understood. The term is often used in this book, both when expressing my own views on the issues under discussion and when citing the arguments of others.

It is widely accepted that the terms 'chronic illness' or 'chronic disease' refer to long-term and incurable medical conditions. Chronic illnesses may be relatively stable but are often degenerative, and are sometimes marked by acute episodes and exacerbation. Particularly prevalent in late capitalist societies are heart diseases, cancers and neurological conditions – associated mainly with later life. Medicine continues to offer little by way of curative or even ameliorative treatments for many chronic illnesses and their symptoms; indeed chronic illness 'frustrates the project upon which medicine's prestige rests'. In the UK, chronic diseases became the major health scourge from the mid-twentieth century, largely replacing the infectious diseases so deadly to both young and old in earlier decades.

## Sociology in Public Health

Public health has been and remains a very applied field. It is also characterized by a population-based approach to health, and statistical methods are deemed the appropriate underlying method for the field. It is viewed as a science that seeks to intervene, control, and prevent large-scale processes that negatively affect the public's health. By these criteria, there is a strong logical fit of sociological principles and practices within public health. Nonetheless, sociology has not been the key social science discipline in public health. That position has gone to psychology, where the emphasis on individual behavior resonates more with a biomedical model. Despite this, many of the primary concerns of present-day public health, with large-scale variables such as social capital, social inequality, social status, and health care organization and financing, remain topics best suited to the sociological perspective and methodology. The emphasis in public health is thus shifting toward a sociological perspective.

## Sociological Concepts in Public Health

Sociology in public health is reflected in the myriad of sociological concepts that pervade the practice of public health. More than any other social science, sociology has the discussion of socioeconomic status at its very core. Social-class variation within society is the key explanatory variable in sociology—for everything from variation in social structure to differential life experiences of health and illness. Indeed, there appears to be overwhelming evidence that Western industrialized societies that have little variation in social class experience have far better health outcomes than societies characterized by wide social-class dispersion. In short, inequalities in health are directly related to social and economic inequalities. Much of later-twentieth-century public health is devoted to the reduction of these inequalities.

## Sociological Methods in Public Health

Methodological concerns are critical to sociological research. The great debate in sociology has been on the relative merits and role of quantitative *versus* qualitative approaches. Both approaches are widely used and play a critical role for public health. Sociology has long recognized that the social world comprises both an objective and a subjective reality. For example, the objective reality of having cancer is accompanied by the subjective reality of the experience of cancer by the patient, and the patient's family and friends. Both realities are relevant to the sociological approach. The subjective, qualitative approach is generally discussed in the theory and methods concerned with illness behavior, but qualitative approaches are equally applicable to the understanding of social policy, world systems, and areas of sociology where statistical measurement is difficult or less relevant.

Within public health, surveillance is seen as a key approach to describing the distribution and dynamics of disease. In sociological approaches to public health, the role of social and behavioral factors in health and illness is central. Survey methodology has occupied a central place in sociological research since the middle of the twentieth century. The concern has been with the collection, management, analysis, interpretation, and use of large quantities of data obtained by direct interview with respondents. Social surveys are characterized by large random samples, complicated questionnaires, and the use of multivariate statistics for analysis. By their very nature, most sociological variables are complex to measure and to analyze. For example, the assessment of socioeconomic status of an individual requires the accurate measurement of several variables that sit within a larger social context. Socioeconomic status (SES) is regarded as a product of several components, including income, residence, education, and occupation. Determining the relative weight of each of these components is a major analytical problem. Thus, when considering the role of socioeconomic status on health care outcomes, there is no easy answer to what mechanism actually works to determine the observed relationship between SES and health.

## Sociology and Evaluation in Public Health

Because many sociological variables are at the so called macro level, there is limited opportunity to intervene rapidly, directly, or simply. For example, the SES of a group is affected by complex components, such as education and occupation that are part of the total life course of individuals within the group. Thus, to change the SES of a group would require significant redistribution of resources of the larger social structure. A significant period of time and concerted effort is needed to change such macro variables. This is, however, not dissimilar to many other challenges in public health, such as the long-term and time-consuming effort to change lifestyles and reduce behavioral risk factors related to chronic diseases.

The chief role of sociology in public health remains its evaluation of those macro components of society that affect public health at the population level. Such evaluations provide an understanding of why inequalities in health exist, and they help elaborate upon the mechanisms and processes that sustain these inequalities. This relates to the long-standing theoretical concern with social structure among sociologists. Further, sociology reveals the mechanisms for long-term changes that may lead to a reduction in health inequalities. The product of sociological thinking in public health is not immediate nor easily understood by those who seek quick and easy solutions to the suffering of humanity. Nonetheless, the long-term role of sociology in public health is to change and improve the public health.

## Social and Behavioral Sciences

While it is undoubtedly true that a biomedical perspective dominated public health in the first-half of the twentieth century, there has emerged, largely since World War II, a social science perspective in public health. This perspective has developed in departments of social and community medicine in Europe and in schools of public health in the United States, and it is reflected in the growth of the behavioral and social sciences in the curricula for public health professional and research degrees. This perspective is also evident in the establishment of departments of social and behavioral sciences in universities.

Many social and behavioral science disciplines are relevant to the understanding and articulation of the mission of public health. It would be impossible to document here all the various discipline areas; these include disciplines as diverse as psychology, economics, history, and anthropology. The focus here will be on those disciplines that most directly attempt to describe, understand, predict, and change the public's health.

## Social and Behavioral Sciences Literature

A considerable literature on individual behavior and public health has developed in the second-half of the twentieth century. The general failure of public health to pick up and nurture the more macro social science perspectives to the same degree has limited the full potential of the impact of the social and behavioral sciences on public health, particularly because the historical roots of public health in the latter half of the nineteenth century included a strong social structural viewpoint. Since that time, the theoretical development of economics, political science, sociology, and anthropology has accelerated, but it was often not brought to bear on contemporary public health issues because these issues were often defined in terms of the characteristics of individuals rather than as characteristics of social structure. The argument is, then, that public health picked up the wrong end of the social science stick—the individual micro end rather than the socio cultural macro end. This assertion is supported by any perusal of public health journals or literature on social and behavioral science in public health in the second-half of the twentieth century. Nonetheless, as the end of the twentieth century in public health witnessed increasing concern with social concepts such as social inequity, inequality, and community interventions, the disciplines of sociology, anthropology, economics, and political science had a more important role in public health, for the determinants of health were being defined in terms of a social and behavioral perspective. For example, many individual behaviors were recognized as risk factors for poor health, but were also seen as embedded in a wider social context. In addition, a social science–informed healthful public policy was seen by many as a key to the development of public health strategies to improve health.

## The Scientific Disciplines and Public Health

As noted previously, there are several social and behavioral science disciplines applied to public health. What follows is a brief summary of each of the key disciplines, with attention given to the theory and work of each discipline relevant to public health. In some of the social science disciplines there are large subdisciplinary areas devoted to medicine. For example, there are large subdisciplinary fields such as history of medicine, medical sociology, medical anthropology, health psychology, and medical geography. Most of these subdisciplines have university departments, dedicated journals, and professional organizations. However, most of these subdisciplines are concerned with medicine in the very broadest interpretation, including health promotion, clinical care, disease prevention, and biomedical research. Only a part of a subdiscipline such as medical sociology is concerned with public health. Similarly, most of the subdiscipline of history of medicine is concerned with the development and evolution of clinical medicine rather than public health. Thus, the interpretation of the role of the social and behavioral sciences in public health is very much tied to one's definition of public health.

## The Social and Behavioral Science Disciplines

The social sciences are concerned with the study of human society and with the relationship of individuals in, and to, society. The chief academic disciplines of the social sciences are anthropology, economics, history, political science, and sociology. The behavioral sciences, particularly psychology, are concerned with the study of the actions of humans and animals. The key effort of the behavioral sciences is to understand, predict, and influence behavior. The chief academic disciplines of the behavioral sciences are anthropology, psychology, and sociology, with the distinction between social and behavioral science often blurred when these disciplines are applied in public health research and practice, particularly in schools of public health and governmental agencies. Many, if not most, public health approaches are problem focused and lead to a multidiscipline solution encompassing several social and behavioral science disciplines and combinations of them such as social psychology, in addition to other public health disciplines such as epidemiology and biostatistics.

## Anthropology

Anthropology is a broad social science concerned with the study of humans from a social, biological and cultural perspective. Historically it is a Western-based social science with roots in Europe and North America. It includes two broad areas of physical and sociocultural anthropology; both are relevant to public health. Physical anthropology divides into two areas, one related to tracing human evolution and the study of primates, and the other concerned with contemporary human characteristics stemming from the mixture of genetic adaptations and culture. Medical anthropologists with this perspective are often concerned with the relationships between culture, illness, health, and nutrition. Socio-cultural anthropology is concerned with broad aspects of the adaptation of humans to their cultures—with social organization, language, ethnographic details, and, in general, the understanding of culturally mitigated patterns of behavior. In recent decades this perspective has taken a more ecologically focused view of the human species. From a public health perspective, this approach to anthropology is probably most salient in terms of the methodological approaches used by anthropologists. They have a critical concern with understanding communities through participant observation. Indeed, participation is probably the key concept linking modern-day anthropological approaches to twentieth-century concepts of public health community interventions. Although the methodology of rapport-based structured interviews and observation is a highly developed methodology among anthropologists, it has had limited application in public health. More recent efforts in public health to address issues of inequity at the community level have created more attention to anthropological approaches.

## Economics

Economics is perhaps the oldest of the social sciences, with its concern with wealth and poverty, trade and industry. However, current economic thinking generally dates from the last three centuries and is associated with the great names in economic thinking, such as Adam Smith, Robert Malthus, David Ricardo, John Stuart Mill, and Karl Marx. Present-day economics is an advanced study of production, employment, exchange, and consumption driven by sophisticated mathematical models. Basically, the field breaks into two distinctive areas: microeconomics and macroeconomics. Microeconomics is largely concerned with issues such as competitive markets, wage rates, and profit margins. Macroeconomics deals with broader issues, such as national income, employment, and economic systems. The relationship between economics and health is obvious because in developed countries the percentage of Gross National Product consumed by the health care industry is significant, generally ranging from 5 to 15 per cent of the gross national product. In the poorer countries, the cost of disease to the overall economy can prohibit the sound economic development of the country. In recent years there has been a concern with both the global economic burden of disease as well as with investment in health. That poverty is highly related to poor public health is a widely accepted tenet of modernday thinking in public health. However, economic systems ranging from free enterprise through liberal socialism and communism offer quite differing alternatives to the reduction of poverty and the distribution of economic resources.

## Psychology

Psychology is probably the most common disciplinary background found in the application of the social and behavioral sciences to public health. Modern psychology is a large field that encompasses physiological psychology, concerned with the nervous and circulatory systems, as well as social psychology, and concerned with the behavior of individuals as influenced by social stimuli. In general, psychology is concerned with the relationship of living organisms to their environment. In addition to studies focused on physiological mechanisms, psychology is concerned with the broad area of human cognition, including learning, memory, and concept formation. The subfield of abnormal psychology is concerned with mental disorders, ranging from psychoses to neuroses. The subfield of clinical psychology offers direct patient care mechanisms to treat mental problems in individuals. Thus the application of psychological approaches to health is quite apparent. However, the most salient branch of psychology for public health practice, and particularly for the task of understanding the determinants of health, is probably social psychology. A major focus of social psychology is on attitudes, opinions, and behaviors. Thus, there is an emphasis on understanding how groups and individuals interact with one another. The degree to which many interactions are easy or difficult can play a major role in determining the stability of groups and individuals. Therefore, broad concepts such as stress, social cohesion, peer influence, civic trust, and others derive strong theoretical and research support from social psychology.

## The Social and Behavioral Sciences Working Together

Many social and behavioral scientists who work in public health have strong, disciplinary-based, undergraduate and graduate training in one of the social sciences. However, the practice of academic and governmental public health involves disciplinary bases that are seldom as narrow as they would be in traditional, university-based academic departments. Indeed, in many government institutions of public health such discipline-trained social scientists may be simply referred to as health scientists or even as social epidemiologists. Public health practice is largely problem-focused, and whatever, disciplinary base is appropriate to the problem will be used. Thus, it would not be uncommon for a person trained as a psychologist to be involved with a program addressed at community change or for an anthropologist to be involved with individual behavioral change. Nonetheless, all of the social and behavioral sciences share a commonality in approach to public health that differs from that of the biomedical approach. Disease is usually seen as a distal outcome, the focus being on those social and behavioral processes that prevent and reduce disease in people. Generally, the social sciences take a view that health and sickness are only one part of people's lifestyle.

The social and behavioral sciences have varied and broad-based methodologies. Discussions of methodological approaches to knowledge attainment are at the heart of many discipline-based discussions. Perhaps the greatest ongoing debate is that over the role of qualitative and quantitative approaches to understanding. Many researchers and practitioners in public health consider data to be the sine qua non of public health. Often data are perceived as being quantitative and numerate. The social and behavioral sciences take a much broader view of what data is. Data can be personal accounts and stories as well as statistical presentations. Nonetheless, the rigor underpinning the appropriate collection of good data applies to both the quantitative and qualitative approaches. There is a strong appreciation that many quasi scientific cognitive ideas, such as race, poverty, or trust, cannot simply be quantified and understood numerically, yet still play a key role in determining health outcomes.

## The Determinants of Health

In discussing the determinants of health it is useful to distinguish between the health of individuals and populations. The determinants of health for any individual relate highly to the unique characteristics of that individual. In the first instance, these characteristics are highly determined by biology—the gender, age, and genetic background of the individual. These characteristics play a primary determining role and are usually not modifiable. For example, it is obvious that a man cannot die from ovarian cancer, or a woman from testicular cancer. Generally, only an older person will suffer from Alzheimer's disease; only a person with a genetic deficit will suffer from Down syndrome. Medical science and public health can do little to change these powerful determinants of health in the individual. However, it is also anticipated that most individuals born in the Western World of the twenty-first century are biologically equipped to have a life expectancy of some seventy to eighty years.

The health of populations is a different concept from that of the health of individuals, and the determinants of the health of populations may be conceptualized very broadly. The following is just a short list of some of the hypothesized determinants of population health: health care services, sewers and drains, potable water, sanitation, adequate nutrition, shelter, transportation networks, supportive social environments, healthful public policy, stable child-rearing environments, healthful work environments, and peace and tranquility. What is apparent in such a broad list is that most of the hypothesized determinants are outside of the traditional medical care sector of clinics and hospitals. Many determinants of population health are determined by human conditions at the broadest level of political interaction, such as the protection from the ravages of poverty, war, and refugee status. Most important, the individual has relatively little direct control over these determinants. Even in those arenas where the individual believes he or she has control, such as in pursuit of education, occupation, and income through the life span, the reality remains that access to education, occupation, and income is socially determined.

People suffer disease and illness due to social processes that are only remotely related to personal health care. As public health moves away from personal health care as the major determinant of public health to a position where it is merely one of many determinants of public health, the role of the social and behavioral sciences becomes more important in understanding population health. The World Health Organization European Office lists ten social determinants of health that are supported by strong research evidence: (1) the social gradient people's relative social and economic status and circumstances strongly affect their health throughout life; (2) stress harms health (3) early life the effects of early development last a lifetime; (4) social exclusion social exclusion creates misery and costs lives; (5) work stress in the workplace increases the risk of disease; (6) unemployment job security increases health, well-being, and job satisfaction; (7) social support friendship, good social relations, and strong supportive networks improve health at home, at work, and in the community; (8) addiction individuals turn to alcohol, drugs, and tobacco and suffer from their use, but use is influenced by the wider social setting; (9) food healthful food is a political issue; and (10) transport healthful transport means reducing driving and encouraging more walking and cycling, backed up by better public transport.

## The Role of the Social and Behavioral Sciences

In contributing to the understanding of the determinants of health, there are two chief challenges for the social and behavioral sciences. The first is to continue to build in greater depth the knowledge and evidence base for the role of socioeconomic factors in health. The second is to develop appropriate best practices for addressing the role of socioeconomic factors in order to improve the health of the public. These are related challenges, but the first is perhaps more of a challenge for the academic world, and the second for the world of public health practice. Despite the enormous complexity inherent in these challenges, there is a large and growing literature to address both of them. There is a very large literature in Western languages addressing the role of socioeconomic status (SES) and its relationship to mortality and morbidity in infants, children, adolescents, and young and old adults. In general the available evidence is more extensive for working-aged adults, where multiple studies from many countries show powerful evidence linking low SES to increased chronic disease mortality and morbidity among males and a consistent gradient of the association between levels of SES and levels of health.

Conceptually, this is a very complex and extensive area for research because of the large number of variable combinations in any research approach. Thus, if one takes SES as the determinant of interest, it needs to be studied for its impact on every age group, gender, and ethnic or racial group, in relation to many possible outcomes, including chronic disease morbidity and mortality and risk factors for each disease. The resulting matrix of variable combinations is indeed exceedingly complex. Even though research has looked at many of the relationships possible, they clearly have not all been explored in the detail to bring surety in conclusions. That is why the research challenge is so great—there is much more basic research that needs to be undertaken to fully understand the complexities associated with the social determinants of health.

The second challenge is even more critical and is at the heart of public health ideology. Public health is predicated on the idea that one wants to take action to prevent or control disease; at the same time public health is also concerned with promoting health and preventing disease at the population level. Thus, the ideal strategies for public health practice call for action at the population level. It is, however, one thing to understand the complex mechanisms that link social determinants to health, it is quite another to try and alter them. At first glance it would appear that the solution is simple. If poverty causes poor health, then elimination of poverty should increase the overall population health. Few could disagree; nonetheless poverty itself is the result of many contributing factors. Furthermore, many in public health might well argue that large-scale programs to eliminate poverty, such as equal income distribution policies, are well beyond the scope of public health practice and carry with them political risks and an adverse impact on economic aspects of a society.

One socialscience approach is to look at the scope and characteristics of the problem and then determine what is a feasible course of action to maximize benefits within the restraints of a given social system—an approach that is based on the realities within any given country's sociopolitical system. Such an approach recognizes the diversity and variability both within and between sovereign countries, but at the same time recognizes the global interdependence of all countries. Nonetheless, when public health researchers and agencies within countries have addressed the socioeconomic determinants of health from the standpoint of interventions, several common themes emerge. First, there is the recognition of the need to pursue macro-level economic and social policies that create investment in the physical and social determinants of health. In general, this means an effort to address broad issues to improve health care infrastructure, education, transportation systems, and housing, as well as participation in a just society. It also means addressing inequities and issues of poverty. Such approaches are made explicit in documents such as Healthy People 2010.

Second, there is a strong attention to the community as the setting for public health interventions. That is, the everyday living and working conditions must be improved, particularly when these are accompanied by poverty and the plight of disadvantaged groups. Increasing control of the environment by those within it is a strong component of a participation-based intervention approach.

Third, behavioral risk factors remain a critical component of interventions to address the social determinants of health. Although the social setting and milieu may produce many barriers to behavior change, there remains considerable latitude at the individual level for change.

Particularly in the addictive behaviors, the role of the individual remains powerful and inescapable. Evidence-based interventions need to combine the knowledge of the social and behavioral science disciplines to address the complexity of behavioral change.

Fourth, the personal health care system is seen as a critical component of the determinants of health and is the system closest to the professions of most of those who labor in the field of public health. The critical issue for the personal health care system is to address the inequities in access to quality care. These inequities stem from many determinants, including poverty and prejudice. Socio-demographic factors such as geography and urbanization also play a key role. Adequate and equitable distribution of health care resources remains a challenge for the entire globe, as does humane treatment and attention to social and psychological factors in the overall well-being of patients and families seen in these settings.

**Behavior, Health Related**

Health-related behavior is one of the most important elements in people's health and well-being. Its importance has grown as sanitation has improved and medicine has advanced. Diseases that were once incurable or fatal can now be prevented or successfully treated, and health-related behavior has become an important component of public health. The improvement of health-related behaviors is, therefore, central to public health activities.

Behavioral factors play a role in each of the twelve leading causes of death, including chronic diseases such as heart disease, cancer, and stroke, which are the major causes of death in the United States and other developed countries. The most common behavioral contributors to mortality, or death, in 1990 included the use of alcohol, tobacco, firearms, and motor vehicles; diet and activity patterns; sexual behavior; and illicit use of drugs. Behaviors such as these are thought to contribute to almost half of the deaths in the

United States, and, according to J. McGinnis and W. Foege (1993), they were responsible for nearly 1 million deaths in the United States in the year of 1992 alone. The social and economic costs related to these behaviors can all be greatly reduced by changes in individuals' behaviors.

The last two decades of the twentieth century saw a rising interest in preventing disability and death through changes in health-related behaviors, particularly changes in lifestyle habits and participation in screening programs. Much of this interest was stimulated by the change in disease patterns from infectious to chronic diseases as leading causes of death, combined with the aging of the population, rapidly escalating health care costs, and data linking individual behaviors to increased risk of morbidity and mortality. The AIDS (acquired immunodeficiency syndrome) epidemic also contributed.

Although there is more information about what constitutes healthy behavior and risk factors than ever before, this information has not always led to healthier behaviors. There have been some positive changes, however. Between 1988 and 1994, the average daily intake of dietary fat in the United States dropped from 36 percent to 34 per cent of total calories; seat belt use increased from 42 per cent to 67 per cent; and the number of women over the age of forty who had breast exams and mammograms doubled. Cigarette smoking has decreased among men by as much as 50 per cent in some countries. Unfortunately, during this same period, the number of obese adults rose, sexual activity among adolescents increased, more teenage girls began smoking, and the incidence of HIV (human immunodeficiency virus)/AIDS reached epidemic proportions.

## Definitions of Health Behavior

There are many questions about health-related behavior or health behavior that are not yet well understood.

Therefore, both public health workers and scientific researchers continue to attempt to understand the nature and causes of many different health behaviors. Health behavior encompasses a large field of study that cuts across various fields, including psychology, education, sociology, public health, epidemiology, and anthropology.

In the broadest sense, health behavior refers to the actions of individuals, groups, and organizations, as well as the determinants, correlates, and consequences, of these actions—which include social change, policy development and implementation, improved coping skills, and enhanced quality of life. This is similar to the working definition of health behavior that David Gochman proposed, which includes not only observable, overt actions but also the mental events and emotional states that can be reported and measured. Gochman defined health behavior as "those personal attributes such as beliefs, expectations, motives, values, perceptions, and other cognitive elements; personality characteristics, including affective and emotional states and traits; and overt behavior patterns, actions, and habits that relate to health maintenance, to health restoration, and to health improvement." Interestingly, this definition emphasizes the actions and the health of individuals. A public health perspective, in contrast, is concerned with individuals as part of a larger community. These perspectives are interrelated, as the behaviors of individuals determine many of the social conditions that affect all people's health.

Gochman's definition is consistent with the definitions of specific categories of overt health behavior proposed by S. Kasl and S. Cobb. In two seminal 1966 articles, Kasl and Cobb define three categories of health behavior:

- *Preventive health behavior* involves any activity undertaken by individuals who believe themselves to be healthy for the purpose of preventing or detecting illness in a asymptomatic state. This can include self-protective behavior, which is an action intended to confer protection from potential harm, such as wearing a helmet when riding a bicycle, using seat belts, or wearing a condom during sexual activity. Self-protective behavior is also known as cautious behavior.

- *Illness behavior* is any activity undertaken by individuals who perceive themselves to be ill for the purpose of defining their state of health, and discovering a suitable remedy.
- *Sick-role behavior* involves any activity undertaken by those who consider themselves to be ill for the purpose of getting well. It includes receiving treatment from medical providers, generally involves a whole range of dependent behaviors, and leads to some degree of exemption from one's usual responsibilities.

These classic definitions have stood the test of time, and continue to be used by students and public health workers alike. However, the lines between these three categories have blurred somewhat over-time, and there are also several categories of behavior that warrant specific definitions.

## Behavior *versus* Lifestyle

Health behavior can be something that is done once, or something that is done periodically—like getting immunizations or a flu shot. It can also be something that one does only to oneself, such as putting on sunscreen, or a behavior that affects others, like putting up a shade cover so that children at a playground are protected from the sun. Other health behaviors are actions that are performed over a long period of time, such as eating a healthful diet, getting regular physical activity, and avoiding tobacco use. It is these latter types of behaviors, which are sustained patters of complex behavior that are called "lifestyle" behaviors. A composite of various healthful behaviors is often referred to as "healthy lifestyle." However, most people do not practice either healthful or risky behaviors with complete consistency—someone might get regular, health-promoting exercise several times a week but be a cigarette smoker who seldom brushes his or her teeth; or someone might quit smoking, only to begin eating chocolate as a substitute. In the ideal, the person who practices a variety of behaviors in a health-enhancing manner can be described as living a healthy lifestyle. More realistically, though, many people practice some, but not all, lifestyle behaviors in a consistently healthful manner.

## Health-Related and Health Directed Behavior

Health-related behavior is any action that is related to disease prevention, health maintenance, health improvement, or the restoration of health. This type of behavior can be either voluntary or involuntary, and can be undertaken explicitly for health purposes, as a matter of habit, or to comply with a law or requirement. For example, a child who runs 800 meters in a physical education class is performing a health-related behavior, but only because the teacher requires it to get a passing grade. In contrast, an adult who exercises to reduce the risk of heart disease is engaging in that behavior for the express purpose of restoring, maintaining, or improving his or her health. This type of action is called "health-directed behavior." Sometimes these two types of health behavior coexist—a toddler buckled into a safety seat is participating in health-related behavior, but for the parent this is a health-directed behavior.

## Self-Care Behavior

Self-care behavior involves taking actions to improve or preserve one's health. Self-care is often thought of in terms as prevention or self-treatment of definable health problems or conditions, but it can also include primary prevention in the absence of any symptoms. Self-care includes the actions taken to treat symptoms before or instead of seeking professional medical attention, such as eating chicken soup, drinking liquids, or taking over-the-counter medications for cold or flu-like symptoms. It also includes treating minor injuries such as bruises, scrapes, and twisted ankles when a person does not think a health care professional is needed. Self-care is also a continuum whereby a patient may complete home treatments such as changing a bandage or wound dressing, doing rehabilitation exercises, or avoiding foods that inflame an allergic reaction. The use of alternative and complementary medical treatments, without medical supervision, is also self-care behavior. An important feature of self-care behavior is that it involves active participation in the health care process.

### Health Care Utilization Behavior

Health care utilization is the use of health services, whether it be clinical public health services or the services of medical care professionals. Health care utilization behavior is a continuum that ranges from using preventive services, such as getting immunizations or early detection and screening tests, to elective surgery or involuntary hospitalization after an injury. Health care utilization is influenced by many different factors, and, therefore the study of utilization behavior includes examining who uses medical services, when and why they use these services, and how satisfied they are with the services. Because health care utilization behaviors, like lifestyle behaviors, are quite complex, various factors need to be examined to understand them. A framework for understanding these factors that has been widely used is the model devised by R. Andersen and L. A. Aday. According to their model, among the factors influencing health care utilization are: characteristics of individuals and populations at risk, the availability and quality of availability services, economic factors such health insurance, and additional access factors such as the location of health services and the availability of transportation.

In addition, the level of "health need" is very important in terms of motivation and/or choice about using medical care. This approach provides an important and robust model for studying health care utilization behavior.

## Dietary Behavior

Dietary behavior refers to eating patterns that people engage in, as well as behaviors related to consuming foods, such as shopping, eating out, or portion size. Dietary behavior differs from some other types of health behavior in that it is, in its basic forms, essential for life. Of course, some dietary behaviors, such as drinking alcoholic beverages or smoking cigarettes, are not necessary to sustain life. It is recognized that dietary behaviors influence the development of many chronic diseases, including coronary heart disease, some cancers e.g. breast, colon, prostate, stomach, and cancers of the head and neck, type II diabetes mellitus, and osteoporosis. Recommendations for healthful dietary behavior include limiting consumption of high-fat foods, having a high intake of fruit and vegetables, increasing fiber, and controlling caloric intake to prevent obesity. Although most people know about the health consequences of unhealthful diets, many of the public health goals for dietary behavior have not been met. The prevalence of obesity and type II diabetes mellitus increased markedly in the United States and Canada during the last decade of the twentieth century.

Dietary behaviors play a role in preventing or managing disease when they are sustained over the long-term. Behavioral considerations are key to any attempts to promote healthful dietary behavior. Several core issues about dietary behavior have been recognized. First, most diet-related risk factors are asymptomatic and do not present immediate or dramatic symptoms. Second, health-enhancing dietary changes require qualitative charge, not just changes in the amount of food consumed. Third, both the act of making changes and self-monitoring dietary behaviors require knowledge about foods. Thus, information acquisition and processing may be more complex for dietary change than for changes in some other health behaviors, such as smoking and exercise.

**Substance-Use Behavior**

Substance-use behavior focuses on the use of both licit and illicit mood-altering substances. This category of substances, typically referred to collectively as "drugs," includes tobacco, alcohol, caffeine, marijuana, cocaine, heroin, "designer drugs," and prescription medications taken improperly. These substances are ingested for various reasons, but they are similar in that they are all taken without the advice of a physician. Substance abuse, which occurs when substance use behavior is at an extreme and unsafe level, is sometimes associated with addiction, which makes it difficult to stop using the substance. Substance use and abuse are responsible for many social and health problems, and for an enormous burden of avoidable injuries in the United States each year.

**Sexual Behavior**

Sexual behavior may or may not involve sexual intercourse. Sexual behaviors have health implications that range from reproduction and childbearing to sexually transmitted diseases and, the most serious of these, HIV/AIDS. Taking precautions or avoiding sexual contact with multiple partners can help prevent sexually transmitted diseases (STDs) and prevent unwanted pregnancies. Sexual freedom due to social changes, a broadening of women's participation in society, and the availability of effective birth control has increased the prevalence of sexual behavior bringing with it significant health and social problems. Attention toward this area of health behavior has increased greatly over the last two decades of the twentieth century, especially due to the AIDS epidemic.

### Reckless Behavior

Reckless behavior involves individuals putting themselves in situations not normally required in daily living that substantially increase their chances of illness, injury, or death. It is often used synonymously with the terms "risk taking behavior" and "risky behavior." Reckless or risky behavior is observed in adolescents and young adults, especially young males, more often than in other demographic groups. Examples of behaviors considered risky or reckless include drinking and driving, drag racing, substance use, carrying a concealed weapon, engaging in unprotected sex, and playing extreme sports. Reckless behaviors have been shown to be strongly related to an individuals' tendency toward impulsivity and sensation-seeking.

## UNDERSTANDING AND IMPROVING HEALTH BEHAVIOR

The best way to design programs to achieve positive changes in health behavior is to have an understanding of why people behave as they do and what might motivate them to change? Theories and models of health behavior have been developed for this purpose. A theory is a set of interrelated concepts, definitions, and propositions that present a systematic view of events or situations by specifying relations among variables in order to explain and predict the events or situations. Theories can be useful during the various stages of planning, implementing, and evaluating interventions. They can, for example, be used to guide an exploration of why people are or are not consuming a healthful diet or adhering to a therapeutic dietary regimen. Theories can guide the search to understand why people do or do not follow medical advice; to help identify what information is needed to design an effective intervention strategy; and to provide insight into how to design an educational program so it is successful. Thus, theories help to explain behavior, as well as suggest how to develop more effective ways to influence and change behavior. A theory about why a person chooses the foods he or she eats is one step toward successful nutrition management, but some type of change model will also be needed to guide the person toward a healthful diet.

The most widely accepted theories about health behavior have been tested in research and found to be helpful in understanding or predicting health behaviors. Health behavior is, however, far too complex to be explained by a single, unified theory, and some professionals have devised models that draw on a number of theories to help understand a specific problem in a particular setting or context.

## THEORETICAL MODELS OF HEALTH BEHAVIOR

No single theory or model dominates research or practice in health-related behavior. Four of the most frequently mentioned theories of health behavior in the late 1990s were the health belief model; social cognitive theory; the stages of change/transtheoretical model; and community organization. These theories focus on a range of factors influencing behavior determinants, including factors within an individual such as thoughts, feelings, and beliefs, factors in groups or relationships, and factors that exist in organizations, communities, and governments such as structures, regulations, policies, and laws.

The health belief model was originally developed to explain why people did or did not take advantage of preventive services such as disease screening and immunizations. Its central thesis is that health behavior is determined by two interrelated factors: a person's perception both of the threat of a health problem and of his or her accompanying appraisal of a recommended behavior for preventing or managing the problem. The model works well, especially for early detection or for some conditions, such as infectious diseases, that people might find frightening, especially if they are uncertain about the effects of treatment methods.

The stages of change model concerns an individual's readiness to change, or to try to change, unhealthful behaviors. Its basic premise is that behavior change is a process and not an event, and that individuals are at varying levels of motivation, or readiness, to change. This means that people at different points in the process of change can benefit from different programs for change, and the programs work best if matched to their stage of readiness.

Social cognitive theory (SCT) is very complex. From this theory's perspective, people and their environments are thought to interact continuously. A basic premise of social cognitive theory is that people learn not only through their experiences, but also by watching the way other people act and the results they achieve. SCT also takes the view that, while people are influenced by the world around them, they can also actively change that world. SCT provides a foundation for several strategies for behavior change, for example the use of role models who carry out a behavior and achieve good results. Another way SCT applies to behavior change is by emphasizing that individuals change their situations by changing their own behavior.

Community organization articulates the process by which community groups identify problems or goals, mobilize resources, and develop ways to reach their goals. It includes several ways of bringing about change, including developing resources and skills; getting specialized help from outside experts; and social action, which involves people joining together for a cause, especially one that involves a particular group that is being greatly affected by a particular problem. Examples of this are AIDS activists, women's health activists working for more research on breast cancer prevention and treatment, and youths developing coalitions to fight the tobacco companies' efforts to attract customers among teenagers.

## IMPORTANT CROSS CUTTING ISSUES AND CONSTRUCTS

The various theories of health-related behavior often overlap. Not surprisingly, these explanations for behavior and models for change share several constructs and common issues.

### Behavior Change as a Process

One central idea that has gained wide acceptance is the simple notion that behavior change is a process, not an event, which is the major tenet of the stages of change model. It is important to think of the change process as one that occurs in stages. It is not a question of someone deciding one day to stop smoking and the next day becoming a non-smoker for life. Likewise, most people won't be able to dramatically change their eating patterns all at once. The idea that behavior change occurs in a number of steps is not particularly new. In fact, various multistage theories of behavior change date back to the 1940s. This theory gained wider recognition toward the end of the twentieth century, however. One example is the diffusion of innovations theory, which distinguishes the diffusion or spread of new behaviors from their adaptation or use by increasing numbers of people.

### Changing Behaviors *versus* Maintaining Behavior Change

Even where there is good initial compliance to a health-related behavior change, a relapse to previous behavior patterns is very common. Undertaking a behavior change and maintaining the change, therefore, require different types of programs and self-management strategies. For example, someone could quit smoking by going "cold turkey," but he or she will probably be tempted again, perhaps at a party where friends are smoking. Maintaining cessation involves developing self-management and coping strategies, as well as establishing new behavior patterns that emphasize perceived control, environmental management, and improved confidence in one's ability to avoid temptation.

A model called the relapse prevention model focuses very specifically on this issue.

### Barriers to Actions and Decisional Balance

The concept of barriers to action, or perceived obstacles, is often mentioned in theories of health behavior. An extension of this concept involves what is known as "decisional balance." This idea is called the "net benefits of action" in the health belief model and "pros minus cons" in the stages of change model. These terms all reflect the idea that individuals engage in a relative weighing of the pros and cons of a prospective behavior change. This notion is basic to models of rational decisionmaking, in which people intellectually think about the advantages and disadvantages of engaging in a particular action.

## IMPLICATIONS FOR PUBLIC HEALTH

Understanding and improving health-related behavior is critical to the future of public health and to the well-being of individuals, and has become central to public health activities. While policies, laws, and regulations can affect health behaviors, there are also many individual factors that must be considered in these public health efforts.

Change is incremental. Many people have practiced a lifetime of less than optimal health behaviors of one sort or another. It is unreasonable to expect that significant and lasting changes will occur during a short period of time. Public health programs need to identify and maximize the benefits of positive change, pull participants along the continuum of change, and consider changes in educational programs and environmental supports to help people maintain changes over the longterm.

### Chronic Illness

A chronic illness is a disease that has a prolonged course, does not resolve spontaneously, and rarely is completely cured. Typical examples include cancer, heart disease, diabetes, and arthritis. These illnesses are usually more common as a population ages. In the United States, as in most developed countries, chronic diseases account for approximately 70 per cent of all deaths, and a similar proportion of all health care costs. Recent analyses have shown chronic illnesses to be a more important cause of the burden of disease in developing countries than was previously recognized.

The commonly held belief that chronic illnesses have noninfectious origins has become blurred. A few chronic illnesses, including cervical cancer, liver cancer, and some forms of arthritis, now appear to have infectious causes. Given the large chronic disease burden and the aging population, efforts to reduce the burden, arrest or slow deterioration, and prevent disability from these illnesses will be among the paramount issues in public health for the foreseeable future.

### Psychology, Health

Psychology has various definitions most of them stating that psychology is the study of behavior. Health psychology is the application of psychology to health-related problems and behavior. Most psychological applications in health are from the discipline of social psychology. The contribution of health psychology to public health is in such areas as psychological processes in prevention, health maintenance e.g., not smoking, and patient education, particularly in helping people cope with an illness e.g., mastering the use of the peak flow meter to control asthma.

## HEALTH PSYCHOLOGY PERSPECTIVES

Health psychology deals with individual behavior in a social context. However, within the public health sector, behavior is not restricted to behavior of atrisk persons, but also includes behaviors of peers, parents, health professionals, employers, politicians, and others. Unfortunately, while there is a large amount of empirical data available regarding individual behavior of the atrisk person or patient, there is very little data available about behaviors at other social levels.

Health psychologists try to understand behavior by describing psychosocial determinants for individual behavior. But health psychologists also try to understand and promote behavior change. One basic assumption in health psychology is that to change people's behavior—at least through health promotion interventions—it is necessary to understand the psychosocial determinants of behavior. For example, when a smoker fails to stop smoking because of a lack of motivation, another type of intervention is required than for a smoker that fails because of a lack of social support.

The first public health applications of psychology were strongly focused on risk perception and risk taking. The best example may be the health belief model, where the perception of the severity of the risk and the susceptibility for the risk were seen as the primary determinants of health-protective behaviors. Over-time, it became clear that people have many reasons for health-related behaviors, of which risk perception is often not an important one. In this multicausality approach, there is also a growing recognition of the many psychosocial and environmental influences on individual behavior. Changes in psychosocial determinants e.g., self-efficacy are most effective in creating behavior change when paralleled by changes in the social and physical environment e.g., removal of barriers.

The application of psychological theories to public health is not without debate. Some professionals state that psychological theories will never be able to fully help us understand behavior and behavior change; other professionals claim that in practice there is nothing so helpful as a good theory. Both perspectives are justified. Theories are, by definition, a reduction of reality, but they do help people organize their thoughts and ask the right questions. The interesting contribution of theories is that they can generalize findings from one area of behavior to be of use in another.

## PSYCHOSOCIAL DETERMINANTS OF BEHAVIOR

The most often applied theories to explain the psychosocial determinants of behavior are Icek Ajzen's theory of planned behavior and Albert Bandura's social cognitive theory. Social cognitive theory (SCT) specifies the following determinants of behavior: outcome expectations, self-efficacy expectations, behavioral capability, perceived behavior of others (modeling), and the social and physical environment.

The theory of planned behavior (TPB) is an extension of the earlier theory of reasoned action. TPB postulates that intention, the most proximal determinant of behavior, is determined by three conceptually independent constructs: attitude, subjective norms, and perceived behavioral control or self-efficacy. The attitude towards the behavior is determined by salient beliefs, or outcome expectations, about that behavior. Beliefs are weighted by evaluations or judgments about the value or importance of the expected outcome. For example, the expected outcome of going on a low fat diet might be a lowering of blood pressure, which could be judged to be important and worthwhile.

Subjective norms, or perceived social expectations, are beliefs that specific, important individuals or groups approve or disapprove of the behavior. These beliefs are weighted by the motivation to comply with the referent person or group—that is, how important is a friend's or group's approval or opinion. Note that Ajzen's perceived social expectations are different from Bandura's perceived behavior of others, where the social environment does not necessarily expect certain behavior. Other authors have broadened the TPB social influence construct to include perceived behavior of others, perceived expectations of others, social pressure, and social support. Perceived behavior control or self-efficacy refers to the subjective probability that a person is capable of executing a certain action e.g., going on a low-fat diet might be perceived to be difficult.

Since the theory of planned behavior was introduced in the 1980s, other determinants have been suggested, including: personal moral norms, anticipated regret, identity concerns, and self-evaluation. Another development is an increasing attention to the relation between intentions and behavior. Studies on implementation intention show that helping people to make plans to behave in a certain way can improve the intention-behavior link. Intentions, however, may be overruled by habits. Behaviors become habitual when performed frequently and when performed in a stable environment. Under conditions where habits conflict with intentions, intentions become poor predictors of behavior. It is possible, however, to break bad habits by replacing a habitual sequence with an alternative sequence.

TPB is most often applied at the individual level. However, it has been applied to higher ecological levels as well, such as the voting behavior of legislators regarding a cigarette tax increase, or the adoption behavior of school teachers and principles for HIV human immunodeficiency virus prevention programs.

## THE PSYCHOLOGY OF BEHAVIOR CHANGE

The most prominent psychology theories of behavior change are the social cognitive theory, James Prochaska and Carlo DiClemente's transtheoretical model, Richard Petty and John Cacioppo's elaboration likelihood model, and various theories on coping and self-regulation by authors like Richard Lazarus. Social cognitive theory suggests the following methods for change: active learning, reinforcement, and modeling and guided practice including feedback.

The transtheoretical model (TTM) has two major sets of constructs: stages of change and processes of change. In the stages of change, people are thought to move from a state of no motivation to change to one of internalization of new behavior. The first stage is "precontemplation," in which people have no intention to change their behavior. In a successful change process, people make a transition to "contemplation," in which they are thinking about changing the problem behavior. Ideally, people then move to "preparation," in which they are planning to change this behavior in the short term. People who have recently changed their behavior are in the "action stage," whereas, people who have performed the behavior for a longer time are in the "maintenance stage." People in the action stage may lapse and then recycle to an earlier stage. TTM can be used to describe and to change behavior. An important contribution of the model is the specific tailoring of educational efforts to include different models and processes of change for individuals in different stages of change. For instance, a re-evaluation of outcome expectations is used to make the change from precontemplation to contemplation; and a guided practice for skills improvement can help with the change from action to maintenance.

Social psychology has a long tradition in persuasion research. Petty and Cacioppo have a new perspective on persuasion effects with their elaboration likelihood model (ELM). The basic idea of ELM is that people differ in their ability and motivation for thoughtful information processing of persuasive messages. These authors explain two ways of information processing, central or peripheral also called systematic *versus* heuristic. Central processing occurs when a message is carefully considered and compared against other messages and beliefs. Peripheral processing occurs when a message is processed without thoughtful consideration or comparison. A variable—for instance, the credibility of a sports hero as a model—may have a positive effect when the receivers process the message through the peripheral route, but a negative effect when they follow the central route, because people might realize that their behavioral capabilities are different from those of the sports hero. Research findings suggest that thoughtful information processing is related to a higher persistence of attitude change, a higher resistance to counter-persuasion, and a stronger attitude behavior consistency. ELM suggests two ways to stimulate central processing: Make the message more personally relevant and unexpected, and repeat the message.

Self-regulatory or self-management conceptualizations, including coping theories, have to do with how individuals function to behaviorally self-correct. Various authors describe this process. The general procedure is: (a) monitoring of some aspect of behavior or health, (b) comparing one's observation with normal or desired outcomes or behavior, describing a problem or divergence from normal, and analyzing the causes of the problem, and (c) trying a behavioral correction. This entire process recycles with a return to monitoring. Self-regulatory theories are useful for the designation of health-promoting behaviors for the self-management of chronic diseases, such as asthma, diabetes, or cystic fibrosis.

## Social Determinants

Any case of a disease results from a long and complex chain of characteristics, circumstances, and events. The terms used to refer to the stages in this causal chain are not well agreed upon, however. Causal factors are loosely grouped into precipitating causes, which refer to agent factors, such as a virus, and some aspects of the host, such as inadequate nutrition which increases susceptibility. The events and environmental factors that give rise to the immediate causal factors are often termed "determinants." These include biological, physical, and social circumstances. Determinants account, in some measure, for the underlying rates of disease in a population, while variations in these rates are explained by risk factors. The social determinants of health include socioeconomic circumstances, social structure and function, and cultural factors. Social determinants refer to broad patterns and not to individual details—the state of being married would constitute a risk factor for some conditions, while the cultural and economic circumstances that lead to high divorce rates might form a social determinant of mental health in a particular population.

The use of the term "determinants" deserves some clarification. In most instances it does not imply a deterministic relationship, as might hold in chemistry, for example. Nor does it imply the absence of free will. Instead, determinants refer to macro social influences that affect health, such as poverty or social strife, and that would prove very difficult for an individual to alter. Perhaps the broadest social determinant of health is a country's level of social and economic development. This is related to patterns of longevity, health, and disease, but the relationship is dynamic and far from simple, and economic development and health status influence one another. Patterns of disease shift as a country's economy grows, producing the epidemiologic transition from a pattern of short life expectancy and high mortality due to infectious disease, to a pattern of long life expectancy and deaths due mainly to noninfectious chronic diseases that are typical of industrial countries. Social determinants influence health through many intervening factors, such as the quality of sanitation, medical care, or food distribution systems. Examples are provided by the twentieth-century adverse impact on health seen in Eastern European countries in the former Soviet bloc.

While social determinants undoubtedly exert much of their influence through individual behaviors that promote or prevent disease, it is also clear that disease patterns cannot be fully explained in terms of individual behaviors.

Health behaviors form the tip of an iceberg of social forces that also include contextual variables such as social mores, urbanization, and political changes, which seem to exert direct effects on health. Our understanding of the social determinants of health remains in its infancy; there is little understanding of many details relating to how health is determined. Social epidemiology is still looking for its Pasteur to explain the processes involved. Current explanations are akin to stating that a car works when you put gasoline in and turn the key.

### Cultural Factors

Culture encompasses the set of beliefs, moral values, traditions, language, and laws or rules of behavior held in common by a nation, a community, or other defined group of people. Culturally determined characteristics include: the language spoken at home; religious observances; customs including marriage customs that often accompany religious and other beliefs; acceptable gender roles and occupations; dietary practices; intellectual, artistic, and leisure-time pursuits; and other aspects of behavior. In the United States, and in other nations with large immigrant populations, there is a wide range of cultural diversity, religious beliefs, customs, and values, reflecting the scattered origins of the people. The "melting-pot" concept of nationality reduces this diversity with successive generations, but considerable variation remains—distinguishing rural from urban, African American from European, East Asian from South Asian, and religious believers from secularists.

Anthropoligists and epidemiologists have identified many associations between culture, customs, and risks to health. Those who, for religious reasons, abstain from tea, coffee, alcohol, and tobacco have smaller risks of getting cancer of the gastrointestinal or respiratory tract than others of similar social, economic, and residential background. Seventh-day Adventists, who are strict vegetarians and are very health conscious have low death rates from coronary heart disease when compared to neighbors of similar socioeconomic backgrounds. Though often called "lifestyle factors," in such cases these differences are culturally determined because the related behaviors are associated with religious beliefs and practices. Jews who practice circumcision have lower incidence and death rates than gentiles from cancer of the male genital tract, perhaps related to sexual hygiene and reduced risk of infection with carcinogenic viruses.

Many cultural characteristics, and the health states related to them, are associated with education, occupation, income, and social status. These factors influence one's awareness of the world, and whether one will seek improvement or accept things as they are. Well-educated white-collar workers may be more aware of the benefits of exercise than those lacking education—they are more likely to play than watch sports, and are more likely to have better-paying jobs that enable them to afford sporting equipment. Values related to these perceptions also shape the relative priority accorded to intellectual *versus* athletic pursuits, motivating some working-class parents to encourage their children to study and remain in school in hopes of a better life for the children than the parents have had. The clash of competing values between environmental sustainability and economic development also has a cultural component. Appreciation of the fact that health is ultimately dependent on the integrity of the earth's life-supporting ecosystems is part of a value system. Such values may sometimes be over-ridden by short-term priorities such as job security or financial gain.

Much can be learned about the linkages between culture and health by studying migrant populations, whose culture of origin is often very different from the culture into which they migrate. Japanese migrants to California and Hawaii were found to have higher rates of coronary artery disease than their counterparts in Japan. Part of this difference could be attributed to changes in risk factors such as diet, weight, and cholesterol levels. However, loss of a stable, cohesive social environment also appears to have contributed to the rise in prevalence of coronary artery disease in the migrant groups. In another study, blood pressure values among African Americans from the Southern United States who migrated to an urban environment were compared with that of urban born African Americans. The longer the period of city life, the higher was their blood pressure. Many studies have shown that immigrants have higher rates of mental illness, probably due to the tremendous stresses of living in a new cultural environment. Cultural groups that have a strong group identity and cohesion seem to be somewhat protected against this type of stress.

Culturally shaped illnesses are disorders that reflect the social, political, and moral worlds of the patient. They also often represent ways in which deep cultural messages are transmitted through the medium of the human body. For example, among Latino populations in Central America and the United States, anthropologists describe "ataques de nervios," an illness characterized by symptoms such as shaking, a feeling of heat in the chest, difficulty in moving the limbs, and parasthesias. Among Latino immigrants in the United States, anthropologists have linked the illness to the sense of social and political disempowerment that these people experience. Other culturally shaped illnesses include: "heart distress" in Iran; "semen loss" in South Asia; and "susto" in Latin America. Anthropologists study the symbolic meaning of symptoms within specific cultural contexts in order to understand the cultural messages these illnesses express.

Cultural context can profoundly affect the transmission of disease. A tragic example is the spread of HIV/AIDS (human immunodeficiency virus/acquired immunodeficiency syndrome), particularly in Africa, where economic necessity shapes choices that are often hazardous to health. The combination of limited education, migratory labor that separates men from their wives and families, and the breakdown of traditional family networks creates a context in which men may seek multiple sexual partners. Women often lack the social power to negotiate condom use, and their need for economic and social survival outweighs the risk that they know they are taking by having unprotected intercourse. In Thailand, where culturally condoned intravenous drug use is widespread among the large population of sex workers, HIV/AIDS and other blood-borne viral diseases became epidemic in the 1990s, creating a national public health emergency.

The health of girls and women is particularly sensitive to cultural influences. In societies where women are able to make decisions for themselves, especially about their education and their reproductive choices, have longer life expectancy, lower fertility rates, and better overall health. When political totalitarianism and religious zealotry flourish, women usually suffer oppression disproportionately compared to men, and this can adversely affect their health and longevity.

Patriachal values can also be harmful to the health of girls and women. Such values have a pervasive influence in many settings, mainly in traditional agricultural societies, but also in some urbanized economies. In some strict Islamic societies where girls and women are segregated and allowed to appear in public only if totally covered from head to toe, deprivation of sunlight can impair the cutaneous synthesis of vitamin D, causing a deficiency of this vitamin and putting the women at risk for rickets or osteomalacia.

Another cultural practice with severe health consequences is female genital mutilation, which is performed on young girls in many African and Middle Eastern nations. In its most extreme form, the procedure can be life threatening. It deprives women of sexual fulfillment and makes childbirth a hazardous process for both mother and infant. While performed in many predominantly Islamic countries, this procedure is not a religious ritual, and is not condoned by any Islamic scripture. Anthropologists have described the complex cultural meanings of ritual purity associated with female genital mutilation that serve to perpetuate this practice despite its serious adverse effects on health. The majority of women and men in cultures that perform genital mutilation support the continuation of the practice which makes change all the more difficult. Both international and national efforts are underway to stop or change this practice, with some of the most promising initiatives coming from within the cultures themselves. Female genital mutilation was banned in the United States in 1995, and is also outlawed in Britain, France, Canada, Sweden, Switzerland, and some African countries.

In Western societies the female body is often altered for cultural reasons. Women in the nineteenth century constricted their waists and compressed their breasts with rigid corsets. Many women today wear high heels and tight shoes that deform their feet, with painful consequences in old age. Some undergo painful cosmetic surgery in the quest for an idealized physical form, with reshaped ears, eyes, and nose; facelifts; liposuction; and breast implants. Some girls and women strive to achieve a very low body weight, a modern, culturally shaped notion of beauty that has supplanted the former "ideal"—the plump female form depicted in the paintings of Rubens and Renoir. The pursuit of very low body weight may be associated with the development of anorexia nervosa, an illness that can be fatal. Men in Western society in the late twentieth century also began seeking an "improved" body image by taking muscle-enhancing steroids or having muscle grafts to enlarge pectoral and calf muscles.

In modern industrial societies an adolescent culture has developed. This culture often fosters rebelliousness and defiance of adult authority figures, leading some young people to smoke, take drugs, and expose themselves to dangerous and unhealthy practices. Such actions have, unfortunately, often been encouraged by the tobacco industry and advertisers of beer and other alcoholic drinks. The pervasive influence of the media, especially television, in almost all contemporary societies projects cultural values and behavior that emanate from the American entertainment industry. Many of these messages, such as encouraging the use of mood-altering substances and sexual promiscuity, are potentially harmful to health.

Public health specialists must be aware of these and other cultural trends, and they must endeavor to mobilize beneficial cultural influences while discouraging unhealthy ones. The task of public health professionals is particularly challenging when influential and economically motivated interests glorify aspects of culture that are harmful to health.

### Ethnicity and Health

The issue of cultural sensitivity is central to ethnicity and health, and to developing health-promotion and disease-prevention programs for different racial and ethnic populations. We provide definitions and a conceptual framework for understanding cultural sensitivity and the rationale for tailoring health-promotion programs for different cultural groups. Most of the examples provided relate to African Americans and Hispanic/Latino populations. Nonetheless, the principles discussed are applicable to other racial, ethnic, and socio demographic sub-populations.

## CULTURAL SENSITIVITY

Cultural sensitivity goes by many names, including cultural competence, culturally appropriate, culturally consistent, multicultural, cultural diversity, cultural pluralism, cultural tailoring, and cultural targeting.

Although definitions and distinctions for these terms have been offered, the terminology has no accepted standards. In response to this need, the following definitions are proposed:

**Cultural Sensitivity** the extent to which ethnic and cultural characteristics, experiences, norms, values, behavioral patterns, and beliefs of a target population, as well as relevant historical, political, environmental, and social forces, are incorporated in the design, delivery, and evaluation of targeted health-promotion materials and programs.

**Cultural Competence** the capacity of individuals to exercise interpersonal cultural sensitivity. "Culturally competent" refers to practitioners, whereas "culturally sensitive" relates more to intervention programs, materials, and messages.

**Multicultural** incorporating and appreciating perspectives of multiple racial and ethnic groups without assumptions of superiority or inferiority. In this sense, culturally competent individuals and culturally sensitive interventions are implicitly multicultural. Cultural pluralism is a synonym.

**Cultural Tailoring** the process of creating culturally sensitive interventions; often involving the adaptation of existing programs, materials, and messages to racial/ethnic sub-populations.

**Culture-Based** This term refers to programs and messages that use culture, ethnicity, history, and core values to motivate behavior change.

**Ethnic Identity (EI)** Ethnic identity involves the extent to which individuals identify with and gravitate to their own racial or ethnic group. Ethnic identity includes elements such as racial and ethnic pride, affinity for group culture e.g., food, media, and language, attitudes toward majority culture, involvement with group members, experience with and attitudes regarding racism, attitudes toward intermarriage, and the importance placed upon preserving one's culture and aiding others of like background. For immigrant groups, ethnic identity includes aspects of acculturation i.e., adoption of values and practices of the host country.

Cultural sensitivity can be conceptualized in terms of two primary dimensions: "surface structure" and "deep structure." Surface structure involves matching intervention materials and messages to characteristics of a target population. For audiovisual materials, this may involve using people, places, language, music, and foods familiar to, and preferred by, the target audience. Surface structure includes identifying the channels e.g., media and settings e.g., churches, schools that are most appropriate for delivery of messages and programs. It also entails understanding characteristics of the behavior in question. Surface structure refers to the extent to which interventions correspond to the needs of the target population and to how well interventions fit within the culture, experience, and behavioral patterns of the population.

The second dimension of cultural sensitivity, deep structure, reflects how cultural, social, psychologic, environmental, and historical factors influence health behaviors in different populations. This includes understanding how members of the target population perceive the cause, course, and treatment of illnesses; as well as perceptions regarding the determinants of specific health behaviors. Specifically, this involves appreciation for how religion, family, society, economics, and the government—both in perception and in fact— influence the target behavior. Among many African Americans, for example, there is a belief that the U.S. government may be covertly encouraging the spread of HIV/AIDS (human immunodeficiency virus/acquired immunodeficiency syndrome), guns, and drugs in their communities. Some

Hispanics feel that certain illnesses are a punishment from God or the result of the "evil eye." Messages that incorporate, though not necessarily accept or refute these beliefs, will likely enhance program acceptance and effectiveness.

Core cultural values for African Americans include: communalism, religion and spiritualism, expressiveness, respect for verbal communication skills, connections to ancestors and history, commitment to family, and intuition and experience rather than empiricism. African-American culture is also characterized by a unique sense of time, rhythm, and communication style. The use of oral communication i.e., interpersonal *vs.* print interventions, as well as stories, religious spiritual themes, and historical references to convey messages in health-promotion programs for African Americans can improve the success level of programs. For Hispanics, core cultural values include *familismo* importance of family, *respecto* respect for elders, *dignidad* the value of self-worth, *caridad* the value of rituals and ceremonies, fatalism, and *simpatía* the importance of positive social interactions. The novella format i.e., the use of stories may be a particularly effective mechanism to convey these concepts to motivate health behavior change among Hispanic populations. Whereas, surface structure generally increases the receptivity, comprehension, or acceptance of messages, deep structure conveys salience: Surface structure establishes feasibility, whereas deep structure determines program impact.

## CULTURAL SENSITIVITY IN HEALTH PROMOTION

The rationale for targeted and tailored health-promotion programs derives from essentially three observations: (1) differences in disease prevalence rates among racial and ethnic groups; (2) differences in the prevalence of the behavioral risk factors among racial and ethnic groups; and (3) differences in the predictors of health behaviors among groups. Whereas, the first-two factors provide the rationale for targeted delivery of programs to sub-populations prevention programs, it is the latter that provides the basis for tailoring adapting programs and messages for subpopulations programs.

## SOCIOECONOMIC FACTORS

Because African Americans tend to have lower socioeconomic status than whites, and because numerous health indicators are related to socioeconomic variables, it is important when examining between-group differences in health indicators to account for socioeconomic differences. Failure to do so may lead to inappropriate attribution of differences to ethnic, racial, or genetic factors rather than socioeconomic disparities, which in turn may perpetuate views of racial inferiority as well as misdirect health care research and service dollars. Total mortality and cancer rates, as well as some chronic-disease risk factors, are inversely related to income and education among both African Americans and whites. The magnitude of the association appears similar among both groups, at least with regard to all cause mortality, cancer rates, and smoking prevalence. Any differences that exist diminish, or even reverse, after controlling for socioeconomic status, further suggesting that racial and ethnic differences may be related more to socioeconomic factors than to ethnic, cultural, or biologic factors.

On the other hand, infant mortality rates, as well as other health indicators such as obesity, body-image preferences, high blood pressure, sedentariness, smoking quit-rates, diabetes markers, and poor diet, remain higher among African Americans, even after adjustment for education and/or income factors. Conversely, African-American adolescents appear less likely to smoke cigarettes than whites, and adult African Americans have a higher dietary carotenoid intake after adjusting for education and income. Thus, some ethnic differences in health indicators appear independent of socio-demographic factors.

One explanation for these inconsistent results is that there is often an insufficient number of middle and upper socioeconomic-level African-American participants in epidemiologic studies, and conclusions regarding the effects of socioeconomic status on health indicators across ethnic groups are often based on small samples and unstable parameter estimates. Another explanation is that socioeconomic factors function differently among African Americans and whites. For example, African Americans reap a lower increase in income per year of education and they have lower net worth at all income levels than whites. It is also possible that ethnicity, genetics, and socioeconomic factors can each independently influence the same health indicator.

Racial and ethnic differences in the prevalence of socioeconomic and environmental risk factors associated with health behavior are also evident. These include, for African Americans, higher school dropout rates, low socioeconomic status, and a more chaotic family life. For Hispanics, acculturation stress is a major factor. Compared to whites, African Americans experience a greater number of stressful events. They also experience different types of stressors and employ different types of coping strategies in response to stress, and they derive social support a buffer against stress from different sources. African-American adolescents are more likely than their white counterparts to be the victims of, or witnesses to, violence; to experience death of a parent or sibling; to be involved in the criminal justice system; and to have parents whose income has recently decreased. African-American youth also rate the impact of stressful events differently than white adolescents.

Another important source of stress for African Americans is racism, which can increase feelings of anger, hostility, alienation, and helplessness—all of which have been associated with negative health outcomes. The higher levels of risk would appear inconsistent with the lower rates of alcohol, tobacco, and other drug use among African Americans. One explanation for this apparent paradox is that the predictors of substance use, both risk and protective factors, function differently among racial and ethnic subgroups.

## THE IMPORTANCE OF HETEROGENEITY

Failure to appreciate the heterogeneity *within* ethnic groups can lead to what has been called "ethnic glossing," and ultimately to insensitive and ineffective interventions. Thus, to achieve cultural sensitivity it is essential to understand the heterogeneity of the target population. For example, among African-American youth living in low—income public housing complexes a seemingly homogeneous population, there will be considerable variability with regard to important predictors of behavior, including parental attitudes and behaviors, religiosity, educational attainment, and political beliefs. For Hispanic and other populations, there may also be variability in levels of acculturation. Whereas, it may not be feasible or desirable to develop interventions segmented to each of these parameters, interventions can nonetheless incorporate multiple perspectives that appeal to a broad spectrum of the target population. In effect, through audience segmentation, even materials designed for a single racial or ethnic group can be multicultural in design. A related phenomenon is the fluidity of racial or ethnic group membership. Different populations may be defined by external parameters established by researchers, rather than by any indigenous cultural ethos. For example, an African-American group defined by church membership will yield a different cultural subgroup than one defined by income status.

Culturally sensitive health-promotion programs are necessitated by differences in disease rates, risk-factor distribution, and behavioral predictors. Controlled research demonstrating how these factors can be incorporated into prevention interventions and what impact, if any, they have on outcomes is lacking, however. While the ethical or philosophic arguments for cultural sensitivity may not require scientific evidence, there are nonetheless several key empirical questions regarding feasibility and effectiveness that merit investigation.

With regard to surface structure, some of the assumptions are *a priori* valid. For example, it is largely self-evident that interventions should be written in the language of a population or at an appropriate reading level. However, other surface structure issues, such as whether materials should portray role models exclusively from the target audience or if images should reflect the same socioeconomic background as the target audience, require empirical examination. Some bilingual populations may prefer interventions in English, while others may prefer a mix of languages.

A key phenomenon that remains under-researched is the substantially lower substance—use rates that have been documented among African-American and Asian youth. Rather than approaching minority populations from a deficit model, these lower rates provide an opportunity to use African-American culture as the exemplar. The possible protective role of parental monitoring, family bonding, spirituality, and other positive attributes of African-American family life and culture that may buffer African-American youth from use have not been adequately explored. Other avenues of exploration include how exposure to drug use, as well as the crime and violence associated with the sale and use of drugs in the home and the community may discourage use among minority youth.

Even less is known about the efficacy of deep structure messages. Controlled trials comparing the efficacy of culturally sensitivity materials *versus* standard non–culturally sensitive materials are needed. To a great extent, it is not known if culturally sensitive programs are, in fact, more effective.

## Environmental Determinants of Health

An environmental determinant of health is, in general, any external agent biological, chemical, physical, social, or cultural that can be causally linked to a change in health status. However, since virtually everything that is not genetically determined could be considered "environmental," this general definition is too all—encompassing to be useful. Rather, environmental epidemiologists have narrowed the term to include only those environmental influences that are involuntary. For example, breathing second hand tobacco smoke would be an environmental hazard, whereas active tobacco smoking would be considered a behavioral determinant.

In the developed world, environmental epidemiologists are concerned about such things as gene-environment interactions, environment-environment interactions, particulate air pollution, nitrogen dioxide, ground-level ozone, environmental tobacco smoke, radiation, lead, video display terminals, cellular telephones, and persistent organic pollutants (POPs) that act as endocrine disruptors. Exposures to these types of environmental vectors are known as downstream, or proximate, determinants of health that is, the exposures are closely related in time and space to the ill effects they produce, and they impact both health and well-being.

In the developing world, the primary environmental determinants of health are biological agents in the air, water, and soil that account for most deaths, and for most deaths in the world. Four million children die annually from diarrheal diseases acquired from contaminated food or water. Over one million people die from malaria each year. Hundreds of millions of people suffer from debilitating intestinal parasitic infestations. Hundreds of millions of people suffer from respiratory diseases caused by biological and chemical agents in the air, both indoors and outdoors. According to the World Health Organization (WHO), over one billion people are unable to meet their basic needs i.e., adequate food, clean water, and shelter because they lack the necessary income or land. These are environmental hazards that take a far greater toll on human life and suffering in absolute terms compared to those environmental determinants of concern in the developed world.

To understand approaches needed to address environmental health concerns, a distinction is made between infectious and chronic causes of disease. A distinction also is made between short-term, acute exposures resulting in epidemic outbreaks of illness, and long-term, low-dose exposures resulting in chronic diseases. Such classifications are necessary to ensure appropriate methods for researching and understanding the extent of health problems in the world. The workplace often serves as a laboratory for understanding the relationship between environmental exposures and health. It serves as a laboratory because, in their occupational environment, workers tend to be exposed to measurable amounts of pollution. This fact allows occupational health researchers and epidemiologists to link adverse health outcomes to these environmental factors. If no link between a workplace pollutant and worker ill-health can be demonstrated, then that pollutant is unlikely to have measurable consequences for human health beyond the work environment owing to comparative lack of frequency and concentration of exposure experienced by those not working in that specific environment. One notable exception, however, is that class of people who are more susceptible to ill-effects even from low levels of exposure.

An emerging concern with great potential impact on public health relates to upstream, or distant, determinants of health the exposures are far apart in time or space from the witnessed ill-effects including as policies that drive current levels of population growth, consumption and waste issues, and the uses of technology. For example, the environmental, transboundary transport of contaminants through the food chain has resulted in global chemical contamination. Other transboundary issues include acid precipitation, ozone, greenhouse gasses, and hazardous wastes. Global ecological integrity i.e., the ability of life-support systems to sustain themselves in the presence of polluting forces and global change including concerns about climate change from global warming, ozone depletion, and the loss of biodiversity have given people reason to adopt the WHO maxim: "Think globally, act locally." Reducing wastes and consumption at the local level can have positive effects on the entire earth's ecosystems.

## Epidemiologic Transition

Epidemiology is the study of the distribution and determinants of health-related states or events. It has traditionally been associated with the study of external agents of disease microbial infectious agents. Events such as the Black Death, which killed about one-third of the population of Europe during the Middle Ages, have left their trace in the collective unconscious and are still largely perceived as being caused by external environmental agents. Progress in medical science, however has changed the perceptions of epidemiology as new patterns of illness and disease are confronted.

The first transition in epidemiology occurred over a period of about one hundred years during the nineteenth and twentieth centuries, when humankind progressively curbed the major epidemics of infectious diseases. Some, such as smallpox, were completely eradicated, while some, such as measles, diphtheria, and tetanus, have been significantly reduced. Even taking into account the emergence, or reemergence, of diseases like AIDS acquired immunodeficiency syndrome, Ebola fever, and malaria, infectious diseases, in many parts of the world, are not the immediate universal threat today that they once were.

The reduction of epidemics and infectious diseases has led to a considerable increase in life expectancy. As a result, there has been an increased appearance of manifestations linked to aging the so called degenerative, or chronic, diseases, e.g., some cancers, cerebrovascular disease, and certain mental disorders such as Alzheimer's disease. Major changes in behavior and lifestyles have also appeared, albeit more recently, including driving cars, changes in smoking and diet, and an increased pressure related to work or unemployment. These changes have led to new patterns of disease, distinguished by the growth of the "human-made" diseases such as lung cancer, coronary artery disease, and motor-vehicle injury. Many of these diseases, of course, are not new and have complex etiologies, but the shift from the prevalence of infectious diseases to the prevalence of chronic diseases defines this second transition that has occurred in every part of the developed world. In the developing world, this transition is rapidly emerging, putting these countries under a new burden while they are still suffering from the ongoing—and in some cases increasing—onslaught of the acute communicable diseases.

The next transition may be brought about by changes in how individuals relate to disease. Patterns of usage of health services, ranging from the limitation of services on economic grounds to the provision of technologically advanced services such as organ transplantation and *in vitro* fertilization, are continually shifting. At the same time, efforts made by individuals to manage the consequences of nonfatal impairments and disabilities are also likely to bring changes in the distribution and determinants of health-related states or events. Epidemiologic transitions are, in fact, an ongoing phenomena, with one phase overlapping another. These transitions will continue as the face of disease continues to change.

## Theories of Health and Illness

Theories about health and illness deal with the ideas people use to explain how to maintain a healthy state and why they become ill. Ideas about illness causation may include such ideas as breach of taboo, soul loss, germs, upset in the hot-cold balance of the body, or a weakening of the body's immune system. Theories of illness causation derive from the underlying cognitive orientation of a cultural group, and therapeutic practice usually follows the same cultural logic.

Anthropologists often divide theories of illness into two broad categories: personalistic and naturalistic. In a personalistic system, illness is believed to be caused by the intervention of a sensate agent who may be a supernatural being a deity or dead ancestor or a human being with special powers a witch or a sorcerer. The sick person's illness is considered to be a direct result of the malign influence of these agents. In naturalistic causation, illness is explained in impersonal terms. When the body is in balance with the natural environment, a state of health prevails. However, when that balance is disturbed, illness results often, people invoke both types of causation in explaining an episode of illness, and treatment may entail two corresponding types of therapy.

According to personalistic theories of illness, illness may be linked to transgressions of a moral and spiritual nature. If someone has violated a social norm or breached a religious taboo, he or she may invoke the wrath of a deity, and sickness—as a form of divine punishment—may result. Possession by evil spirits is also thought to be a cause of illness in many cultures. This may be due to inappropriate behavior on the part of the patient—failure to carry out the proper rituals of respect for a dead ancestor, for example—or it may be simply due to bad luck. Sometimes, one person's envy of another's good fortune is believed to exert a malign influence through the "evil eye," which can result in illness or other calamities. Witches and sorcerers are malevolent human beings who manipulate secret rituals and charms to bring calamity upon their enemies. Recovery from an illness arising from personalistic causes usually involves the use of ritual and symbolism, most often by practitioners who are specially trained in these arts.

Naturalistic theories of disease causation tend to view health as a state of harmony between a human being and his or her environment; when this balance is upset, illness will result. The humoral system is a naturalistic approach to illness whose roots are over two thousand years old. Humoral concepts of health and illness are widely found in India, South-East Asia, China, and, in a somewhat different form, in Latin and South America. Maintaining humoral balance involves attention to appropriate diet and activity, including regulating one's diet according to the seasons. Illnesses may be categorized into those due to excess heat and those due to excess cold. Treatment of an illness of overheat would involve measures such as giving cooling foods and application of cool compresses.

In India, the ancient system of Ayurveda is based on naturalistic ideas of illness causation. Therapy in Ayurveda includes a vast pharmacopeia of preparations made from herbs and minerals, and dietary advice also forms part of every prescription. Ayurveda is actively practised in India today and has shaped the way Indians think about their bodies in health and in illness.

An important set of theories about health and illness, often called "vitalist" theories, is widespread in China, South Asia, and South-East Asia. When vital forces within the body flow in a harmonious pattern, a positive state of health is maintained. Illness results when this smooth flow of energy is disrupted, and therapeutic measures are aimed at restoring a normal flow of energy in the body. In China this vital force is known as "chi"; in India it is called "prana." In China the ancient art of acupuncture is based on this understanding of the body. Acupuncture needles are inserted at various points along the "meridians," or energy orientations, of the body. The stimulation of the needless helps to restore a proper flow of energy within the body. In India, Yoga particularly hatha yoga, the physical form of yoga is used therapeutically to restore a balanced energy flow through body and mind.

Biomedicine modern traditional medicine is founded on a naturalistic set of theories about the body, and these theories are continually evolving. One of the core theories of contemporary biomedicine, the germ theory of disease, is of relatively recent origin. According to an older biomedical concept, the miasma theory of disease, poisonous emanations from rotting vegetation or carcasses were believed to cause disease. By the mid-1800s, controversy still raged as to whether miasma or a waterborne pathogen was the cause for cholera. The "body-as-machine" metaphor has been a powerful way of conceptualizing the body within biomedicine, and a core assumption of the value system of biomedicine is that diagnosis and treatment should be based on scientific data. However, treatment approaches are often not rigorously analyzed scientifically before being employed therapeutically. For example, angina pectoris has been treated in a variety of ways, including with the use of xanthines, khellin, vitamin E ligation of the internal mammary artery, and implantation of this artery. These treatments were used for many years before controlled trials finally showed that the efficacy of these treatments were no better than placebo alone (Helman). Ritual and symbolism play important roles in the healing process in biomedicine, as they do in other healing systems. Taking a prescribed medication, for example, has a symbolic as well as a pharmacological effect. Symbolically, taking the medication may indicate to others that the person is unwell and is deserving of concern and sympathy. Surgical treatments such as coronary bypass surgery employ complex equipment and are performed in specialized settings. These settings and equipment all have powerful symbolic associations as well as technical functions. Rituals are patterned forms of behavior that have symbolic significance, that often help to provide a context of meaning in a strange or frightening situation. Both patients who undergo the surgery and surgeons who perform the surgery are involved in rituals that serve to order a life-changing event i.e., major surgery. The processes of obtaining informed consent, getting a patient prepped for surgery, and complex stages of post-operative care all have ritual as well as technical functions.

Alternative therapies also called complementary therapies have been rapidly gaining in popularity worldwide. These therapies are diverse, ranging from traditional treatments adapted from their lands of origin, such as acupuncture and shiatsu, to newly developed forms of therapy such as therapeutic touch. Many alternative therapies have underlying theories of illness causation that are quite different from that of biomedicine. In therapies such as acupuncture, reiki, and shiatsu the concept ot vital energy, or chi, is the basis for the practice. Successful therapy is that which regulates and harmonizes energy flows. In iridology, particular areas on the iris of the eye are thought to correspond to specific body organs, and a diagnosis of malfunction of the organs can be made by an examination of the iris. Conceptually, this theory of illness links to an ancient philosophical system of "homologies" that makes connections between the cosmic and the terrestrial; between the outer environment and the inner; and between the external body and the internal body.

All theories of health and illness serve to create a context of meaning within which the patient can make sense of his or her bodily experience. A meaningful context for illness usually reflects core cultural values, and allows the patient to bring order to the chaotic world of serious illness and to regain some sense of control in a frightening situation.

# 4

# Medical Social Theory

In the intimacy of the medical encounter, patients present to their doctors a variety of personal troubles. From Mills' perspective, these troubles often have roots in social issues that go beyond the individual level. Yet the social issues themselves tend not to receive critical attention in conversation between patients and doctors. In trying to help their patients, doctors often find ways that patients can adjust to troubling social condition. Seen from this vantage point, medical encounters are "microlevel" processes that involve the interaction of individuals. These interpersonal processes, however, occur in a social context, which is shaped by "macrolevel" structures in society. For example, when patients and doctors discuss problems at work, they take their bearings from the organization of work in society, social expectations about work, social class relations pertaining to work, and so forth. Similarly, when problems pertaining to family life arise in medical encounters, the conversation must deal in some way with such issues as women's and men's roles in the family, expectations about reproduction and the maintenance of households, and social patterns affecting children, elderly people, and individuals at different stages of the lifecycle. Patients also raise other kinds of social problems when they talk with their doctors, and macro-level structures in the society shape the context of those problems as well.

One challenge for social theory has been to clarify how macro-level social structures and micro-level processes affect one another. Many schools of thought have dealt with this theoretical challenge. Some theorists have argued for the importance of macro-level structures like social class and political power in determining what happens in interpersonal processes at the micro level. Others have claimed that micro-level processes are primary, and that macro-level structures emerge only as a reflection similar terms include integration, aggregation, gloss, repetition, and transformation of micro-level processes occurring routinely in everyday life. A compromise position holds that macro-level structures profoundly influence interpersonal processes, but that micro-level processes cumulatively reinforce social structures at the macro level as well.

## MEDICAL IDEOLOGY

Ideology, while difficult to define, is in general an interlocking set of ideas and doctrines that form the distinctive perspective of a social group. Through such ideas and doctrines, ideology represents—on an imaginary level-individuals' relationship to the real conditions of their existence a critical appraisal of Althusser's contribution. This imaginary quality of ideology, which patterns how individuals perceive and interpret their experience, contributes to ideology's impact in society. Because it helps shape a population's perceptions and interpretations, ideology can achieve a most profound effect on social life. As a macro-level structure in society, ideology impinges on patients and doctors as part of the social context of medical encounters. At the micro level of interpersonal interaction, elements of ideology appear in doctor-patient communication. What patients and doctors say when they meet reinforces their particular ideologic conceptions about social life. Although ideology has received wide attention in social theory, several previous theoretical contributions are helpful for clarifying ideology in medicine.

Ideology, work, and the family: perspectives from early Marxist theory. In classic Marxist theory, ideology is an important though inconsistently developed notion. According to the principle of economic determinacy, the events of history emerge chiefly from economic forces and the conflicting relations of social class. From this viewpoint, economic forces affect the ideologies of a specific historical period. Despite the primacy of economic forces, ideology is crucial in sustaining and reproducing the social relations of production, especially patterns of domination.

Marx called attention to the mechanisms by which ideology reinforces capitalist relations of production and the interests of the capitalist class. While ideologies arise in many different areas, including religion, aesthetics, and politics, early Marxist analyses did not discuss in depth the ideologic components of medicine.

The Marxist perspective, however, leads to questions about how elements of ideology in medical encounters relate to economic behavior. Ideologic conceptions of work, as they are transmitted in doctor-patient interaction, reflect more general ideologic notions about economic activities in a given society. When they are spoken in medical encounters, these notions reinforce a society's dominant ideologic conceptions about the nature of work and of economic production.

For instance, among the many definitions of "health" that have appeared during the twentieth century, modern medicine has emphasized in practice an interpretation of health as ability to work. There are several ways that this definition of health has been reinforced and diffused in the population. The public health policies that large philanthropies and government agencies have initiated in the United States and other countries consistently have emphasized the importance of a healthy work force. Images of health conveyed by the mass media also have supported the symbolism of health as the capacity to do productive work. These images have communicated a message that the healthy person is one who produces economically. Moreover, a widely touted standard by which to judge medicine's cost-effectiveness is its contribution to patients' subsequent work productivity.

Doctor-patient interaction, health as the ability to work. In certain encounters with patients, doctors communicate explicitly or subtly a message that works is preferable to idleness. When people become sick, they often stop working, and doctors get involved in this process in several ways. Frequently doctors certify that a patient is physically disabled and thus unable to work. By the certification of disability, a doctor in effect decides when a patient must return to the job. When judging the seriousness of a patient's complaints, a doctor investigates whether the patient's problems interfere with work. Doctors write letters to employers, insurance companies, and government agencies about patients' work limitations and discuss this correspondence to a greater or lesser degree with the patients themselves. During their routine talk with patients, doctors inevitably convey attitudes about work, usually to encourage patients' continued performance on the job. In these instances and many others, the impact of the doctors' words is to define health as the capacity to work productively.

The family becomes a second important focus for ideologic elements in medical encounters, and theorists in the Marxist tradition have emphasized the connections between the family and economic production. For example, Engels claimed that the family, by "propagation of the species," plays a key role in reproducing the labor force. Women's subordinate position in the family, according to Engels, helps maintain the family's reproductive role. However, the family's importance goes beyond the physical reproduction of labor. The family also helps reproduce the ideologic framework of the economic system. For instance, patterns of sexuality and child rearing in the family reinforce personality characteristics and attitudes that tend to accept hierarchies of class and authority. By sustaining such patterns, Engels argues, the family becomes an important institution for ideologic reproduction, which helps achieve the population's acquiescence to and participation in current relations of economic production.

Medicine also mediates the family's reproductive role. As noted already, medicine tends to define health as the ability to work. However, a secondary and related definition is that health is the ability to reproduce labor. Women's activities as homemakers, wives, and mothers are crucial in the family's reproductive activities. Even when women do not work outside the home, they often care for working husbands and for children who later will take part in production and reproduction. Although a greater proportion of women have entered the labor force since World War II, they still face the social expectation that they remain primarily responsible for these reproductive activities. That is, "healthy" women do these things, and doctors predictably help many women in sustaining their reproductive capabilities. For their male clients, doctors also may interest themselves in the stability of family relations. For both men and women, adequate functioning in familial responsibilities thus becomes another criterion in doctors' assessment of health. It could be observed that doctors are among the expert professionals who increasingly have regulated family life during the twentieth century. How doctor patient interaction conveys ideologic notions about family life is a question of some interest.

## Later Theories of Ideology

The examples of work and the family lead to a consideration of how certain other theorists-Gramsci, Lukacs, Althusser, and Habermas – have treated the question of ideology. A unifying theme among these theoretical positions, all of which are influenced by classical Marxism, is that ideology serves as a subtle mechanism which helps win a population's consent to the ways a society is organized.

These theorists also emphasize that ideology helps maintain the economic system and that supporting institutions like the family are key elements in reproducing a society's dominant ideologic patterns. Although the theorists to be considered do not deal specifically with medical encounters, one purpose of reviewing these theories is to apply them to the question of ideology in medicine.

From Gramsci's viewpoint, groups in power use two types of sociopolitical control to maintain and reproduce relations of economic production. In the first place, there is direct coercion; by holding the legal means of violence—in the armed forces, police, prisons, courts, and related institutions—the state protects the established order partly through force and repression. However, Gramsci claims, no regime can hold power for long periods of time strictly by authoritarian rule. Ideologic hegemony, according to Gramsci, is a second and ultimately more important mechanism of control. Such institutions as the schools, churches, mass media, and family inculcate a system of values, attitudes, beliefs, and morality. This ideologic system supports the established order and the class interests that dominate it. The same ideologic forces achieve consent and mute resistance from disadvantaged groups.

While Gramsci did not consider medicine's ideologic impact, a similar theoretical perspective would ask to what extent medicine reinforces the dominant ideologic system of a society. When doctors convey ideologic notions about desirable behavior, especially as these notions help shape patients' roles in work and the family, medical encounters contribute to the broader hegemonic impact of ideology, In this sense, medicine exerts ideologic effects that parallel those of such institutions as schools, churches, and the mass media.

Lukacs' conceptions of class consciousness and reification also are pertinent to medicine's ideologic impact. Regarding class consciousness, Lukacs, like Gramsci, explores how a society's dominant ideologies are conveyed and reinforced. In discussing literature and other forms of cultural expression, Lukacs emphasizes the ways that these materials both reflect and strengthen broad ideologic patterns. According to Lukacs, such ideologic patterns shape the consciousness of individuals and, cumulatively, of social classes. In this process, the *totality* of social relations in an entire society becomes mystified and blocked from conscious thought. Reification, Lukacs argues, involves the transformation of social relations into things or thing-like beings that take on their own separate reality in people's consciousness. Shaped by ideology, consciousness focuses on the concrete problems and objects of everyday life, especially economic commodities, rather than on the totality of social relations that lies behind these routine concerns. Attention becomes focused on the concrete objects of daily life, and in this process of reification the totality of social relations escapes conscious attention.

Reification contributes to medicine's impact. In medical encounters technical statements help direct patients' responses to objectified symptoms, signs, and treatment. This reification shifts attention away from the totality of social relations and the social issues that are often root causes of personal troubles. Instead, attention gets paid to problems of individual pathophysiology and personality. By reifying problematic social relations, medicine reduces the potentiality for effectively criticizing those relations. Symptoms, signs, and treatment take on an aura of scientific fact, rather than subjective manifestations of a troubled social reality. The medical processing of social problems invests them with the symbolism of objects, relatively immune from criticism or change. This same process constricts the level of attention to the disturbed individual, rather than social structures impinging on the individual. For instance, when the organization of work or tension in the family creates personal distress, expression of that distress in a medical encounter tends to reify the social structural roots of the problem. Under these circumstances, it is the objectified symptom or sign that requires treatment—not the institutional sources of individual distress.

Influenced by Gramsci and Lukacs, Althusser further analyzes the structures of control in modern societies. Althusser considers the interconnections among repressive and ideologic institutions, as well as their relationships to government. Repressive state apparatuses, Althusser argues, include the army, police, prisons, courts, and other institutions that maintain control through violence or repression. Ideologic state apparatuses are institutions that instill dominant ideologies in the population.

Althusser's analysis of the wide-ranging repressive and ideologic effects of many institutions in society, though controversial, pertains to medicine as well. In rare instances, medicine exerts directly repressive effects — as when physicians helped implement policies of genocide in Nazi concentration camps. Less obvious instances of medicine's repressive impact include doctors' roles in involuntary mental hospitalization, prison health care, capital punishment in some cases administering lethal injections or otherwise assisting in executions, involuntary sterilization, and so forth.

Medicine's ideologic impact, however, is doubtless much more important than its repressive role. In their encounters with patients, doctors may interpret personal problems and encourage individual behaviors in directions that are consistent with the society's dominant ideologic patterns. From the perspective of Althusser's theory, when medical encounters convey a definition of health as the ability to work, they encourage workers' participation in economic production. Doctor-patient interaction also predictably transmits notions about family life that strengthen the family's ideologic impact. In these ways, medicine exerts ideologic effects consistent with those of other institutions like the educational system and mass media.

Another quite different theoretical approach also pertains to medical ideology. The "critical theory" of Habermas and other analysts of the Frankfurt School provide a link between ideology and science—and by extension, scientific medicine. Although Habermas's and Althusser's theories both have roots in classical Marxism, these two schools of thought diverge in fundamental ways. In particular, the Frankfurt School usually assumes that individuals have the capacity to reflect critically about society and to take "purposive" political action; Althusser diminishes the potentiality for effective criticism and political action by individuals. Both approaches, however, emphasize the impact of ideology. While Althusser focuses on the ideologic effects of various social institutions in reproducing the relations of production, Habermas stresses the ideologic components of science.

For Habermas, science is ideology par excellence precisely because it claims to be above ideology, that is, objective and value neutral. Habermas argues that scientific ideology has defined an increasing range of problems as amenable to technical solutions. In this way, scientific ideology tends to depoliticize these social issues by removing them from critical scrutiny. According to Habermas, science legitimates current patterns of domination, including the class relations of production:

> Technocratic consciousness is, on the one hand, "less ideological" than all previous ideologies. . . . On the other hand today's dominant, rather glassy background ideology, which makes a fetish of science, is more irresistible and farther-reaching than ideologies of the old type. For with the veiling of practical problems it not only justifies a ***particular class's*** interest in domination and represses ***another class's*** partial need for emancipation, but affects the human race's emancipatory interest as such.

What are the specific processes by which scientific ideology provides legitimation? One problem in Habermas' account is that it remains on an abstract level and rarely grounds theoretical claims in empirical reality. Habermas conveys an impression that scientific ideology creates legitimation through cultural symbols in the mass media, educational system, and technical organization of the workplace. He also argues that ideology and domination appear in the face-to-face interaction of individuals. Distorted communication, Habermas argues, arises in both the macrolevel realm of politics and the microlevel realm of interpersonal relationships. Domination creates distortion in communication, and undistorted communication is impossible, according to Habermas, under conditions of domination. In a major part of his project, Habermas encourages resistance against domination and aims toward the creation of new, less distorted forms of communication. Concrete examples of scientific ideology, however, rarely appear in Habermas' work; for this reason, his account remains abstract and utopian regarding directions of change. On the other hand, his analysis causes one to look for specific instances of scientific legitimation and distorted communication in face-to-face interactions. These considerations are pertinent to medical encounters to the extent that doctor-patient interactions convey ideologic message under the rubric of scientific medicine. From Habermas' perspective, such messages legitimate current problems in society and further depoliticize these issues by deflecting critical attention from them. In addition, medical interactions show features of distorted communication, fostered for instance by devices of language that reinforce professional domination. In actual encounters between patients and doctors, then, one can ask how and to what extent medical discourse transmits scientific ideology?

## PROFESSIONAL SOCIAL CONTROL

Social control—again to offer a simple definition of a complex concept-refers to mechanisms that achieve people's adherence to norms of appropriate behavior. In medicine, ideology and social control are closely related. When doctors transmit ideologic messages that reinforce current social patterns—at work, in the family, and in other areas of life—they help control behavior in ways that are defined as socially appropriate.

Dealing with problems outside the narrow realm of technical medicine tends to "medicalize" a wide range of psychological, social, economic, and political problems. Historically, numerous—areas gadually have fallen under medical control. Examples include sexuality and family life, work dissatisfaction, problems of the lifecycle including birth, adolescence, aging, dying, and death, difficulties in the educational system learning disabilities, maladjustment,— and students' psychological distress, environmental pollution, and many other fields. By participating in these areas. Practitioners tend believe that they are extending the caring function of the medical role.

On the other hand. medicalization has become the subject of a critique that focuses on heath professionals' expanding role in social control. As medical management of social problems has increased, the societal roots of personal troubles become mystified and depoliticized. That is, by responding in limited ways to some of patients' non-technical problems, medical practitioners tend to shift the focus of attention from societal issues to the troubles of individuals.

***The history of professional social control: Foucault.*** The intrusion of the scientific discourse into many areas of social life has preoccupied Foucault in his work on the history of the professions. Through his studies of what he calls the human sciences, Foucault has conveyed the connections between knowledge and power.

While Foucault's early work traces the history of medicine's diagnostic and therapeutic ideas, his more recent studies emphasize how professional control has widened into everyday life. Although modern punishment is more hidden than prior techniques like torture and public execution, Foucault argues, it orients itself to surveillance and professional control over the deviant population. Through new technologies of power, according to Foucault, the criminologic profession could create what appeared to be a humane reform over prior forms of gross corporal punishment. Further, he argues, the administrators of penal institutions have achieved surveillance of people who deviate from society's expectations about appropriate behavior.

Most important from Foucault's viewpoint, criminology has become a standard for professional practices throughout society. According to Foucault, similar technologies of surveillance also have emerged to achieve professional power in mental institutions, hospitals and clinics, workplaces, and schools. Foucault's examples show that social control has become more subtle, professionalized, and oriented to surveillance of deviant behavior.

Although Foucault's studies of prisons touch on medicine mainly by analogy, his work on sexuality pertains directly to medical encounters. Foucault's colorful account of modern sexuality begins in the seventeenth century. Until that time, Foucault argues, religious institutions took an interest in sexuality, mainly through the confessional. When people confessed their sexual activities, priests commented on what liaisons and positions were appropriate and what actions required penance? After the Reformation and Counter Reformation, according to Foucault, concern gradually shifted from bodily activities to thoughts, fantasies, intentions, and other mental processes related to sexuality. Especially during the nineteenth century,

Foucault notes, surveillance and regulation of mental processes pertaining to sex became a preoccupation of science and particularly medicine. Professional practitioners then assumed a measure of control over the activities and psychological meanings of sexual life.

In discussing sexuality, Foucault emphasizes professional discourse and links discourse to power. That is, what professionals have said about sexuality has deepened professional power in everyday life. What previously was a concern for the clergy has become a challenge for professionals, who assume various degrees of control over their clients' sexual expression. Medical doctors mediate sex, according to Foucault, but so do psychoanalysts, social workers, educators, bureaucrats in social welfare agencies, and other professionals who lay claim to expert knowledge. The discourse through which professionals communicate their special knowledge, from Foucault's perspective, enhances their ability to intervene in and to control others' behavior.

Where does one find such professional discourse? Foucault of course looks for discourses on sex in the books, articles, and other documents that professionals have written and published. However, for Foucault, unpublished discourse becomes as important as publications in achieving professional power, if not more so. For this reason, a variety of materials are appropriate sources for study. These sources include the brochures and files of medical institutions treating sexual disorders, the records of public welfare bureaucracies, therapists' notes, and professional correspondence concerning individuals who are considered deviant. Perhaps most important for the purposes here, one also may look for such discourse, whenever possible, in the face-to-face talk of professionals and their clients. Predictably, for instance, what doctors say to their patients about sex comprises a concrete expression of professional discourse and its power in daily life, probably to a greater extent than what doctors write about sex in textbooks and scientific articles. Although Foucault alludes to the usefulness of oral materials, however, he does not use them himself in developing his arguments.

*On the unintentionality of medical social control.* As noted earlier, social control in medicine is generally an unintended process, dimly if at all perceived by participants in doctor-patient encounters. Health professionals seldom consciously view their activities as contributing to social control. In listening to words of distress from their clients, doctors usually do not see their responsibility as preserving the current organization of economic production or the stability of the family. Nonetheless, by focusing on individual troubles rather than social issues, doctorpatient encounters may reinforce the social order as presently constituted. Why do these processes tend to occur without the participants' conscious awareness?

To help explain the unintentionality of medical social control, one may look first to the class origins and position of health professionals. Since the beginning of the twentieth century, the vast majority of doctors have come from upper-middleclass families. In 1920, 12 per cent of North American medical students came from working-class families, and this percentage has stayed almost exactly the same until the present time. The extremely limited recruitment of doctors from working-class families has persisted despite recent increases in the proportion of women and racial minorities entering the profession. For the small numbers with working-class roots, as for the rest of the profession, the acquired class position of physicians is one of relative privilege. Their predominantly comfortable lifestyle does not encourage professionals to criticize the social structural roots of their clients' distress, especially the sources of suffering in class structure. Instead, professionals' life experiences predictably leads them to help clients adjust to things as they are.

Professional education and socialization further contribute to the unintentionality of medical social control. A critique of power in society is, needless to say, seldom part of the medical school curriculum. On the contrary, professionals in training receive many lessons about individual pathophysiology and treatment. Within progressive instructional programs, trainees hear information about emotional disturbance and social problems. This training, however, consistently emphasizes the importance of psychological and social knowledge in responding to the needs of the individual patient. Such an approach seeks to help the patient cope with stresses arising in work, the family, and other key institutions. It does not, even in its more progressive and enlightened versions, foster social criticism or social change as part of the medical mission.

There are also situational constraints that leave medical social control below the level of consciousness. When a client is in trouble, a professional usually feels that something should be done. Yet the professional also senses the limits of what he or she as an individual can do. For instance, when a patient's symptoms reflect stress at work, a doctor tends to feel that changing the workplace is beyond the responsibility or even the capability of the medical role. With rare exceptions, such as those involving physical abuse, disruption of familial relations is not an appropriate goal of medical intervention. Wanting to help but unable personally to change the social structure, a health professional typically seeks a solution within the existing institutional context. Relaxation techniques, tranquilizers, counselling, family therapy, and related methods are all feasible approaches for the professional who wants to do something. For a patient in crisis, a doctor cannot do everything. What can be done tends to encourage coping and accommodation. Conscious recognition of these choices, or consideration of more critical alternatives, seldom occurs.

These situational constraints contribute to the generally conservative effects of the medical role. On the one hand, medical discourse usually does not attend to institutional causes of suffering. This orientation leads health professionals to overlook social change as a possible therapeutic option. On the other hand, when doctors do consider institutional problems in their encounters with patients, this intervention frequently serves to support the *status* quo. When a professional encourages mechanisms of coping and adjustment, such communication conveys a subtle political content. By seeking limited modifications in social roles—at work and in the family, for instance—which preserve a particular institution's overall stability, the practitioner exerts a conservative political impact. Despite the best conscious intentions, the practitioner thus helps reproduce the same institutional structures that form the roots of personal anguish. This contradiction is one source of pathos in the helping professions.

Medical social control also involves the management of potentially troublesome emotions. Doctors, for instance, regularly deal with patients' anger, anxiety, unhappiness, social isolation, loneliness, depression, and other emotional distress. Often these feelings derive in one way or another from patients' social circumstances, such as economic insecurity, racial or sexual discrimination, occupational stress, and difficulties in family life. Such emotions, of course, are one basis of political outrage and organized resistance. How health professionals manage these sentiments is an interesting question. One of medicine's effects may be the defusing of socially caused distress. Medicine is not the only institution in which such processes occur, nor do these phenomena necessarily occupy a major part of medical encounters. Still, it is worth asking how such largely unintentional microlevel processes take place. This question leads us to an analysis of the structure of doctor-patient interaction.

## THE TRADITIONAL FORMAT OF THE MEDICAL ENCOUNTER

The traditional format of the medical encounter is as follows:

Chief complaint (CC) + present illness
(PI) + past history (PH) + family history
(FH) + social history (SH) + systems

review (SR) + physical examination (PE)
+ other investigations (01) + diagnosis
(Dx) + plan (P).

During a typical encounter, the doctor tries to cover some or all of these components in his or her spoken interaction, and by examination of the patient. In addition, the doctor provides a written version of the encounter, in the medical record. There, the doctor usually labels each component of the encounter with the same abbreviations that I am using here. This traditional format appears in most textbooks that provide instruction on clinical methods for trainees and practitioners of medicine. Research on doctor-patient communication, reported previously, has confirmed that medical practitioners actually do use the traditional structure as an organizing framework for their encounters with patients.

To define and to comment on each of these elements, we focus first on the components of the medical history (Hx), which comprises CC, PI, PH, FH, SH, and SR in the above scheme. In the chief complaint (CC), the physician elicits what is bothering the patient, in the briefest possible terms? The physician leads into the chief complaint usually with an opening question like: "Hello, what brings you in today?" or "Well, what's bothering you today?" or "How can I help you?" To these or similar questions, the patient might answer, "Headaches" or "My back hurts" or "I've got pain in my chest" or "I can't sleep" or "I want a check-up" and so forth. In asking for the CC, the physician seeks to elicit the patient's foremost concern.

Through the present illness (PI), the patient elaborates on the chief complaint. He or she tells the doctor when the problem began, what the specific characteristics of the symptom might be, which medications or other measures relieve the symptoms, what prior medical attention he or she has received for the problem, and similar details that may contribute to the doctor's attempts to reach a diagnosis.

Guiding the patient to elicit the CC and PI purportedly is the greatest skill that doctors develop in taking a medical history; some commentators argue that this is the most important skill in medicine. Doctors in training presumably learn a comfortable and effective balance between open-ended listening to the patient's story and more directive questioning that clarifies the patient's problem in terms of medical diagnoses.

Interruptions by doctors commonly begin to occur during the PI. Such interruptions basically are attempts to cut off story-telling by patients, for the following reasons among others the story may not contribute to a *doctor's cognitive process of reaching a* diagnosis; the patient's version of the story may be confusing or inconsistent; telling the story may take more time than is perceived to be available; or parts of the story may create feelings that are uncomfortable for the doctor, the patient, or both. The circumstances under which the doctor interrupts the patient's story to focus the PI that is, what is interrupted, when it is interrupted, what reason is given for the interruption, and so forth are important, especially to the extent that they cut off concerns about the social context of the medical encounter. Predictably, the PI is a critical juncture, during which certain elements, though they may be quite important in the patient's experience, come to be excluded from discourse, while other elements are included.

What is the relations between the spoken PI and the version—that the doctor writes in the medical record? While writing a comprehensible PI may involve skillful effort by a doctor, its orderliness invariably gives a false sense of what happens during the spoken PI. For example, the doctor never writes, "I interrupted the patient at this point," or "I thought the patient's comments about his family here weren't pertinent to his pain, so I asked him about what medications he was taking," or "I was in a hurry to get my daughter from child care so I cut off the patient at this point," and so forth. Instead, the written PI represents the doctor's interpretation of a disorderly series of spoken exchanges. The orderliness of the written version belies what actually gets said during the PI, which is my chief focus here. This is not to say that the written PI is uninteresting, and others have documented the enormous differences in content between the spoken and written versions. I am mainly concerned, however with the spoken PI in all its disorderliness.

While the CC and PI are almost always present in medical encounters assuming the patient is awake and conversant, other components may appear or not, depending on time, the doctor's desire to complete a comprehensive evaluation, financial issues such as the chiatient's insurance and how extensive an evaluation it permits, and other situational constraints. A doctor may choose to defer some or all the remaining components to future visits, or not cover them at all, although there is usually some attempt initially to develop a diagnosis and plan. In the past history PH, the doctor gathers information about past medical events in the patient's life that are not directly pertinent to the PI. These events typically include prior hospitalizations and surgery, other major illnesses, medications, allergies, immunizations, smoking, drinking habits, and recreational substance use. The family history FH includes data about illnesses and deaths in the patient's immediate family: mother, father, sisters, brothers, spouse, and children. Additionally, in this section many doctors routinely elicit information about family occurrences of cancer, heart disease, hypertension, diabetes mellitus, and other common problems that may carry an increased risk in certain families.

Although one might expect the social history (SH) to be important for a contextual analysis of medical encounters, it is usually a perfunctory listing of demographic data. For instance, the doctor typically asks about birthplace, occupation, educational attainment, living situation, and insurance status. The contextual concerns that retain to a patient's distress usually appear, subject to interruption and cut-off, during the PI, rather than the SH. In the SH itself the doctor traditionally tends not to purse in much depth how the patient's social circumstances might relate to the difficulties for which he or she is seeking medical attention.

Presumably, the systems review (SR) elicits any additional information about the patient that might be left out or missed by other parts of the history. The SR is sometimes very brief and sometimes quite lengthy; scuttlebutt among medical practitioners has it that the SR's length is inversely related to clinical experience. The expectation, however, is that the doctor will ask the patient whether he or she has experienced symptoms in more or less each of the following organ systems: skin, lymph nodes, head, eyes, ear, nose, throat, neck, respiratory system, cardiovascular system, gastrointestinal system, genitourinary system, reproductive system, neurological system, endocrine system, and bones and joints. For instance, under the gastrointestinal system, the doctor would question about symptoms of the esophagus principally swallowing, stomach heartburn, ulcers, cancer, and so forth, duodenum, small intestine, large intestine irregularity in bowel habits, bleeding, infections, rectum hemorrhoids, fissures, bleeding, liver jaundice, hepatitis, toxic exposures, and pancreas. In other words, the systems review can be quite exhaustive, even more so if the patient happens to be a "yea-sayer." Then, doctor and patient enter potentially endless labyrinths of questions and answers, leading to frustrating excursions through a welter of symptoms and diseases that have little to do with the current purposes of the medical encounter. Gradual recognition of these pitfalls during a medical career accounts for the exhaustive efforts that medical students devote to the SR, while their supervising physicians often truncate the SR to a very brief series of questions, for which they do not expect to hear "yes" as a frequent answer.

The physical examination (PE) involves the laying on of hands, whose impact in medicine has been so highly touted. Without intimate touch, medical encounters would not differ nearly so much from other types of professional client interactions. If time is available and if it has not already been done, a doctor will examine the body's entire external surface during the PE, as well as its internal orifices. When time is not available, or if the doctor is not inclined toward comprehensiveness, he or she does a more focused PE, concentrating on those parts of the body that might be related to the CC and PI.

After the PE, the doctor sometimes initiates one or more other investigations (OI)-lab tests, x-rays, electrocardiograms, and so forth—whose purported aim is to clarify the diagnosis or to gather data that may be useful for treatment or prevention. OIs also seem to communicate something. They may convey an impression of thoroughness and concern. A scientifically oriented intervention may be reassuring because of the technical knowledge it presumably reflects. Further, when an OI leads to a negative finding, it doubtless produces a feeling of relief and well-being. In fact, one research study has shown that normal lab results lead to improvement in symptoms, even when OIs are not ordered for a specific clinical reason from a doctor's point of view. Thus, a doctor's act of recommending an 01 may have several meanings in a medical encounter, aside from the specific results that are obtained.

With the data gleaned from the various components of the medical history, the PE, and the results of OIs, the doctor reaches a diagnosis (Dx), that may be provisional or confirmed. The cognitive operations involved in making a diagnosis undoubtedly are complex and poorly understood. Essentially the doctor takes the patients' comments in the medical history, observations made during the PE, and data from OIs, and shapes this information into one or more diagnostic categories.

The drive to reach a diagnosis is extremely strong. Practitioners and doctors in training view the facility of diagnostic categorization as one of the most important professional skills in medicine. The "differential diagnosis" involves a list of all possible categories into which a patient's physical problems might fall. Most practitioners would acknowledge that the tendencies to interrupt, cut off, or otherwise redirect the patient's story during the PI derive at least partly from the drive to make a diagnosis. That is, a doctor wants to hear those words that are consistent with previously defined diagnostic categories. Parts of patients' stories that do not fit neatly into these categories function as unwanted strangers in medical discourse and tend to be shown to the door.

While the drive to make a diagnosis is strong, diagnostic reasoning tends to be both limited and exclusionary. True, doctors and doctors-in-training must learn to deal with an awesome number of diagnostic categories and subcategories. Yet this set of diagnoses corresponds to no more than a tiny fraction of human experience. In large part, the cognitive process of reaching a diagnosis involves excluding a substantial part of a patient's experience that—no matter how relevant to the patient—is not relevant to the diagnosis. Features of patients' social context may be very troubling to patients and actually may affect their physical conditions in fairly direct ways. These contextual issues, however are almost always difficult to define with precision, are loaded with ambiguity, and are not completely consistent with the technical categories of differential diagnosis. The exclusionary drive, so much — a part of reaching a medically proper diagnosis, profoundly affects what is spoken and recorded during medical encounters. Contextual concerns that do not lend themselves to the technical lexicon of diagnostic possibilities tend to gravitate toward the margins of medical talk.

The medical plan (P) constitutes the interventions that the doctor suggests, usually toward the end of an encounter.

Traditional teaching about the medical plan holds that it contains two components. First, there is a diagnostic plan, which involves the OIs that the doctor wishes to obtain after the present encounter ends. Second, in the therapeutic plan, the doctor recommends the medication, surgery, diet, rest, exercise, counselling, relaxation, attitude change, and so forth that he or she believes the patient's diagnosis warrants. A substantial part of medical education involves learning and keeping up with current vogues of preferred diagnostic and therapeutic plans.

Just as it affects diagnostic reasoning, the exclusionary drive also shapes the plan that is formulated. Among the infinitely varied possibilities for human action, the limited range of medical diagnoses encourages relatively few options. Usually these options involve OIs that create more technical data, or treatments that use medication, surgery, or similar technical intervention. Alternatively, a doctor may suggest nonintervention, which involves reassurance that a problem is not serious enough to require technical action, or a schedule of follow-up to be sure that the problem does not become worse. Sometimes, a doctor recommends other maneuvers such as dietary improvement, changes in habits such as smoking and alcohol consumption, counselling, psychotherapy, or behavioral change. In such situations, the problems underconsideration often have roots in the social context of the encounter.

Partly because the medical diagnosis rarely provides a technical name for such contextual problems, the plan does not generally call for a contextual intervention. Instead, the medical plan tends to accept the social context as a given. Even the limited behavioral changes that doctors may encourage generally aim at a patient's less troublesome reconciliation with his or her context, rather than change in the context itself. For the medical plan, given the power and limits of the diagnostic process, the range of the possible becomes quite restricted.

Where does giving information to the patient fit in the traditional format of the medical encounter? Remarkably, this format—as taught to generations of doctors in training-lacks a specific niche for providing information. It is probably for this reason that giving information has often been catch-as catch- can in medicine. Similarly, the absence of a specific place to give information in the encounter's format doubtless has contributed to the very problematic deficiencies and dissatisfactions that have arisen in this arena. Suffice it to say, the traditional format also does not guide the doctor in communicating information about contextual issues.

## BENEATH THE TRADITIONAL FORMAT: PROCESSING IDEOLOGY AND CONTEXT

By questioning, by interrupting, and by otherwise shifting the direction of conversation from non technical problems to technical ones, doctors ***exclude*** certain topics from talk and *include* others. Of particular interest here are the verbal techniques that divert attention from sources of personal distress in the social context. Such techniques cut off the possibility of considering the context critically, let alone changing it. How medical encounters convey ideologic messages and how they invoke social control, sometimes involve doctors' explicit pronouncements about what patients should or should not do. It is also likely that ideology and social control emerge from what doctors and patients exclude from their talk, and how it comes to be excluded.

Several studies of communication in medicine have suggested that medical encounters contain common structural features. In a sociolinguistic analysis of doctor-patient conversations, West has found typical "troubles" that arise in encounters (1984). When patients express concerns about events in their lives that are not amenable to doctors' technical intervention, West argues, questions and interruptions are mechanisms by which doctors steer patients', concerns back to a technical track. As West notes, other studies also have observed that doctors interrupt patients frequently and initiate more questions than patients do. In West's taperecorded sample of medical interactions, male doctors tended to interrupt patients more often than did female doctors. West interprets interruptions and frequent questioning as gestures of dominance, by which doctors control the flow of conversation. She also postulates a connection between social power and sexual differences in language use, in conversations generally, and more specifically in professional- client encounters,

Further, in his study of medical encounters, Mishler demonstrates how medical discourse cuts off contextual issues and redirects the focus to technical concerns (1984). Mishler presents detailed transcripts from recordings of doctor-patient communication and describes two "voices" that compete with each other. The "voice of medicine" involves the technical topics of physiology, pathology, pharmacology, and so forth which concern doctors in their professional work. Alternatively, the "voice of the lifeworld" comprises the everyday, largely non technical problems that patients carry with them into the medical encounter. According to Mishler's analysis of transcripts, patients often try to raise contextual issues through the voice of the lifeworld. Doctors, however, are ill-equipped to deal with such issues and, therefore repeatedly return to the voice of medicine. For instance, patients raise personal troubles that do not pertain to technical problems. Or, although related to technical problems, these personal troubles do not seem amenable to technical solutions. Or, the raising of personal troubles leads to discomfort for the professional, the client, or both. Under these circumstances, doctors typically introject questions, interrupt, or otherwise change the topic, to return to the voice of medicine.

Although Mishler's approach conveys how medical language encourages the saying of somethings and the leaving unsaid of others, the "lifeworld" remains rather general. Mishler implies that patients' concerns about contextual issues in the lifeworld are very important to them and that cutting off these concerns is undesirable. When the voice of medicine gains sway, however, this achievement also has much to do with ideology and social control. Diverting critical attention away from the lifeworld, doctors subtly reinforce the ideas that pattern the lifeworld and may help win acquiescence to those features of the lifeworld that patients find most disconcerting. In short, a re-reading of Mishler's materials might emphasize that the voice of medicine not only tends to suppress the voice of the lifeworld but also reinforces the reasonableness and acceptability of the lifeworld in its present form.

What is left silent, unsaid, or hidden in medical encounters has fascinated other researchers, who have interpreted rich textual materials but with little or no contextual theory. For instance Katz provides an extensive account of the "silent world" of the doctor-patient relationship (1984). He shows how medical language overlooks or downplays some important features of doctors' and patients' experience. Thus, Katz argues, doctors often gloss over their patients' concerns, and patients tend to leave these concerns unsaid. In Katz's account, doctors and patients tend to remain silent about many topics, especially those that would require patients' informed consent. Similarly, Cassell interprets the confusions, misunderstandings, insensitivities, and communication lapses in transcripts of doctor-patient interaction (1985). He reiterates a viewpoint frequently expressed, that doctors in training should learn better communication skills to avoid such gaffes in practice. Commenting on the unsaid socio-emotional content of medical encounters, Cassell urges that health practitioners pay more attention to what is excluded from conversation, as well as the reasons why?

These accounts of the unsaid in medical language do not emphasize enough the pertinence of the unsaid for the context of professional encounters. Doctors do not simply overlook or downplay or suppress patients' contextual concerns. The exclusion of social context from critical attention is a fundamental feature of medical language, a feature closely connected to ideology and social control. Inattention to social issues, especially when these issues lie behind patients' personal troubles, can never be just a matter of professional inadequacy, or the inadequacy of professional training. Instead, this lack is a basic part of what medicine is in our society?

What elements of social context help shape the ideologic content of discourse? Social class, of course, is a key contextual element. Relationships of social class are crucial parts of the context in which discourse arises and in which ideology is transmitted. To the extent that doctors and patients occupy different class positions, this class difference patterns the ideologic content of their discourse. Predictably, doctors sometimes voice explicit ideologic messages that legitimate the current class structure of society; or the transmission of ideology occurs more subtly, conveyed by the absence of criticism about class structure and its various injuries. In medical encounters, marginalization constrains an oppositional voice, perhaps that of a patient in distress, through interruption, cut-off or de-emphasis. This way of looking at medical discourse provides a slightly different theoretical prism to see the same problems uncovered by sociolinguists who observe a "diffidence" of working-class patients in medical encounters, or who note contention between the "voice of medicine" and the "voice of the lifeworld". Such observations confirm that social class relations, as an element of context, pattern ideology within discourse.

But social class is not the only contextual element that affects discourse; other crucial elements include gender, age, and race. All these contextual elements can become the basis of dominance and subordination, and they are closely linked to social class. Ideologies of gender pertain in large part to the roles men and women occupy in the family and at work. Through ideologies of gender, expectations about what men and women appropriately should and should not do enter everyday language. Arising in the context of discourse, these ideologies profoundly affect what is or can be said, what appears at the center of discourse, and what slips in at the margins. Similarly, as people age, they encounter a changing set of expectations and demands, which vary a great deal among societies. In the United States, for instance, ideologies of aging can convey the image of a trash heap, where elderly people actually or symbolically move when their productivity, or reproductivity, is used up. Other societies tend to be more lenient, or even respectful, in ideologies of aging. Ideologies of race have entered discourse, whenever societies have encountered the contrast between majority and minority groups. Expressions of racial ideologies have ranged from the master-slave vernacular to the only slightly more subtle versions of modernity. Why highlight these contextual elements here? Class, gender, age, and race are some of the contextual elements that pattern ideologic language in face-to-face discourse, as well as medical discourse. It is not enough to acknowledge that ideology may be reproduced in medical discourse; the question is how this happens. That is, in concrete examples of discourse, the critical reader needs to seek specific places where ideologic reproduction occurs, and where context impinges on discourse.

## CRITICAL THEORY OF MEDICAL DISCOURSE

Now let we turn to three summaries of actual doctor-patient encounters. Transcripts of these encounters were prepared as part of a large study of doctor-patient communication that involved random sampling from private practices and hospital outpatient departments. The encounters are summarized here because they illustrate typical patterns in the sampled interactions. In each encounter, doctors and patients deal with personal troubles that derive largely from broader contextual issues.

A man comes to his doctor several months after a heart attack. He is depressed. His period of disability payments will expire soon, and his union is about to go on strike. His doctor tells him that he is physically able to return to work and that working will be good for his mental health. The doctor also prescribes an antidepressant and a tranquilizer. A woman visits her doctor because of irregularities in her heart rhythm. She complains that palpitations and shortness of breath are interfering with her ability to do housework. The doctor checks an electrocardiogram while she exercises, changes her cardiac medications, and congratulates her in her efforts to maintain a tidy household. A man goes to his doctor for a premarital blood test. The doctor questions him closely about his drinking problem, his smoking, his job, his family, and his plans for married life. Then the doctor encourages attendance at Alcoholics Anonymous and orders a test of liver function, in addition to the premarital blood test that the patient requested.

Figure 4.1 shows some structural elements of discourse in the first encounter. Seen in this way, the contextual issue of uncertain employment initially presents itself (A). Depression is a personal trouble that the patient experiences in anticipation of a return to uncertain employment (B). Coming to the medical encounter (C), the patient tentatively and briefly expresses concern about his impending return to work when his union intends to go on strike (D). He repeats these concerns at several points, but the doctor de-emphasizes them (E). Rather than pursuing the contextual problem, the doctor reassures the patient that work is good for his mental health; further, the doctor prescribes both an antidepressant medication and a tranquilizer (F). After the encounter, one assumes, the patient continues to prepare himself for a return to work.

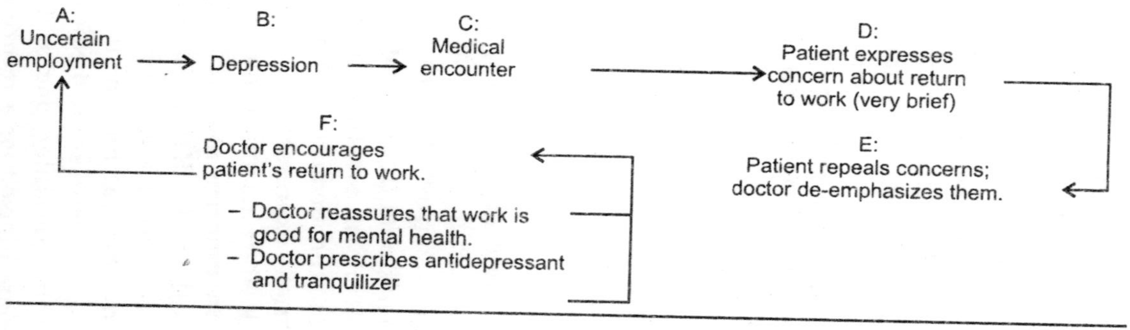


**Fig. 4.1:** Structural Elements of Medical Encounter with a Man Anticipating Return to Work After a Heart Attack

Structural elements of the second encounter appear in Figure 4.2. Here the contextual issue involves expectations about women's social role in the family (A). Housework, as many have noted, is an important activity in economic "reproduction," which traditionally is the responsibility of women. Because this patient's heart symptoms interfere with her housework, she experiences emotional distress (B). When she sees her doctor (C), the patient mentions this concern (D). Rather than exploring her concern in depth, the doctor does an electrocardiogram while the patient exercises (E). Based on the results, the doctor changes the patient's cardiac medications. He also encourages her efforts in at least trying to maintain a tidy household (F). The patient thus returns to her personal challenge of doing housework in the face of serious heart disease.

Figure 4.3 gives some structural elements of the third encounter. This patient faces a contextual issue that derives from the patterning of role expectations that affect men (A). Like most men, this patient finds that he must hold a job steadily to support himself and his family—to use a convenient term, he must earn the "means of subsistence." Further, as he approaches marriage, he also faces an expectation that he stably perform as "head" of a family. Such expectations about work and the family, however are not simple ones, since the patient is something of a lush. The patient, therefore experiences a personal trouble that pertains to actual or potential conflicts deriving from alcohol use (B). During the medical encounter (C), the doctor takes the lead in expressing concern about alcohol (D). The doctor questions the patient closely about alcohol, as well as his heavy smoking, his job, family, and plans for married life. In pursuing these questions, the doctor interrupts the patient frequently (E). Beyond voicing strong encouragement that the patient attend Alcoholics Anonymous, the doctor also orders a test of liver function. In this discourse, the doctor encourages the patient's stable functioning at work and in the family (F)

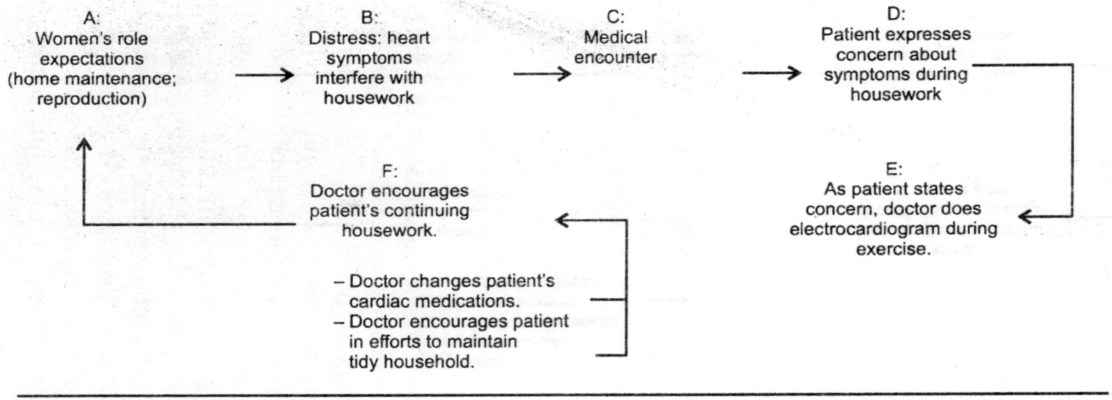


**Fig. 4.2:** Structural Elements of Medical Encounter with a Woman Whose Heart Symptoms Interfere with Her Housework

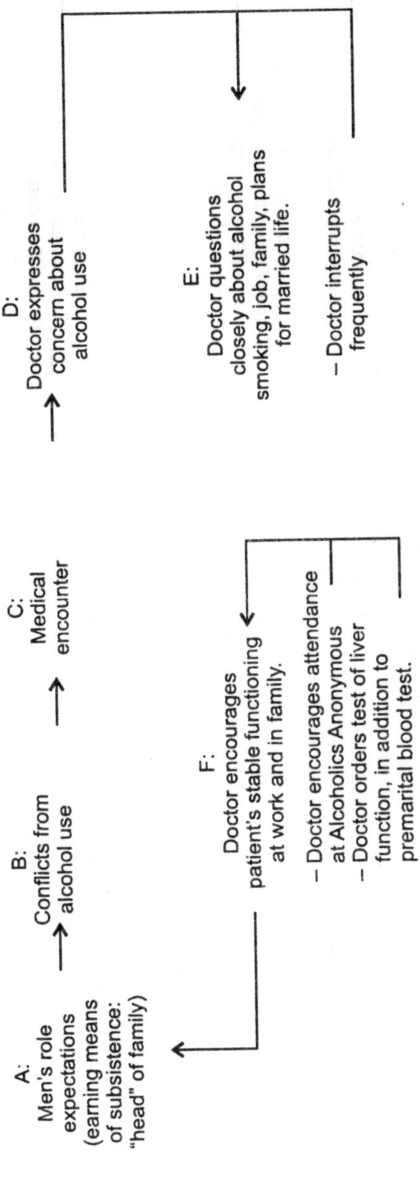


**Fig. 4.3:** Structural Elements of Medical Encounter with a Man Whose Alcohol Problem Potentially Interferes with Work and Family Relations

In the paragraphs that follow, reasoning from these and other encounters, I map some from these and other encounters, I map some from these and other encounters, I map some islands around which medical discourse seems to flow (Figure 4.4). I interpret these islands as underlying structures in the flow of medical discourse, rarely discerned consciously by the doctors and patients who travel there.

***A. Social issue as context:*** The economic, social, and political context of society contains many difficult conditions. These social issues often lie behind and help create some of the personal troubles that clients experience in their everyday lives (Mills 1959, pp. 3-24). (In the three encounters above, the pertinent social issues are: uncertain employment, women's role expectations, and men's role expectations.)

***Personal trouble:*** Clients tend to experience these troubles privately, as their own individual problems. They are unlikely to recognize consciously the social issues that lie behind their personal troubles. In the same three encounters, personal troubles include: depression, distress that heart symptoms interfere with housework, and conflicts from alcohol use.

***The medical encounter:*** Clients come to medical professionals with complaints that very often though not always have economic, social, and political roots. Such contextual sources of personal troubles include class structure and the organization of work; family life, gender roles, and sexuality; aging and the social role of the elderly; the patterning of leisure and substance use; and limited resources for dealing with emotional distress.

***Expression of contextual problems in medical discourse:*** The traditional and technical sequence of the medical encounter does not facilitate the expression of contextual concerns. Regarding patients' own characteristics, the relations between language and social structure predictably make the expression of contextual concerns more difficult for working-class people, women, and racial minorities. Certain humanistic or progressive doctors encourage patients to talk about the non-technical components of their problems that pertain to their lifeworlds. These patients can express concerns and vent emotions about such personal troubles. Less humanistic or progressive doctors tend to discourage patients from expressing such concerns or to ignore them when expressed.

**Counter textual tensions deriving from social context** Contextual problems, however, create tensions in medical discourse. Periodically such tensions that derive from troubling social issues erupt into the course, or appear at its margins, and create a countertextual reality that cannot be resolved in the framework of a medical encounter. Doctors tend to suppress such tensions by dominance gestures like interruptions, cutoffs, offs, and de-emphases that get the discourse back on a technical track.

***Management of contextual problems:*** Whether such tensions are expressed or suppressed, the language of medicine leaves few options for action. Limited options for action apply to both humanistic encounters, when doctors encourage patients to talk about non technical components of their personal troubles, and to less humanistic encounters, where such concerns are discouraged. Generally, doctors respond with technical solutions and counsel patients how best to adjust to their previous roles. The language of medical science can convey ideologic content, especially when it converts social problems into technical ones. Ideologic language also arises at the margins of medical discourse or achieves its impact through absence. That is, by a lack of criticism directed against sources of distress in the social context, medical discourse ideologically reinforces the *status quo*. The discourse of medicine thus tends to exclude basic social change as a meaningful alternative. In accepting the present context as given, and in remaining

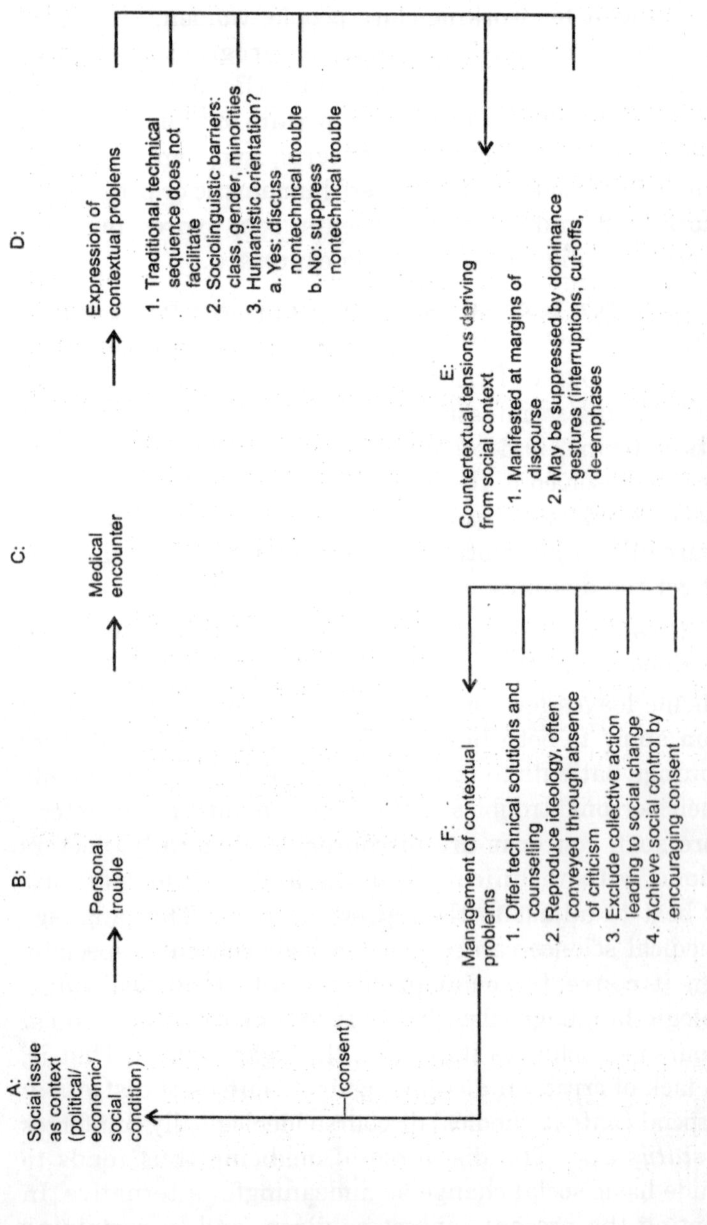


**Fig. 4.4:** The Micro political Structure of Medical Discourse

silent about collective political action, medical discourse encourages consent by rendering social change unthinkable. This latter accomplishment of medicine may be its main contribution to social control. Further studies will show how this structure helps us understand what is happening as doctors and patients deal with problems of work, the family and gender roles, aging, sexuality, leisure, substance use, other "vices," and troublesome emotions. In addition, medical discourse in which this structure is not apparent will become a matter of particular interest.

To, whatever extent this theory is persuasive, other questions immediately suggest themselves: Can the structure of medical discourse be reformed? Can medical discourse include a criticism of the sources of personal distress in the social context of the professional encounter? A critical discourse in medicine, one might argue, would no longer encourage consent to contextual sources of personal troubles. By suggesting collective action as a meaningful option, medical professionals might begin to overcome the impact that its exclusion exerts. Can this be done without further medicalizing social problems? If so, critical discourse in medicine also would recognize the limits of medicine's role and the importance of building links to other forms of praxis that seek to change the social context of medical encounters. Moving beyond the current structure of medical discourse then becomes a major goal of this attempt to analyze it.

# 5

# Social Workers in Public Health

Social workers have been involved in the health care field since the turn of the 20th century. The profession's earliest concerns were with making health care services available to the poor and with improving social conditions that bred infectious diseases such as tuberculosis. As the social work role expanded, social workers joined other health professions in the delivery of high quality services. Today, social workers can be found in every component of the health care system.

## Social Work Guiding Principles

The basic values of social work, from promoting an individual's right to self-determination to having an attitude of empathy for the individual, are the foundation of social work practice. When confronting dilemmas or needs in health care, social workers can use the principle of client self-determination in matters where clients or their proxies are faced with such issues.

Social workers have skills in cultural awareness and cultural competence, in which social work practice respectfully responds to, and affirms, the worth and dignity of people of all cultures, languages, classes, ethnic backgrounds, abilities, religions, sexual orientation, and other diverse features found in individuals. Social workers look at the person-in-environment, including all of the factors that influence the total health care experience. Social workers practice at the macro and micro level of health care and thus have the ability to influence policy change and development at local, state, and federal levels and within systems of care. Social work research in health care benefits not only individuals and families, but also the very existence, effectiveness, and validation of the profession. These standards offer a guide for social workers practicing in any health care setting.

## Definitions

### *Bioethics*

Bioethics is the analysis and study of moral, legal, social, and ethical considerations involving the biological and medical sciences. Many health care settings have organized forums such as bioethics committees, institutional review boards, or consultation processes to address ethical dilemmas and questions.

### Biopsychosocial–Spiritual Perspective

The biopsycho social–spiritual perspective recognizes that health care services must take into account the physical or medical aspects of ourselves (bio); the emotional or psychological aspects (psycho); the sociocultural, sociopolitical, and socioeconomic issues in our lives (social); and how people find meaning in their lives spiritual. This approach draws from the strengths perspective of social work practice. The strengths perspective recognizes an individual's strengths and abilities to cope with problems; and awareness and use of the client's strengths is part of the foundation of social work theory and practice. The strengths perspective is seen in social work practice through our role of enhancing personal strengths and resources, helping clients solve both interpersonal and environmental problems, and helping clients mobilize for change. The strengths perspective helps clients use their past successful choices and behaviors, skills, and insights to resolve or "work through" a current crisis.

## Case Management

Case management, sometimes used interchangeably with care management, is the collaborative process of assessment, planning, and facilitation for options and services to meet an individual's complex needs. When appropriate, this would include arranging, coordinating, monitoring, evaluating, and advocating on behalf of the client and/or his or her family for the multiple services needed from a variety of social service and health care agencies. Case management addresses both the individual client's biopsychosocial-spiritual status (micro level) as well as the state of the social systems in which the services operate (macro level).

## Client/Patient/Consumer

These terms refer to the person receiving care and treatment from physicians and allied health care personnel. Social workers generally use the term client to identify the individual, group, family, or community who seeks or is provided with professional services. The client is often seen as both the individual and the client system or those in the client's environment. The term consumer is also used in settings that view the client as the consumer, that is, one capable of deciding what is best for her or himself and encourages self-advocacy and self-judgment in negotiating the social service and welfare system? The term *patient* is more commonly used by social workers employed in health care settings.

## Continuum of Care

The care continuum includes the specialized health, social work services, rehabilitative, and home-based services that a seriously or chronically ill or injured person might need. This continuum addresses both the medical care and the other services that promote the patients' well-being.

### Continuity of Care

Continuity of care ensures the coordination of care within an organization or across different agencies or settings to reduce duplicate services, to address gaps in existing services, and to ensure consistent and continuous services for the client as they transition in care or are discharged.

### Disabling Condition

A disabling condition is considered a temporary or permanent reduction in a client's capacity or functioning based on the inability to perform some activities that most others can perform. A disabling condition can be congenital, can be the result of an accident or trauma, or more frequently is the result of chronic illness that is, diabetes, hypertension.

### Health Care Settings

Health care settings are practice areas in which assessment, care, and treatment address the physical, mental, emotional, and social well-being of the person; and address prevention, detection, and treatment of physical and mental disorders with the goal of enhancing the person's biopsychosocial and spiritual well-being. The health care setting includes personnel who provide the necessary services for example, physicians, social workers, nurses, hospital attendants; appropriate service delivery facilities for example, hospitals, hospice, assisted living, medical centers, and outpatient clinics; and educational and environmental facilities that work to help prevent disease.

## Health Planning

Health planning is conducted in government organizations, medical and research organizations, and educational institutions and in prevention, early intervention, treatment, and follow-up. Planning should involve determining and ensuring the number of necessary health care personnel presently and in the future, and how to both finance and control costs. It includes where to locate facilities, how to provide the most effective means of service delivery, and how to provide services in a cost effective manner.

## Managed Care

Managed care is a process designed to manage health care costs primarily through the private sector, although Medicaid's or Medicare's capitated systems are a form of managed care. It is a technique used by insurance carriers and characterized by preauthorization to qualify the patient for particular services; preauthorization for a given amount of care; review of treatment and patient response(s); utilization review; predischarge planning to ensure the patient is ready to be released having received the care required and has an aftercare plan. Managed care plans include preferred provider organizations, health maintenance organizations, or a combined version through a point-of service plan.

## Medicaid

Medicaid is a government-funded health insurance program that provides payment for hospital, nursing home, home care, dental, and medical services to people who meet disability guidelines and income eligibility requirements.

## Public Health Model

The Public Health Model of services focuses on the health of the individual, the family, and the larger community or general public and is administered by federal, state, and local agencies. The goal of programs, policies, and health care personnel is to prevent and treat disease, identify and eliminate environmental hazards, prolong life, and promote better health.

## Standards for Social Work Practice in Health Care Settings

Ethics and Values Social Workers shall have knowledge the primary mission of the social work profession is to enhance human well-being and help meet the basic human needs of all people, with particular attention to the needs of people who are vulnerable, disenfranchised, oppressed, and living in poverty. The mission is rooted in a set of core values. These core values, embraced by social workers throughout the profession's history, are the foundation of social work's unique purpose and perspective: Service social, justice dignity and worth of the person, importance of human relationships, integrity and competence.

In a health care system increasingly driven by technological advances, the ethical and moral questions and dilemmas raised for clients, families, and health care professionals are numerous and complex. Health care settings have designed a number of different systems to ensure ethical behavior among health care practitioners. Ethics committees are often used to provide "objective" reviews to health care providers and clients and families, when there is conflict between providers or providers, clients, and families. Institutional review boards are used to protect clients from the potential of experimentation in research projects. Social work supervision and peer consultation can also be used to discuss. Health Disparities Social Workers practicing in local, state, national, and international health care settings require knowledge and skills to help them recognize and address inequalities and injustices directed toward clients, organizations, and communities related to access to care and provision of health services.

Many social workers have historically delivered services as part of community-based organizations and public health programs to address health disparities among those who are least likely to be able to gain access to adequate care. Social workers have an ethical obligation to address the health care needs of these groups and advocate for change to ensure access to care. Training of health care professionals to achieve a level of cultural competence—an understanding of practice patterns and attributes of diverse groups—is an essential part of basic and continuing education for all health care professionals, including social workers. Health is a matter of both economics and social well-being. Both domestically and internationally, health care social workers strive to gain knowledge about health care: behavior, expenditures, reforms, systems, teams, insurance, health maintenance organizations, health protective behaviors, and more. Social workers also help clients to gain access to health care as they navigate between and among complex service delivery systems and entitlements.

Different entities shape public and global policies in every country. Therefore, social workers must keep abreast of policies to competently help clients and to assess physical, environmental, historical, situational, cultural, and structural factors that affect health care systems. Accessibility to preventive, palliative, and curative health care depends largely on the client's ability to pay, and often, people cannot afford existing fees. In many nonprofit community-based clinics, services are provided on a "first come-first serve" basis often with a long wait or long lines and are limited by a shortage of supplies and equipment. Increasingly, private systems of care emerge alongside public systems and other health care providers to care for the uninsured or underinsured who need health services, yet prefer to care for those who can pay fee for services. When these realities exist, social workers shall act as brokers, advocates, and mediators for clients.

## Cultural Competence

Social workers shall develop and maintain an understanding of the history, traditions, values, and family systems of client groups as they relate to health care and decision-making. The importance of recognizing, respecting, and understanding other cultures and related health beliefs lays a foundation to build therapeutic alliances with clients and families. Social workers are responsible for self-reflection regarding the impact of their own cultural beliefs on their professional and personal life. Social workers in health care shall approach each client and family interaction from a perspective of cultural respect and awareness. This implies reluctance to stereotype individuals based on assumed group similarities and seeks instead to ask individuals what aspects of their cultural experience are meaningful in understanding a particular health care need? Social workers recognize that ethnic, cultural, spiritual, and religious factors can have an impact on health care choices and adherence to regimens of care.

## Confidentiality

Appreciation of cultural influences is especially important for clients at critical health junctures, such as birth, diagnosis of a major illness, and facing the end of life. Social workers have a responsibility to assist the client and family system in observing culturally meaningful practices, whenever possible. Confidentiality Health care social workers shall maintain appropriate safeguards for the privacy and confidentiality of client information. Social workers must be familiar and comply with local, state, and federal mandates related to confidentiality. Professional judgment in the use of confidential information shall be based on best practice, ethical, and legal considerations regulations. Clients, families, and other professionals should be informed of the confidentiality limitations and requirements before services are initiated and in all phases of the health care experience.

**Knowledge**

Knowledge social workers in health care settings shall demonstrate a working knowledge of current theory and practice and integrate such information into practice. The social worker uses knowledge about, and psychosocial implications of, illness, injury, and health conditions to provide social work services to clients and families to help them manage and cope with the impact of such health matters. Social workers have expertise in communication; navigating systems of care, resources, client and family coping skills; and the comprehensive impact of health conditions on the client. With the person-in-environment perspective, social workers look at all of the influences and aspects of a person's life to complete a thorough assessment and treatment plan with the client, family, and other health care professionals.

Essential areas of knowledge and understanding about health care include: the roles and functions of social work in health care the biopsychosocial needs of clients and families the physiological elements of illness and their impact on psychosocial functioning the psychological and spiritual needs of clients and families and how to ensure that they can be addressed community resources to assist clients and families the disparities across cultures and economic groups in gaining access to and funding for health care ethical and legal questions and dilemmas laws, regulations, and policies affecting clients, families, and social work practice the accreditation and regulatory standards governing settings providing health care evidence-based practices and social work research in health care and the needs of special populations.

**Assessment** social workers shall provide ongoing assessment, including gathering comprehensive information to use in developing interventions and treatment strategies. Assessment is a fundamental process of social work practice. Treatment and intervention strategies/plans require that social workers both assess and reassess client needs and modify plans accordingly. Social work assessments in health care settings include considering relevant biomedical, psychosocial, and spiritual factors and the needs of the individual client and the family (as defined by the client).

A comprehensive, culturally competent assessment includes: past and current health status including genetic history of family health the impact of health conditions or treatments on cognitive, emotional, social, sexual, psychological, or physical functioning the impact on body image, intimacy, and sexuality social history, including current living arrangement and household environment work, school, or vocational history stage in the life cycle and related and relevant developmental issues cultural values and beliefs, including views on illness, disability, and death family structure and the client's role within the family social supports, including formal and informal support systems behavioral and mental health status and current level of functioning, including history, suicide risk, and coping styles and financial resources, including access to and type of health insurance.

Comprehensive assessments shall address unique needs relevant to special populations, including children, people with severe and persistent mental illness, immigrants and refugees, people with substance use disorders, victims of violence or trauma, homeless people, and people with physical or psychiatric disabilities.

## Intervention and Treatment Planning

Intervention and Treatment Planning Social Workers implement intervention and treatment plans that promote client well-being and ensure a continuum of care. Planning shall be based on a comprehensive, culturally competent assessment with interdisciplinary input. Intervention and treatment plans are steps identified by the health social worker, in collaboration with the client and with other members of the team, to achieve objectives identified during assessment. Social workers shall be able to adapt practice techniques to best meet client needs within their health care setting to work effectively with individuals across the life-span, with different ethnicities, cultures, religions, socioeconomic and educational backgrounds, and across the range of mental health and disability conditions.

Intervention or treatment plans may include: strategies to address needs identified in the assessment information, referral, and education individual, family, or group counseling vocational, educational, and supportive counseling psychoeducational support groups financial counseling case management discharge planning interdisciplinary care planning and collaboration client and systems advocacy and goals and objectives.

**Case Management Social Work** case management shall optimize client functioning. Case management facilitates collaboration among providers to address the client's biomedical and psychosocial needs to better provide efficient, appropriate, and beneficial health care services to a client with (often) multiple needs. Social work case management requires the professional social worker to develop and maintain a therapeutic relationship with the client, which includes linking the client with resources that provide a range of services, resources, and opportunities to enhance successful quality outcomes for the client. Culturally competent case management is both micro and macro in nature and requires interdisciplinary care planning and collaboration with other professionals to maintain a team-oriented approach. Case management may include having regular meetings with the client and family and assisting the client to navigate systems.

**The scope of services would include the following:**

Psychosocial assessment, including diagnoses, interventions, and treatment plans, financial assessment, planning, and intervention, case facilitation, patient and family counseling, crisis intervention, quality improvement, resource brokering/referral/development, continuity of care planning, system integration, outcome/practice evaluation, teamwork/collaboration, patient/family education and patient/family advocacy.

## Empowerment and Advocacy

Empowerment and Advocacy Social Workers have a responsibility to advocate for the needs and interests of clients and client systems in health care, including advocating for larger system change to improve access to care and improved delivery of services. Social workers have a special responsibility to advocate for the needs of the disenfranchised or the most vulnerable of the population at both the micro and macro levels. Social workers will identify barriers to services and actively seek to resolve them. The responsibility to advocate for quality improvement also implies a responsibility for health social workers to act as advocates to expand the role of the profession, develop leadership programs, and mentor new professionals. Client and Community Education Social Workers Act as educators for clients, families, the community, and other professionals regarding disease prevention, impact of illness and disease progression, advocacy for benefits, health maintenance, and adherence to treatment regimens. Social workers have a formal role as educators. Social workers gain knowledge and expertise in the health practice setting from other professionals and from formal education, work, or teaching experience. They have the knowledge and skill to implement the principles of learning theories in education programs, activities, and resources. They communicate and collaborate with departments and other staff to foster client education. They serve with other members of the health care team for program and resource development, planning, implementation, and evaluation.

Social workers use a variety of methods to define and identify learning needs of individuals and families. Assessment identifies the educational needs based on the expressed needs of individuals, family members, and significant others. The social worker identifies deficiencies in the knowledge base of the client and works with the client to obtain the needed information and resources. Social workers collaborate with the health care team to design educational activities to meet the client's needs, to deliver the activities in a method that facilitates the learning needed, and to evaluate the process in an integral, ongoing, and systematic manner.

## Teamwork and Collaboration

Teamwork and Collaboration Social Workers shall participate in care teams, and collaborate with other professionals, volunteers, and groups in and outside of their practice setting to enhance all aspects of the client and family system's care. Social workers participate in multiple care teams, which are typically interdisciplinary. These teams often provide comprehensive care and information in a client's home, in outpatient or inpatient health, and mental health care settings.

As part of such teams and collaborations, social workers shall demonstrate the ability to: understand the mission and functions of the service organization or group for which the social worker is employed understand the role of other relevant professions and organizations communicate and cooperate appropriately with other disciplines and agencies ensure that the social work role and responsibilities are clearly delineated and communicated to other members of the team ensure that the roles and responsibilities of each collaborating organization are clearly delineated and communicated advocate for changes in care that reflect the interests of the client and client system communicate the client's information in a respectful and objective manner and protect the client's confidentiality and privacy and share leadership and decision-making functions

Workload Health Care Social Workers shall maintain a workload that allows for efficient and quality social work service delivery. The size of the social work staff shall represent the scope and the complexity of the organization and the nature and numbers of the populations served. Both the health care organization or setting and the social work leader and staff have joint responsibility for establishing and maintaining a workload that allows for adequate and appropriate interventions and monitoring of services and outcomes. A workload consists of any social work function performed for the purpose of the social work position, including direct practice, administration, policy, research, or education. The workload also reflects the demands of the population served and may include social work coverage outside of regular office hours. It is the joint responsibility of the organization and the social worker to resolve issues of workload concerns. Documentation Social workers shall maintain records or documentation of social work services, which reflect the client and client systems' pertinent information for assessment and treatment; social work involvement and outcomes with and for clients; and in accordance with care goals and legislative and administrative regulations and policies. The importance of clear, concise, and organized documentation reflects the hallmark of quality social work services and often serves as the mode of communication between a social worker and other professionals and clients. There are core elements that need to be included and responsibilities to follow in record keeping. The elements and responsibilities of thorough and comprehensive documentation include the following: comprehensive assessment and services delivered to the client and client systems, including the development of a plan of care ongoing assessments, interventions, and treatment planning goals and planning that reflect an explicit statement of agreement with client, client systems, and team input referral sources and collaborations dates, times, and descriptions of client and client system contacts documentation of outcomes reason for case closure or transfer written permission to release and obtain information, where appropriate documentation of compliance with confidentiality rights and responsibilities and documentation of receipts and disbursements

## Research

Research Health Care Social Workers shall understand research planning, methodology, evidence based outcomes, and program evaluation. Social workers have a responsibility to be familiar with the literature crucial to their area of practice. As professionals, social workers in all settings have a mandate to improve the knowledge of the field, and this can best be accomplished through participation in research activities. Venues where health care social workers might help to develop, implement, or evaluate research include inpatient and outpatient hospital-based settings, community or home health agencies, and federally funded clinical trial research networks. Rich data sources that permit opportunities for quantitative and qualitative research exist within these entities.

Clinical trials (methodological assessments of the safety and efficacy of new treatments or new methods for administering existing treatments) help answer scientific questions and greatly depend on study participants' committed participation. Social workers may help physicians, nurses, pharmacists, and others recruit individuals and encourage study participation and adherence to medication regimens; they can also help clients manage problems that may hinder adherence and retention, such as challenging life circumstances and demands from family members.

## Performance

Performance Improvement Health Care Social Workers shall be a part of ongoing, formal evaluation of their practice to assess quality and appropriateness of services, to improve practice, and to ensure competence. Social workers are trained to facilitate improvements that alter the processes in which health care is delivered. They are ethically charged to promote process improvements that will enhance patient or consumer safety, satisfaction, efficient and effective care, and identify and promote best practices and equitable care on a multidisciplinary basis.

The evaluation of social work practice is a vital part of social work service delivery. The methods to evaluate such practice include peer review, self-evaluation, supervision, and other research methods. Increasingly, social work outcomes from evaluations are used for position justification, performance review, social work standards for practice, goal setting, and research efforts. Evaluation practices may include the following:

Using appropriate tools such as clinical indicators, practice guidelines, consumer satisfaction surveys and measures, and standardized performance assessments, assessing both outcome and process objectives, involving the client and client system and colleagues in the evaluation process, protecting the privacy of the client and client system and other professionals, disseminating evaluative data to clients, payers, and other professionals on request and adhering to privacy rights, using external practice evaluators as appropriate and participating in social work research.

## Access to Information and Technology Health

Access to Information and Technology Health Care Social Workers shall have access to Computer Technology and the Internet, as the need to communicate electronically and to seek information on the Web for purposes of education, networking, and resources is essential for efficient and productive practice. Health care professionals, including social workers, communicate, learn, educate, and document using computer technology on a daily basis. Social workers need initial and ongoing training in technology applications relevant to their practice, including clinical care, research, policy, education, resource finding, and administration. Social workers shall continue to follow guidelines for privacy with regard to confidential information of the client, family, or health care providers.

## Standards for Professional Development

Standards for Professional Development, Education, and Leadership Qualifications Health Care Social Workers shall meet the provisions set for practice. A sufficient number of qualified social work personnel shall be on staff to plan, provide, and evaluate social work services. Health care social workers shall have a social work degree from a school accredited by the Council on Social Work Education (CSWE). As a distinct specialty within the social work profession, health care social work requires specialized knowledge as outlined in these Standards. The social worker should receive this knowledge and skill set from involvement or internship in a health care setting, preferably under social work supervision.

Social workers functioning in leadership roles, such as managers or directors, should be licensed at the advanced practice level and able to provide supervision for licensure. Their experience shall show evidence of advanced practice skills and judgment demonstrating progressively more professional competence and supervisory and management skills. Continuing Education Health Care Social Workers shall assume responsibility for their own continued professional development in accordance with the *Standards for Continuing Professional Education* and state requirements. Social workers shall remain knowledgeable about medical diagnoses and advancements, and the psychosocial implications of illness, injury, disability, and treatment. To accomplish this goal, social workers shall continually seek to improve their practice through education and training, and to share this knowledge with other colleagues.

Social workers shall assist in identifying health care and psychosocial topics for professional development by participating in research; by encouraging organizations and institutions to collaborate, advocate, and provide appropriate education for the field; and from clinical practice.

**Supervision**

Supervision a social work leader or supervisor shall be available to supervise health care social work staff on their responsibilities in practice, research, policy, orientation, and education. The purpose of supervision is to enhance the clinical social worker's professional skills and knowledge, to enhance competence in providing quality patient care. Supervision aids in professional growth and development and improves clinical outcomes. Experienced social workers shall offer guidance and consultation to students, interns, and less experienced peers. Consultation and guidance are separate from supervision, and may be offered in mentoring opportunities.

**Leadership**

Leadership Social workers across all health care settings have a responsibility to provide leadership to ensure access to care and to improve and maintain the quality of care provided by an agency or institution. Leadership skills can be demonstrated in teams and groups across health care settings, and include mentoring others within and outside the social work profession. Social work leaders typically demonstrate knowledge, skills, and abilities in the following areas: management/administration, which includes supervision, consultation, negotiation and monitoring specialized knowledge of how to function within care teams in which various disciplines are involved research and education legal, ethical, and professional standards applicable to health social work practice including standards of documentation (paper and computer) and quality improvement activities ability to prioritize needs for social work services and to recommend adjustments to staffing levels accordingly based on current literature and industry standards social work qualifications, productivity, and continuing education policies and regulations that affect social work practice, and patient and family care information on access to health care for the underserved and marginalized populations consultation to social workers and allied health professionals on relative health social work practice issues and development of and adherence to organizational policies, procedures, and regulations by staff.

# 6

# Hospital Social Work

The hospitals, social workers hold primary responsibility for discharge planning and psycho-social care of the patient. In many hospitals social workers have the formidable task of providing both discharge planning and emotional support to patients and families. Those aspects of practice unique to the community hospital setting, therefore are not fully explored. There are minor differences between systems but the "quick and dirty" list of the main functions of clinical social workers in an academic hospital setting looks like this:

Assessing the family's social situation, dynamics, and capacity to cope with the illness, treatment and hospitalization, consulting with multidisciplinary team members about how to interact most effectively with the patient and family system, identifying or diagnosing the psychological, emotional or social barriers that interfere with treatment, positive outcomes, or discharge-planning, clarifying and addressing conflicts that might arise between providers and the patient, advocating for patients and families, providing medical crisis counseling and emotional support to patients and families, counseling around end-of-life, grief and bereavement issues, consulting around suspected child abuse, elder abuse and domestic violence, in pediatrics, social workers may also be involved with divorce, custody and adoption cases, addressing substance abuse issues, performing mental health evaluations and crisis intervention and writing, teaching and research, especially in academic medical centers.

Hospitals are active, noisy places with staff rushing between units, pagers beeping, alarms sounding and visitors coming and going. Social workers are rarely found in quiet offices; instead they spend most of their time with patients, on rounds or in team meetings. There is often a sense of urgency and excitement in the air. In academic medical centers there are also lectures and Grand Rounds on a variety of medical, social and behavioral topics. The environment is stimulating but can also be intimidating. Simply put there is a lot of activity on a number of levels. Patients, staff and the hospital system make numerous demands on the social worker's time and abilities. There is an expectation to work quickly, efficiently and independently. Social workers have to be able to manage these demands as well as the changes that can occur on a weekly or even daily basis. For instance, when organizational and reporting structures within the institution change it can affect the focus or standing of the department as a whole. Individual social workers may experience reassignments and changes in workload. Even the members of the multi-disciplinary team change as doctors rotate through services. Referral patterns and treatment plans also vary between physicians perhaps requiring the social worker to adjust her practice as well.

There is considerable variety in the types of cases seen by hospital social workers as well as in the pace of work. Days are usually unpredictable with no set schedule. Actually, predictable "chaos" may be the order of the day as the social worker "helps patients and families make sense of situations that have placed their lives in crisis and shifted the ordinary to the chaotic". The workload may be manageable until an unexpected situation requires immediate attention and consumes the remainder of the day.

Although no two days are exactly alike, on a typical day a hospital social worker may be involved with a discussion about withdrawing life support, a child abuse assessment, and crisis intervention with a disruptive patient or facilitating a family support group. To succeed in this type of environment the social worker must be extremely flexible with the ability to prioritize work and change focus in an instant. While talking to a patient and his wife about his prolonged and complicated hospitalization, for instance, a nurse from another area might page to ask for help in dealing with an agitated man who is threatening to leave the hospital against medical advice. On a busy day it is not unusual to get two or three pages within minutes, each requesting immediate social work input or presence. The need to continually reprioritize when several cases "heat up" at the same time can be quite stressful. This is not an uncommon scenario and requires the social worker to make quick decisions and handle the pressure of multiple, simultaneous demands. For instance, perhaps a patient whom the social worker has followed for weeks suddenly dies. En route to see the family, the social worker is paged and asked to evaluate another patient who has just told the nurse about an abusive situation at home. The social worker must decide which case has the most critical clinical, staff or regulatory needs and perhaps also recognize when she needs to call on a colleague for help. Social workers who enjoy stimulation and variety are, therefore most likely to flourish in this type of environment. There are times, however, when periods of high volume or high acuity alternate with slow periods. Motivated individuals or "self-starters" who can utilize "down-time" to work on research, outcome studies or other projects are more likely to be able to tolerate this kind of "feast or famine" pace of work.

The amount of time the social worker spends with patients is yet another variable, as is the intensity of the clinical interaction. Some patients need to be seen only once; others daily during an acute or critical phase of care and then less frequently as the crisis subside. Though not unique to the setting, one of the hallmarks of hospital social work practice is the opportunity and the ability to make a difference in one brief encounter. Even a thirty minute interaction can be effective if in that time the social worker can resolve a misunderstanding between the patient and the treatment team, ease anxiety around impending test results or provide comfort and reassurance to a family after life-support has been withdrawn. And while hospital social workers are highly skilled, interventions need not always be dramatic or sophisticated in nature in order to be effective. Sometime the social worker's presence alone is enough to reassure patients and families that the team recognizes their emotional distress. During a particularly tense and volatile situation in an Intensive Care Unit, one colleague describes his role with a very large group of family and friends as "primarily crowd control with compassion."

**Professional Skills**

Hospital-based social workers face unique circumstances during the assessment and treatment phase of their work. They must be comfortable dealing with unknowns, working quickly and adjusting to patient cues. For example, when they enter the patient's room they may encounter someone who is feeling ill or is in pain. Patients may be disoriented, confused or agitated. Perhaps the patient's illness has brought together family members with long-standing conflict and the atmosphere around the patient is silent but tense. As most patients do not self-refer they are sometimes puzzled by the social worker's presence.

If they associate social workers with financial assistance or child protective services they might be suspicious or guarded. In addition the reason for the referral to Social Work is often vague and the amount of psychosocial information available about the patient is likely to be limited. Therefore, the social worker enters a room filled with unknowns. Hospital social workers must be infinitely skilled at quickly assessing all of these variables: the patient's mental status, emotional state, the family dynamics, the patients' needs and the staff's agenda in seeking social work consultation. They must quickly establish rapport and credibility. They need to simultaneously assess, check and re-assess the situation, developing, refining and implementing a treatment plan while "thinking on their feet."

While the patients' needs are always the first and primary focuses of an intervention, hospital social workers are often called upon to address more than one agenda at a time. Tension between "advocacy and collaboration," between "loyalty to the patient and to the organization" is a constant for a hospital social worker. Before going in to see the patient, it helps to have a good sense of what the treatment team hopes to accomplish by calling for the social worker? To manage the complicated task of balancing the often conflicting and competing needs of a patient, a family, a team or a hospital system requires finesse and critical thinking. For instance, when a family refuses to discuss withdrawing support from someone who has no life-sustainable brain activity, the staff can become angry and frustrated, feeling as though they are being forced to provide futile and invasive care. The social worker's job here is three-fold: to assess the psychological, emotional and cultural factors that contribute to the family's behavior, to support the family, and to act as a consultant to the staff. As a consultant the social worker explains the family's fears and concerns while at the same time validating and supporting the staff's feelings. Successful hospital social workers recognize that the staff is also a "client." They understand that by assisting those to deal with stresses related to patient care, they are enhancing their own value to the institution and are more likely to become fully integrated members of the team.

Sometimes health care providers tend to view patients in a vacuum, forgetting that they exist in a world outside of the hospital. The social worker will often remind the team that the strengths and vulnerabilities of the patient's system follow them into the hospital and should be taken into consideration when developing plans for treatment or follow-up care. Hospital social workers, therefore need to have a good understanding of baseline functioning, family systems theories and a high degree of comfort intervening with family systems.

Another aspect of social work practice in the hospital setting is the need to understand the basics of a patient's disease, the course of the illness and the types of treatment offered. Not only should hospital social workers are experts about the psychosocial issues associated with illness but they also need to develop and constantly update a broader knowledge base about the physiology of disease. Psychiatric social workers for example understand the basics of neurochemistry as well as the side-effect profile associated with atypical antipsychotic. A social worker in Cardiology has a working knowledge of ablation therapy and robotic heart surgery and can discuss the differences and similarities between symptoms of angina and panic attacks. Armed with this specialized knowledge and a wide repertoire of assessment and treatment skills including psychiatric evaluations, crisis intervention, medical crisis

Counseling and supportive psychotherapy to name a few, hospital social workers are evolving into "Clinical Specialists: Sophisticated and adaptable practitioners who work flexibly under minimal supervision".

## The Hospital System: Relationships are Key

Hospitals can be notoriously old-fashioned in their organization and even today remain largely patriarchal and male-dominated institutions. In fact, social workers in this setting have long been confronted with complex and changing systems of authority and have been required to interact and report to various disciplines. These disciplines vary in their knowledge of the Social Work profession and often impose their own definitions on the role. Equally frustrating yet unavoidable is the realization that there is a definite pecking order in the hospital and that social workers are rarely at the top of it. This is one of the challenges inherent to the hospital environment and one which must be acknowledged when planning programs or proposing changes in protocols. For example, a social worker hoping to establish a support group on a unit may not be able to do so without first gaining the backing of key nursing staff in the area. Despite the frustration of dealing with hierarchical power structures, social workers who can work within the system instead of against it are more likely to achieve success and satisfaction. In fact, when social workers are not able to consider the politics of the system they are likely to experience anger, frustration and disempowerment. Understanding how things get done, what works and what doesn't gives the social worker a realistic expectation of the system and minimizes frustrations. Equally important to a social worker's success is her ability to recognize the need to cultivate relationships at all levels within the system. In fact, individual relationships between line social work staff and key physicians or nurses or between social work administrators and hospital leadership create the tenor of the relationship between the entire department and the hospital and often determine the status and scope of social work practice within the institution. When the relationship between the social work department and hospital administration is characterized by mutual respect and recognition the institution is generally more supportive of the department's goals, more willing to maintain or add positions and more open to expanding the role of social work in innovative ways. Successful hospital social workers and administrators seize opportunities to demonstrate their value and versatility by taking on difficult situations, be they individual cases or systems issues. Educating themselves about management and speaking up about how they can help the system thrive may also prove empowering and beneficial for individual social workers. In one hospital, Social Work's standing in the institution was further solidified after the department assumed the task of providing psychiatric evaluations for a busy Emergency Department. At another, the department's response to a horrendous fire highlighted the value of social workers to the hospital and community.

Social work leaders may also capitalize on their knowledge of systems and their expertise in developing alliances when participating in hospital-wide initiatives. Contributing to the change process can help enhance status in the organization. Social workers in settings where the department has been decentralized or merged face a huge challenge. They must retain the desire, energy, commitment and vision to be self-directed, strategizing to promote social work values and ideas without the direction of a social work manager. In the face of managing day to day work loads and administrative tasks, social workers without this structure may be unable or unwilling to "sell the profession".

## Personal Skill Set

Unlike other human service agencies where social workers may be the predominate profession in the staff and administrative structure, hospital social workers play a more consultative role, interacting and collaborating with many disciplines every day. Often these other professionals do not fully understand or appreciate what social workers do? They may feel that social work interventions are not critical to patient care or that social workers do not contribute to the "bottom line." In fact, the profession has been criticized for its inability to articulate social work's contributions to the hospital and it must sometimes struggle to establish credibility. And while some teams welcome social work involvement, quickly integrating them into unit activities, social workers may also encounter considerable resistance and perhaps even hostility. In one area where the clinical social work role was introduced, the social worker was told that "Our patients don't have any problems so we don't need you to come by." It takes considerable self-control and stamina to remain relentlessly professional in such an atmosphere. Overcoming such overt resistance requires a combination of relationship skills and good "customer relations" skills. Responding to requests for consultations quickly, volunteering to take the most complex cases, quickly communicating findings and taking a proactive approach to barriers or conflicts can help establish the social worker with the team. Yet even when there is no resistance to the social work presence individuals often need to actively seek out referrals to ensure a steady referral base. Some people find the constant need to "market" themselves, to educate around the role or to demonstrate positive outcomes to be tedious or frustrating. Certainly it takes patience, perseverance and creativity. One new social worker was accepted and acknowledged by her team only after she came into the hospital at 2 a.m. to observe the team surgeon perform a transplant.

Social workers also encounter resistance of another kind when the prevailing medical model of patient care clashes with the profession's model of patient autonomy and self-determination. A common example: the cocaine dependent person admitted with three cocaine-induced myocardial infarctions refuses substance abuse treatment. The team may become angry at the patient and exasperated with the social worker for failing to get the patient "the help he needs." The social worker understands the frustration but must model respect the patient's autonomy while continuing her efforts to encourage behavior change. Some health care providers remain focused on medical needs and are unwilling to address psychosocial issues within the confines of a brief hospitalization. A social worker on a general surgery service might, for example, identify untreated depression in an elderly man who is hospitalized for a hip fracture. The surgeon may ignore the social worker's recommendation for a psychiatric evaluation or medication believing that the patient will "perk up once he gets back home." The social worker is concerned that the patient's apathy and lack of energy will impact negatively on his rehabilitation and is aware that access to mental health care is very limited in the patient's rural home community.

In these instances the social worker must try her best to advocate for the patient by advising the surgeon about the barriers to recovery.

Hospital social workers have had their share of turf battles and power struggles with other professionals who compete with them to provide psychosocial care. This is especially true during times of restructuring. Professional relationships and alliances that have existed for years, like that between nursing and social work for example, may deteriorate as Advanced Practice Nurses, Psychology, Psychiatry, or Case Managers lay claim to functions that have traditionally belonged to social work. In the clinical arena, keeping the focus on what is best for patient care helps to determine which battles should be fought and which delayed or conceded. Social workers need flexibility when resolving turf battles, sometimes stepping back while at other times asserting their need to remain involved. Here again, social workers must master a delicate balancing act–advocating for their profession while avoiding the appearance of being overly aggressive. Although historically many social workers have felt uncomfortable with promoting themselves, there is a critical need, particularly in a "host" institution for them to talk about their role, claim their areas of expertise and highlight their value to the organization. Social work leaders have noted the need for increased visibility within the institution and recommend accomplishing this by assuming leadership positions, participating in decision-making activities and collaborating with other disciplines and administrators.

## Personal Characteristics

Those who make it as hospital social workers usually have developed strong personal and professional boundaries. This is particularly important because the work they do involves a great deal of loss. Social workers have to learn to manage their own emotions in order to be effective or else risk absorbing patients' pain, and becoming depleted by the suffering they see. Without strong professional boundaries social workers can be distracted by often competing agendas of teams, patients, and departments. They can feel pulled in many directions, conflicted or become overly involved with staff transference issues. When they cannot tolerate the tension between loyalty to the patient and to the organization social workers may become paralyzed, loosing the ability to think critically. On the other hand overly rigid boundaries around role definition or schedules for instance can be detrimental. There are cases that will demand that the social worker stay late or come in to work early. Or he or she may provide a service for a patient that may ordinarily be done by someone else. The social worker needs boundaries that are flexible enough to respond appropriately to the needs of the situation.

A good sense of professional self-worth and self-esteem also helps the social worker weather the inevitable turf battles that are part of the hospital landscape A "thick skin" is also a definite asset, making it easier not to personalize issues. As in other clinical settings hospital social workers must be aware of their own unresolved issues and recognize when these interfere with patient care or lead to decreased job satisfaction or problems with staff.

In Rosalie Pockett's article "Staying in Hospital Social Work" (2003) she describes social workers who succeed and enjoy hospital social work as "self-actualized" individuals with high self-esteem, openness to new experiences and a tolerance of ambiguity. "They tend to be reflective practitioners who are willing to examine their own responses to the challenges of the environment. They expect to succeed and are team players, open to learning and to change." This brings to mind another characteristic that contributes to success in the hospital environment and that is the social worker's willingness to utilize clinical supervision. In this interactive process clinicians can discuss difficult cases, identify issues of counter-transference and become more skilled in understanding the impact of the systems issues on their practice.

The Social Workers have a long tradition of working in hospitals and are always striving to improve the service they offer. The following standards can ensure that people receive a high quality service.

**The Aim is to Work with People**

Help people to remain as independent as possible. Ensure that social works are involved at every stage in the planning and delivery of the service we arrange for people.

We may, of course, ask a member of the ward staff to contact a The social worker on people behalf; or people can contact them directly or ask a member of your family or a friend to contact them.

**Hospital Work Plan**

A named contact in social care services, who will be the person responsible for coordinating the care plan a named contact for each service provider. The name and contact number of people, and people next of kin. The exact services people will receive. The times people will receive these services and when the services will be reviewed.

**The Principles**

The social care services and all service providers will follow these principles:

To provide clear information at all times to provide a service which is: reliable, consistent, private and confidential to take into consideration people needs and wishes and the needs of those closely involved with people to ensure that all employees are highly skilled and knowledgeable and to arrange well coordinated care

## Role and Functions

**Psychosocial Assessment:** Bio-psychosocial assessment of the whole person

Advocacy-advocate for patients needs Medical conditions and their impact social supports family relationships Insurance and financial situation Emotional strengths and deficits housing and environment Life condition prior to hospitalization and Initial discharge and continuity of care planning

## Education

Helping patients and families understand the illness Educating families on levels of care for continuity of care i.e. acute, sub-acute, home care treatments: consequences of various treatments/treatment refusal entitlements resources roles of team members educating staff around the psychosocial issues and responses of friends and/or families consultation to providers and advance directives

## Counseling

Crisis intervention initial adjustment to admission exploring emotional/social responses to illness and treatment using strengths and coping mechanisms to adjust and manage illness and treatment understanding of and adjustment to possible role changes problem definition and potential solution diagnosing underlying mental illness and appropriate referrals.

## Communication

Communicate with team assist patients and families in talking to one another and to members of inter-disciplinary team formulating questions interpreting information-separating emotion from fact promoting communication and collaboration among team members assisting team members in recognizing their responses to particular patients and facilitating decision-making

## Discharge Planning and Continuity of Care

Accessing needed services planning for future needs Ensuring communication and understanding among participants equipment as needed assessing resources-funds, paying for medications, durable medical equipment and Follow-up as needed

## Advocacy

Directly representing patients and their rights in health care championing the rights of patients through direct intervention or empowerment

## High Risk Criteria for In-patients

If a patient meets any of the following criteria, they must be assessed by a The Social Worker. 80 years old and over Undomiciled/homeless Impaired mental status Admitted with trauma, secondary to violence such as assault, rape or elder abuse Current drug, alcohol or psychiatric disorder Chronic medical conditions or surgical treatment that will significantly impair functional capacities post-hospitalization admissions from a nursing home, assisted living, adult home, community residence receiving home care services prior to admission Evidence of lack of sufficient care in the community upon admission, i.e. dehydrated, infested, found lying on the floor, etc. inadequate resources to fund post hospital care needs child who has been abused, neglected, or abandoned or suspected victim of abuse or neglect high risk pregnancy/infant failure to thrive, adult or child mothers admitted with no prenatal care mothers aged 18 and younger and Suspected End Stage Renal Disease or HIV/AIDS.

## Discharge from Hospital

Leaving hospital can be a difficult experience, especially if the person leaving is unable to function as they did before. It can be a difficult time for carers too. Health and Social Services staff are responsible for conducting a joint assessment of the needs of patients whilst they are in hospital in order to determine what care and support services they may need after leaving hospital. Where there are difficulties arising from admission to or discharge from hospital, the hospital social work service should be approached for information and advice.

## Short or Long Term Care in a Residential or Nursing Home

On leaving hospital, it may not be practical or safe for some people to return to their own home in the community and they may require care in a residential or nursing home of their choice in the public or private sector. Responsibility for paying for private and Local Authority Care Homes rests with the individual concerned. However some people may be eligible for financial assistance towards the fees and their eligibility can be established following a financial assessment. The social worker will be able to explain the funding system to parents in more detail and provide parents with further information.

Understanding of the psychological aspects of parents has grown rapidly over the past decade. This increased understanding has resulted in the opportunity to offer informed psychological support as an integral part in management of patients. The course and outcome of severe chronic illness are decisively affected by social, psychological and emotional variables. It is important to understand the individual and the family as all face a series of adaptive tasks in relation to the illness. Each of the three phases of the illness, i.e. the diagnostic, chronic and end stage poses special tasks and requires different defenses and coping capacities from the patient, family and health care personnel.

While assessing the patients, techniques of casework illustrated by Florence Hollis (1964) are used. Each individual comes from a different cultural, religious and educational background, which ultimately guides him/ her in taking crucial decisions about the treatment. The family as such contributes an essential ego sustaining function, for it is the intimate give and take of interpersonal interaction. The family more than any other groups provides the individual with affection, understanding, sympathy, sense of worth and identity. In the family, adults are expected to fulfill certain commitments and carry role tasks. The major vital roles of the responsible family members contain the dynamic experiences that shake and shape the family. Many other factors play a key role in tackling illness, such as economic background, education and emotional interaction between family members.

The training of a social worker includes acquiring skills and knowledge of principles of human growth, behavior and personality development, and interpersonal communication. A social worker with postgraduate medical and psychiatric specialization is ideally suited to undertake this responsibility of assessing the patients. Patients feel the need for psychological support that is neither well nor dying.

## Role of the Social Worker in Dealing Patient

Patient shows decreased functional level due to onset of renal disease or other medical complication. Patient finds difficulty in looking after him-self or performs activities of daily living. Patient and family need information. Patient finds difficulty in understanding the treatment due to language barrier. If patient/family is uneducated he/they find difficulty in understanding implications. Patients' cultural or religious beliefs interfere with adherence to treatment. Patient has poor relationship with health care team that impedes adherence to treatment plan. Patient has difficulty in accepting and adjusting to parent that interferes with adherence to treatment plan. patient is experiencing depression and anxiety. Patient has family/marital problems related to parent and it's treatment patient has sexual problems

1. Patient is having pre-existing psychiatric disorder or organic brain disorder. If patients irregular in follow-up patient has financial problem and requires assistance patient not compliant with diet and medications and requires special certificates for medical reimbursements

**I. Out patient clinic**

The social worker focus should be on:

1. Managing patient's pre-dialysis renal health. Managing or delaying the onset of Chronic Renal Failure
2. Preparing patient for initiation of treatment

**II. Indoor / Admission**

Psychosocial stresses/ changes in self-image

1. Loss of sense of well-being
2. Denial reaction towards disease
3. Loss of physical integrity
4. Possibility of death
5. Uncertainty of the future/ defeat of plans and hopes for the future
6. Trying to find doctors / paramedical, other apathies who "promise cures"

7. Loss of independence
8. Sense of being a burden
9. Coping with tests and hospitalization,
10. Coping with anxiety, discomfort associated with treatment
11. Changes in mobility / freedom
12. Changes in employment/income, exhaustion of savings /mounting debts
13. Changes in financial security / lowering and standards
14. Decreased time/energy for family/socializing
15. Problems in sexual functioning
16. Changes in roles/ responsibility in family

**Social Work Services**

The social worker provides services that support and maximize the psychosocial functioning these services are provided to ameliorate social and emotional stresses resulting from the interaction between the physical, social and psychological aspects of chronic disease. To know the details it is important to obtain family social history by psychosocial evaluation

1. Assessment forms, psychological, life satisfaction, Quality of life, etc.
2. Education: Support groups
3. To obtain co-operation of patient and family in medical management
4. Patient and family counseling to enhance recovery
5. Providing help in decision-making process for the treatment options.
6. Co-ordination with multidisciplinary team members, (being a link between doctors, staff, patient and his family members)

7. Planning intervention strategies / Lifestyle changes
8. Fund raising for patient's treatment liaison with charities and NGOS.
9. Rehabilitation
10. Case evaluation
11. Service outcome
12. On going assessment
13. Staff education
14. Research activities

**Self Management**

Recently researchers have found "setting goals" as an integral part of self-management. This is the way to involve patients by assisting them to set goals through the use of patient centered care plans. Helping patients set goals and work towards achieving them empowers them to take control over various aspects of their lives and manage the impact of chronic illness more effectively.

**Social Workers in Chronic Disease Situation**

To do comprehensive psychosocial assessment of chronic disease patients the social worker should provide on-going comprehensive psychosocial assessment to chronic disease patient and their families to improve their quality of life. The completed psychosocial assessment forms to be attached with patients out patient or Indoor files, which indicates appropriate and timely assessment and the details of interventions done by The Social Worker, helps multidisciplinary team to understand the patient behavior and the social worker will interview the patient the same day the patient is referred, will complete the assessment by mutually convenient time. The complete assessment is ready for the multidisciplinary team meetings/or during treatment plan discussions with the specialists, irrespective of outdoor patient or indoor patient status.

The social worker should do clinical assessment with the following aims at first consultation: Problems related to adjustment to diverge and it's treatment problems related to physical activities of daily living, sexual and emotional relationship problems related to employment, educational and vocational rehabilitation and problems related to financial resources, living situation and transportation

The social worker to record the casework activities in the specified record form. The casework activities should be aimed at: Providing personal counseling services to individuals, families and groups on issues like anxiety and fears associated with chronic kidney disease. The social worker to form and maintain therapeutic relationships with patients and their family members sensitivity to religious and cultural diversity advanced assessment and treatment skills; including individual couple and family therapy the social worker to guide patients in treatment planning, decision-making and availability of "quality care"

The social worker to record all intervention strategies used for patients benefit. The intervention should be aimed to achieve following goals: To provide patient information and education. The social worker refers patients to support group. It is enlightening to meet fellow patients and know more about the disease. The social worker gives encouragement to patients to pursue hobbies, and the social worker counsels patient to follow daily exercise regime tore main fit within one's functional limitations. The social worker encourages patients to continue employment as before or helping to plan new opportunities to make a living. The social worker to initiate mediation in conflict situation and the social worker should handle patient's potential problem behaviors. The social worker should do following activities aimed at achieving patient and his/her family's satisfaction: The social worker to record patient's level of functioning. The social worker to assess patient quality of life through psychological tests like mental health status, marital adjustment. Maintaining liaisons with charitable organizations / NGO'S and other philanthropic sources and should raise funds for patient's treatment. The social worker maintains contact and seeks co-operation from various community services and social organizations the social worker should assess and record status of patient's vocational rehabilitation

The social worker to regularly undertake follow-up, for recording of psychological assessment: Based on the assessment necessary changes in patient's current situation and may be made leading to tailoring the intervention strategies.

The social worker should take appropriate action for implementing recommendations and help patients to achieve set plans: Advocacy on patient's behalf within the setting and with appropriate local, state and central governmental agencies for various programs and development of services. The social worker to help the patient achieve set manageable goals and the social worker to assess and enhance adherence to treatment plan

The social worker should conduct a review of pathological condition and Social Work outcome with multidisciplinary team members: The social worker should primarily deal with challenging patients through effective working relationship with multidisciplinary team members. The social worker works closely with the multidisciplinary treatment team in planning for patient care with long term therapy. The social worker regularly participates in team meetings and communicates effectively for the patient benefit initiates and/aspartic pates in patient, family and staff orientation, education, rehabilitation and treatment programs, such as developing educational materials and providing group services for patients and families and in-services programs for staff. Organizing community based programs for prevention of kidney diseases and spreading more and more awareness. To provide education to staff regarding ramifications of the social worker should participate towards advocacy through presentations and Research Work: The social worker should maintain records, statistics as applicable and participate in continuous quality improvement (CQI) activities the social worker to participate in local, national and international scientific meetings and to undertake clinical practice research projects focusing on social work assessment and treatment strategies with patient, families and staff.

# 7

# Clinical Social Work

Clinical social workers represent the largest group of behavioral health practitioners in the nation. They are often the first to diagnose and treat people with mental disorders and various emotional and behavioral disturbances. Clinical social workers are essential to a variety of client-centered settings, including community mental health centers, hospitals, substance use treatment and recovery programs, schools, primary health care centers, child welfare agencies, aging services, employee assistance programs, and private practice settings.

Clinical social work has a primary focus on the mental, emotional, and behavioral well-being of individuals, couples, families, and groups. It centers on a holistic approach to psychotherapy and the client's relationship to his or her environment. Clinical social work views the client's relationship with his or her environment as essential to treatment planning. Clinical social work is broadly based and addresses the needs of individuals, families, couples, and groups affected by life changes and challenges, including mental disorders and other behavioral disturbances. Clinical social workers seek to provide essential services in the environments, communities, and social systems that affect the lives of the people they serve.

### Goals of the Standards

Clinical social workers are committed to the delivery of competent services to individuals, families, couples, and groups. Therefore, they shall recognize the client's role in his or her treatment planning and the client's right to have a knowledgeable, skilled practitioner who is guided by sound ethical practice. This standard for Clinical Social Work is intended to guide clinical social workers in all clinical settings. Specifically, the goals of the standards are to: maintain or improve the quality of services provided by clinical social workers establish professional expectations to assist social workers in monitoring and evaluating their clinical practice provide a framework for clinical social workers to assess responsible, professional behavior and inform consumers, government regulatory bodies, and others about the professional standards for clinical social work practice.

The scope of clinical social work extends across many practice settings and populations. It is anticipated that these standards will reinforce and support current clinical practice in all settings, while affirming the value of clinical social work services as a discrete practice area.

## DEFINITIONS

### Client Patient Consumer

Social workers generally use the term "client" to refer to the individual, group, family, or community that seeks or is provided with professional services. The client is often seen as both the individual and the client system or those in the client's environment. The term "consumer" is also used in settings that view the client as the consumer, that is, one capable of deciding what is best for her or himself and encourages self-advocacy and self-judgment in negotiating the social service and welfare system. The term "patient" is more commonly used by social workers employed in health care settings. The term patient may also be used for insurance reimbursement purposes in health and mental health settings.

## Clinical Social Work

Clinical social work is the professional application of social work theory and methods to the diagnosis, treatment, and prevention of psychosocial dysfunction, disability, or impairment, including emotional, mental, and behavioral disorders.

## Counseling

This is a procedure that is often used in clinical social work and other professions to guide individuals, families, couples, groups, and communities by such activities as delineating alternatives, helping to articulate goals, and providing needed information.

## Person-in-Environment Perspective

This orientation views the client as part of an environmental system. It encompasses reciprocal relationships and other influences between an individual, relevant others, and the physical and social environment.

## Psychodynamic

This word pertains to the cognitive, emotional, and volitional mental processes that consciously and unconsciously motivate an individual's behavior. These processes are the product of the interplay among a person's genetic and biological heritage, the sociocultural milieu, past and current realities, perceptual abilities and distortions, and his or her unique experiences and memories.

## Psychotherapy

Psychotherapy is a specialized, formal interaction between a social worker or other mental health professional and a client either individual, couple, family, or group in which a therapeutic relationship is established to help resolve symptoms of mental disorder, psychosocial stress, relationship problems, and difficulties in coping in the social environment. Types of psychotherapy include, but are not limited to family therapy, group therapy, cognitive–behavioral therapy, psychosocial therapy, and psychodrama.

**Therapy**

This is a systematic process designed to remedy, cure, or abate some disease, disability, or problem. This term is often used by social workers as a synonym for individual psychotherapy, conjoint therapy, couples therapy, psychosocial therapy, or group therapy.

Standards for Clinical Social Work in Social Work Practice the clinical social workers shall adhere to the values and ethics of the social work profession. The social work mission is rooted in six core values: service, social justice, dignity and worth of the person, importance of human relationships, integrity, and competence. All social workers have a responsibility to embrace these values as a service to clients, the profession, self, colleagues, and society. In delivering clinical social work services, the social worker's primary responsibility is to his or her client. Clinical social workers shall acknowledge the right of clients to receive competent psychosocial services and demonstrate a commitment to act on professional judgment and convictions.

Clinical social workers shall be prepared for the challenges that encompass the assessment and treatment of people with mental disorders and behavioral or emotional disturbances. This includes maintaining a commitment to the client while simultaneously demonstrating responsibility to the practice setting, society, and local, state, and federal policies and regulations governing the social worker's clinical practice. In the event that conflicts arise among competing interests, social workers are directed to the *Code of Ethics* as one of the reference points for decision-making. Services should only be provided in a setting in which the professional relationship can be maintained. Clinical social workers should adhere to the *Code of Ethics* with regard to limits on private and/or dual relationships with clients.

The clinical social workers shall demonstrate specialized knowledge and skills for effective clinical interventions with individuals, families, couples, and groups. Drawing on knowledge of systems theory, person-in-environment orientation, psychodynamic theory, interpersonal dynamics, and family systems, clinical social workers shall be familiar with social, psychological, cultural, and health factors that influence the mental, emotional, and behavioral functioning of the client. They shall have knowledge of theories of personality and behavior and be aware of sociocultural and environmental influences, as well as conditions that have an impact on the physical and emotional state of the client.

In addition to the above, clinical social workers shall have the ability to: establish and maintain a relationship of mutual respect, acceptance, and trust gather and interpret social, personal, environmental, and health information evaluate and treat problems within their scope of practice establish achievable treatment goals with the client facilitate cognitive, affective, and behavioral changes consistent with treatment goals evaluate the effectiveness of treatment services provided to the client identify appropriate resources and assessment instruments, as needed advocate for client services and collaborate effectively with other social work or allied professionals, when appropriate.

When additional knowledge and skills are required to address clients' needs, the clinical social worker shall seek appropriate training, supervision, or consultation, or refer the client to a professional with the appropriate expertise. Clinical social workers shall limit the scope of their practice to those clients for whom they have the knowledge, skill, and resources to serve. They shall be accountable for all aspects of their professional judgment, behavior, and decisions.

The social workers shall be knowledgeable about community services and make appropriate referrals, as needed. To ensure that clients receive optimal psychosocial services, it is sometimes beneficial to collaborate or coordinate services with appropriate community programs to strengthen or improve the continuity of care. Clinical social workers shall be knowledgeable about available community resources and advocate on behalf of the client for appropriate services. The clinical social worker shall maintain collaborative contacts with social work or other related professionals and make appropriate referrals, as needed. The clinical social worker shall not share information about the client without the client's informed consent.

The clinical social workers shall be accessible to their clients. Clinical social workers shall be available to provide clinical services to clients during regularly scheduled appointment times or sessions. In addition, the clinical social worker shall develop emergency plans or be available to the client for emergency coverage during vacations, holidays, illnesses, and at other times when the office may be closed. Arrangements or plans and procedures for emergency coverage shall be made in partnership with competent mental health professionals or reputable institutions and should be discussed with the client at the initial face-to-face interview. In addition, the office setting should be accessible and/or have helping devices for persons with disabilities, or office limitations should be discussed prior to scheduling appointments.

The clinical social workers shall maintain adequate safeguards for the private nature of the treatment relationship. Confidentiality is a basic principle of social work intervention. It ensures the client that what is shared with the social worker will remain confidential, unless there is an ethical or legal exception. All information related to or obtained from the client by the clinical social worker shall be viewed as private and confidential. Clinical social workers shall be familiar and comply with local, state, and federal mandates governing privacy and confidentiality.

Information obtained by the social worker from or about the client shall be viewed as private and confidential, unless the client gives informed consent for the social worker to release or discuss the information with another party. There may be other exceptions to confidentiality as required by law or professional ethics. Social workers should be familiar with national, state, and local exceptions to confidentiality, such as mandates to report when the client is a danger to self or others and for reporting child or elder abuse and neglect. The clinical social worker shall advise the client of confidentiality limitations and requirements at the beginning of treatment. Professional judgment in the use of confidential information shall be based on best practice, as well as legal, and ethical considerations.

The clinical social workers shall maintain access to professional supervision and/or consultation. Clinical social workers should ensure that professional social work supervision is available to them in a clinical setting for the first-five years of their professional experience. If clinical social worker supervisors are not available or accessible, case consultation may be obtained from qualified professionals of other related disciplines. Those clinical social workers with more than five years of clinical experience shall use consultation on an as—needed, self-determined basis. Clinical social workers shall adhere to state and government statutes and regulations regarding supervision and consultation in their states of practice. When appropriate, clinical social workers should offer their expertise to individuals, groups, and organizations, as well as offer training and mentoring opportunities to beginning social workers or those making the transition into clinical social work. In addition, experienced clinical social workers who are able should offer supervision to social workers seeking state licensure for clinical social work practice.

The clinical social workers shall maintain professional offices and procedures. Agencies providing clinical social work services and clinical social workers in private or independent practice shall develop and implement written policies that describe their office procedures, such as the client's rights, including the right to privacy and confidentiality; notices and authorizations; procedures for release of information, fee agreements; procedures for payment; cancellation policy; and coverage of services during emergency situations or when the clinical social worker is not available. These policies shall be made available to and reviewed with each client at the beginning of treatment. Clinical social workers should maintain appropriate liability insurance and have a current working knowledge of risk management issues. In addition to the above, the treatment setting shall be properly maintained to ensure a reasonable degree of comfort, privacy, and security for the social worker and the client.

The documentation of services provided to, or on behalf of, the client shall be recorded in the client's file or record of services. Clinical social workers must document all services rendered to clients and keep the records in a secure location, maintaining them as private and confidential records. Documentation must reflect an accurate account of services. Progress notes, reports, and summaries of services shall be regularly recorded in the client's file and be consistent with all applicable local, state, and federal statutory, regulatory, or policy requirements. Records must meet current federal provisions regarding privacy, security, and electronic transactions standards and code sets.

The clinical social workers shall have the right to establish an independent practice. Clinical social workers may establish an independent solo or group practice. When doing so, they shall ensure that all services, including diagnostic and treatment planning, meet professional standards. When clinical social workers employ staff, they, as employers, bear responsibility for the competency of all services provided; maintaining clinical and ethical standards; and upholding all local, state, and federal regulations. To avoid conflicts of interest, clinical social workers who are both employed by agencies and have independent practices shall not refer agency clients to themselves without prior agreement with the agency and consent of the client. In addition, the clinical social worker shall have offered alternative options to the client, such as transferring the client to another treatment provider within the agency or terminating services.

Clinical social workers in private or independent practice may bill third-party payers or their clients for services rendered. Clients shall be provided with all invoices and receipts in a timely manner. When a client can no longer afford services—or a third-party payer or an agency terminates services—an alternative mutually agreed upon with the client may be instituted, which could include, for example, a referral, termination of services, a sliding scale, or pro bono services. If services continue, consideration must be given to any applicable federal or state laws and regulations as well as insurance or managed care contracts that may limit the type of continuing care.

When a client chooses to terminate treatment, the clinical social worker will offer to aid the client in exploring barriers to treatment and re-examine the treatment plan to help the client reach termination constructively. When appropriate, the clinical social worker shall refer the client to another qualified treatment provider.

The clinical social workers shall demonstrate culturally competent service delivery in accordance with the *Standards for Cultural Competence in Social Work Practice*. The increasingly diverse population seeking psychosocial services requires that clinical social workers raise their awareness and appreciation of cultural differences. Clinical social workers shall have, and continue to develop, specialized knowledge and understanding about history, traditions, values, and family systems as they relate to clinical practice with individuals, families, and groups. In addition, clinical social workers need to be knowledgeable about the deleterious effects of racism, sexism, ageism, heterosexism or homophobia, anti-Semitism, ethnocentrism, classism cartelism and disability-based discrimination on clients' behavior, mental and emotional well-being, and course of treatment. Clinical social workers must also recognize racial, ethnic, and cultural differences that may be interpreted as barriers to treatment and develop skills to ameliorate such barriers.

The clinical social workers shall assume personal responsibility for their continued professional development in accordance with the *Standards for Continuing Professional Education* and state requirements. To practice effectively, clinical social workers must remain knowledgeable about emerging theories and interventions, best practice models in the social work profession; Clinical social workers shall seek to enhance their skills and understanding by staying abreast of research to ensure that their practice reflects the most current knowledge. Clinical social workers should also seek continuing education about risk management and professional liability issues. Numerous opportunities in professional development are available through professional organizations or institutions, coalitions, and service agencies at local, state, and national levels. Clinical social workers should regularly participate in and contribute to professional conferences and training activities and contribute to and promote professional publications.

The clinical social workers shall have access to computer technology and the internet, as the need to communicate via e-mail and to seek information on the web for purposes of education, networking, and resources is essential for efficient and productive clinical practice. Clinical social workers are increasingly using the web, computers, and other electronic technology to improve the quality of services for clients, to communicate with other professionals, and for documentation purposes. Clinical social workers should keep abreast of electronic changes that may affect practice. Technology may be integrated into clinical practice; however, appropriate safeguards for client privacy shall be used. Clinical social workers should engage in ongoing training in technology applications relevant to clinical social work practice including assessment and treatment, research, policy, education, and resource tracking and development.

## Hospitalization Risk Assessment

Home health agencies are in a position to respond to patient and health care system needs by implementing strategies targeted to reduce avoidable hospitalizations. Agencies can identify patients who are at higher risk of hospitalization. Clinicians can partner with these patients to implement strategies, which reduce risk. Patients partnering with clinicians can learn to manage their own health. Experience shows that when agencies partner with patients and physicians, acute care hospitalizations can be reduced. Completing a hospitalization risk assessment at targeted intervals is an intervention used to determine the risk level for hospitalization for patients. Specific interventions are implemented for those patients rated as high-risk to reduce the potential of unplanned hospitalizations.

The completion of the hospitalization risk assessment should be part of a comprehensive assessment to identify those patients who are at risk, especially older adults. A dialogue with the patient and family is necessary to determine their wishes, goals and desires to be met by the interdisciplinary team. The team's responsibility is to commit to achieving the patent's state goals.

Risk assessment forms can be paper-based or integrated into point-of-care systems. A structured communication process must be established to ensure that appropriate staff, including those on-call after business hours are aware of which patients have been identified to be at risk for hospitalization. The risk assessment findings serve as the basis for selection of targeted interventions to be included in the patient's care plan to reduce avoidable hospitalizations and emergent care.

It is the responsibility of the medical social worker to assist with the identification of hospitalization risk factors and assist other care provider disciplines in minimizing those risks to facilitate keeping the patient in his/her home environment, when possible. Discussions between the social worker and patient/family should include the patient's goals for remaining in the home and barriers to doing so. The social worker will assist with the determination of appropriate interventions, providing alternative solutions, making appropriate referrals to help reduce the risk of hospitalization and to find the additional care support or most appropriate placement for the patient. Examples of interventions that an agency may implement include:

| | |
|---|---|
| • Patient emergency planning | • Teletriage |
| • Medication management | • Fall prevention |
| • Front-loading visits | • Immunization |
| • Phone monitoring | • Patient self-management |
| • Telemonitoring | • Disease/case management |

Purpose: to assist the medical social worker in becoming more effective and efficient with using hospitalization risk assessment findings or if the home health agency is not using a risk assessment, to learn to recognize high risk factors. Also, to identify the need for selecting and implementing targeted interventions to reduce avoidable hospitalizations.

Review the completed hospitalization risk assessment and identify areas that need medical social worker intervention. Initiate a discussion with patient/caregiver regarding patient's hospitalization risk factors and his/

her goal to remain at home and avoid emergent care and hospitalization. Utilize risk assessment findings to initiate referrals to community resources to help keep patient safely at home. Learn more about your agency's telehealth program (phone monitoring and/or telemonitoring) and become an advocate for use of these interventions with the patient and family, when appropriate. Participate in case conferences for high-risk patients, discussing high risk factors and offering expertise. Evaluate patient/caregiver cognitive status for potential issues that could impact their ability to remain at home safely. Communicate potential issues and possible solutions to staff, managers and physicians and participate in agency education programs, sharing your expertise related to: patient adherence issues, home safety evaluation, the identification of identifying environmental hazards, community resources, cognitive assessments, anxiety/depression, stress reduction, and patient medication resources.

A risk assessment is conducted at admission and resumption of care post hospitalization. If the patient is determined to be at risk, he/she is seen two to three times a week during the first-three weeks front-loading visits. Because telemonitoring is not available due to financial constraints, the staff use a structured telephone assessment form to make frequent targeted follow-up calls to high-risk patients between home visits phone monitoring. Staff indicate that it is not a burden to conduct additional monitoring of patients, and said that sometimes a simple phone call can make a big difference for the patient and their families.

**Consistent staff assignments** are defined as having the same caregivers whether that is a registered nurse, licensed practical nurse, certified nursing assistant or therapist consistently caring for the same patients every time they are on duty. This is an important part of the plan for patients that are identified as high-risk. High-risk patients are "flagged," which indicates the need for a consistent caregiver.

**Extensive staff education** to be initiated and remains ongoing. Written processes and instructions were developed and each member of the team was assigned staff to review and provide feedback on the processes.

**Patient education** including an emergency contact plan to be initiated. The plan identifies concerns for patients such as when to call the home health agency, when to go to the hospital, and symptoms of problems related to the patient diagnosis. Because of the high, recognized use of the hospital emergency room in this community, physicians are willing to call on the home health staff to visit patients who call the physician for care and/or advice. "Although we use many. In addition, the agency continues its work on telephone triage, also known as teletriage. Teletriage occurs when the patient or family calls the agency with a concern or question. Because teletriage is a patient contact for which agencies can be held legally liable, certain documentation must be included in the patient record. The agency documented patient calls in the past, but not always consistently, according to Smith. The agency is now using a telephone triage documentation form to ensure compliance.

# 8

# Genetics and Medical Social Work Practice

Current and emerging advances in the science of genetics provide significant promise for enhanced health and well-being and an opportunity for social workers to make a major contribution. As rapid discoveries in *genetics* the study of single genes and their effects and *genomics* the study of the functions and interaction of all the genes in the genome continue to identify genetic components of common diseases such as diabetes, cancer, heart disease, mental illness, and even behavioral characteristics, virtually everyone will be affected. Knowledge of the genetic make up of oneself or a family member may present significant dilemmas and may lead to a serious consideration of alternative life plans. A genetic test can alert people to advanced detection and management of some disorders, but currently the ability to test for a genetic disorder often exceeds science's ability to prevent or cure genetic disease. The social worker's role in encouraging clients to become their own advocates in bringing genetic issues to the forefront of quality health care is being defined in part by the completion of the Human Genome Project the international effort to map and sequence all the genes in the human body.

A social worker is often the first to provide psychosocial services to individuals and families with genetic disorders. Therefore, it is imperative that social workers become more aware of the ethical, legal and psychosocial implications of a genetic diagnosis, genetic testing and genetic research in order to empower individuals and families to speak out for their rights as public citizens. In addition, the profession must continue to be active in shaping public policy as well as organizational policy as it relates to genetics and service delivery. Without specialized training, it is inappropriate for social workers to assume the role of genetic counselors, but they have important contributions to make within the social work scope of practice. Social workers can take an active part in ensuring that their clients are protected against genetic discrimination in areas such as health and life insurance, employment, and adoption. There are increasing opportunities for professional development of social workers in the field of genetics, and social workers should take the initiative to seek out those resources.

As critical issues are identified in the field of genetics, such as the benefits and risks of gene therapy, stem cell research, reproductive technology, and tissue cloning, social workers need to become more informed and sensitive to related ethical, legal, and psychosocial considerations to be helpful to their clients. It is also important that they become knowledgeable about genetic resources in the community.

The ongoing knowledge explosion in genetics and its positive and challenging sequelae present considerable opportunities for the social work profession. Increasingly social workers will be called on to develop as well as confront emerging policies related to genetic testing and treatment.

## History of Social Workers and Genetics

For more than 40 years, social work as a profession has recognized the importance of genetic disorders in relation to social work practice and education. The efforts to improve social work education in genetics, the social work practice community have worked to clarify the social work role in genetics. The policy statement on Genetics provided a framework all social workers could use to understand ethical and practical issues in genetic testing and research. The social workers in all fields need to understand the ethical and practical issues involved with genetic testing. These include informed consent, confidentiality, self-determination, equal access, and the implications of knowing one's genetic make-up. The *Practice Update* emphasized the importance of social workers assisting individuals and their families in weighing the positive and potentially deleterious aspects of genetic testing and treatment options. The social work profession is a leader in the field of genetics, to support the development of programs, training, and information that provide social workers with current genetic information for use with clients, and to support policies that provide protection for clients from employment and insurance discrimination.

These standards address genetics as an expanding field of knowledge for social workers and emphasize the need for clarification of, understanding of, and education about this specialized area. The standards are designed to enhance social workers' awareness of the skills, knowledge, values, methods, and sensitivity needed to work effectively with clients, families, health care providers, and the community and to increase their understanding of the impact that the field of genetics has, and will have, on them. It is hoped that these standards can lead to the development of clear guidelines, goals, and objectives for expanding current and future areas of social work practice, research, and policy in genetics.

The specific objectives of the standards are to inform social workers about genetics as an expanding field of social work knowledge to improve the quality of social work services provided to clients with genetic disorders to provide a basis for the development of continuing education materials and programs in genetics to ensure that social work services to clients with genetic disorders to advocate for clients' right to self-determination, confidentiality, access to genetic services and nondiscrimination to encourage social workers to participate in the formulation and refinement of public policy at the state and national levels relevant to genetic research, services, and treatment of populations with genetically identified predispositions or conditions.

Social workers can make a significant contribution to the field of genetics by advancing a humane and ethical approach. Among the current ethical issues of relevance to the social work profession are equitable access to genetic services, including testing and treatment and financial coverage for these procedures privacy and confidentiality of individual genetic information, particularly in relation to the insurance industry and employers self-determination, including allowing the client to select or refuse genetic testing and treatment in a noncoercive, unbiased manner; allowing the client to exercise the right to know or to refuse to know genetic information informed consent, including protecting the right of the client to make decisions with regard to genetic testing and research based on a clear understanding of the risks and benefits voluntary genetic testing and treatment appropriate authority for genetic decision-making on behalf of children and impaired adults protection of the rights of those living with genetically determined conditions.

With its historic commitment to serving and empowering populations at risk and promoting human rights and social justice, social work is well suited to address the ethical challenges that arise from new genetic knowledge. The *Code of Ethics* provides a philosophical framework for ethical social work practice and a set of ethical standards intended to define acceptable professional behavior. Cultural competence is highlighted and practitioners are enjoined to provide culturally sensitive services. Although the genetic make up of all individuals across the spectrum of racial and ethnic groups is remarkably similar, the code acknowledges that members of different cultures have unique norms, traditions, and coping strategies that must be understood and respected. The client's right to privacy and confidentiality, self-determination, nondiscrimination, and social justice are clearly articulated in the Code. Genetic services should be interdisciplinary to achieve a holistic approach to client care. In this context, these standards address mutually respectful relationships among colleagues. The code also acknowledges the complexity of ethical dilemmas, which defy simple answers. The code suggests that the resolution of seemingly contrary mandates is best approached through a reasoned, systematic process that incorporates ethical theory and appropriate peer and interdisciplinary consultation and supervision. Social workers shall acquire a basic understanding about genetics as a science and a field of study, including its biological, psychosocial, ethical, and legal aspects. Advances in the scientific understanding of the human genome leads to better comprehension of diseases, both common and rare, and ultimately leads to better diagnosis and treatment. Because of the rapid increase in genetic knowledge and because most social workers do not have a background in genetics, they need to gain a basic understanding of predisposition to common illness and inherited disease patterns. Social workers must continually update their understanding as new knowledge becomes available.

Social workers need to become familiar with general terminology used in human genetics and basic patterns of biological inheritance and with the role of genetic factors in maintaining health and preventing disease. Because many diseases are now understood to involve a combination of causative factors, including but not limited to genetics, social workers need to understand how social behavioral, cultural, economic, and environmental factors interact with biological factors to influence health. It is important to include a relevant medical history in social work assessments in working with families. A family history is crucial in determining a genetic diagnosis and in predicting how various family members might be affected in the future. Social workers, therefore have an important role to play in this area, particularly in knowing when to refer their families to genetic counselors and genetic clinics.

Although new information on genetics has increased our understanding of the etiology of physical and mental illness, prevention and treatment of genetic disorders are very limited. This creates difficult dilemmas for people who are now in a position to decide whether to get tested themselves or to have their children tested. People who are at risk of genetic disorders will have increased options to use the new information to guide their reproductive behavior. However, many of the possibilities for example, prenatal diagnosis, elective termination of abnormal pregnancies, *in utero* treatments, *in-vitro* fertilization, trait selection combined with selective implantation raise serious moral questions.

As the genetic basis of common diseases becomes better known, it is especially important for social workers to become knowledgeable about indications for genetic testing and referral resources for such testing. In cases where genetic testing is available, social workers need to understand the potential benefits and risks of genetic knowledge to individuals, families, and communities. Social workers involved in the adoption process need to be aware of the impact of genetic testing on all parties, and place the best interests of the newborns and children first. Psychosocial reactions to genetic testing, cognitive responses, and coping strategies are important areas of knowledge for social workers, as are family issues.

A genetic test may provide people with information that can inform both their reproductive decisions and health behaviors. Because environment affects genetic expression, a genetic test may also alert people to a need to change their physical and social environments—something social workers are particularly skilled in assisting people to do. Genetic testing has an uneven history in the United States, and social workers need to be familiar with this and have an understanding of how genetic information can be beneficial or misused. Social workers should understand and advocate for legislation that prohibits genetic discrimination and protects against inappropriate disclosure. Social workers working with clients should make efforts to keep current with legislative and legal developments through continuing education and in-service training.

Social workers need to be able to locate genetic resources in their communities and elsewhere. They need adequate understanding of genetic counseling and how it differs from other types of counseling. This knowledge is helpful in explaining to clients what to expect from genetics professionals and what to expect from social workers? They need to know when referrals are needed and how insurance coverage applies to genetic services.

Social workers shall use appropriate practice theories, skills, and interventions that reflect their understanding of genetic factors in their work with individuals, families, groups, and communities. Basic social work skills can be used to provide genetic services to individuals, families, groups, and communities. A professional commitment to continuing education in genetics is necessary for the integration of current and emerging genetic information and technology into appropriate social work settings. The social workers' biopsychosocial perspective is ideal for their role as liaisons between health professionals and clients, client advocates, and providers of psychosocial support services. Social work interventions can facilitate the identification of individuals in need of medical referral or genetic counseling services, and should include initiating referrals. The social worker should serve as an advocate for these clients, assisting individuals and families in adjusting to chronic health conditions, creating and maintaining appropriate self-help groups, resolving bereavement issues, and taking action at the community level regarding genetic privacy and potential discrimination.

More specifically, social workers should develop skills to gather relevant genetic family history information, including a multigenerational family history that includes parents, children, siblings, grandparents, aunts/uncles, cousins identify clients who might benefit from a referral for genetic services properly communicate to clients the purpose of genetic services and the role of various genetic professionals provide culturally sensitive services to clients with or at risk of genetic conditions seek assistance from and refer to appropriate genetics experts and peer support resources explore with clients the possible range of emotional effects they and family members may experience as a result of receiving or refusing genetic information assist clients and their families in the genetic decision-making process, and in adapting to genetic information throughout the life-cycle discuss costs of genetic services and insurance benefits discuss potential risks of discrimination in insurance, employment, adoption, and other areas safeguard privacy and confidentiality of genetic information of clients to the extent possible facilitate the creation and maintenance of support resources for genetic service clients obtain current genetic information from reliable sources, for self, clients, and colleagues educate clients, professionals and the community about policy issues regarding genetics advocate for client-focused public policy in genetics. Assist clients in the understanding of the limitations and benefits of participating in genetics research and the importance of informed consent.

Social workers shall be able to work with their clients with genetic concerns in a partnership that includes mutual respect, shared information, and effective communication. Individuals and families who have genetic concerns and those serving them have a shared commitment to quality services for everyone. Clients have expert knowledge of themselves and their family situations. Social workers should build partnerships with clients who are affected by genetic diagnoses to create new genetic resources, fight genetic discrimination, and ensure that the needs of individuals and families with genetic concerns are met.

Social workers can be helpful to individuals and families in understanding the information they receive about their genetic make up. Clients need to have a role in the collaborative team when choices regarding health care and other genetic services are being considered. Social workers should be aware of the psychological dynamics that individuals and families experience when making genetic decisions. In addition, social workers and their clients with genetic conditions should pool their knowledge, skills, and experience to advocate for needed programs and services.

Social workers shall participate in multidisciplinary teams that deliver comprehensive genetics services. The complexity of genetic conditions requires a holistic approach to intervention. Individuals and families with genetic disorders, or at risk of them, need to receive services from a variety of health professionals working collaboratively to ensure optimal benefit. Multidisciplinary teamwork is central to the new, dynamic science of genetics. More effective services are provided when an interdisciplinary team shares its expertise with individuals and families with genetic disorders.

By virtue of their education and training, social work professionals are well suited to working as part of a multidisciplinary team. Social workers have expertise in identifying and coordinating services and in bridging gaps in professional communication among service providers. A common goal for all disciplines is to provide quality services to the population of affected persons and their families. In particular, all disciplines must be attuned to the emotional and social needs of individuals with genetic conditions. Health care professionals such as social workers, psychiatrists, psychologists, and nurses who provide psychosocial services to individuals and families can include genetic issues in these services. Other health professionals such as audiologists, speech and language pathologists, nutritionists, occupational therapists, physical therapists, and special educators also provide important services to people with genetic disorders. They have much to learn from one another in helping their clients or patients who must cope with these disorders.

Social workers, with a team approach, can establish bridges between clients and health professionals such as genetic counselors, medical geneticists, and primary care physicians. In addition, the support group/professional partnership is essential in empowering individuals and families living with genetic disorders. Social workers shall have and continue to develop an understanding of their own personal, cultural and spiritual values and beliefs pertaining to genetics and genetic therapies. Genetic knowledge and practices may conflict with basic beliefs, not only in clients, but in social workers themselves. To be able to effectively assist clients, social workers must continually examine their own backgrounds and identify their assumptions, values and beliefs related to human reproduction, medical intervention and the value of life with major disabilities. Social workers must recognize the fact that clients come from a wide variety of religious and cultural backgrounds that may differ from those of the social worker.

Becoming a self-aware and self-reflective practitioner involves the examination of one's own bias about groups with views different from one's own. Social workers need to work to develop an understanding of different views, and to avoid judging clients with different values. They also must understand how a practitioner can subtly influence clients with different beliefs through choice of words and nonverbal expressions and reactions and must learn the skills to avoid doing so in their practice. There may be situations in which social workers will find themselves unable to empathize or remain objective. Self-awareness means taking responsibility for identifying such situations and working on one's issues so that they do not interfere with the client's decision-making. In instances where the social worker is unable to accomplish this, referral should be made to a social worker who can be neutral while assisting clients in this highly sensitive work.

Social workers shall have and continue to develop specialized knowledge and understanding about the history, traditions, values, and family systems of client groups as they relate to genetics. Social workers need to possess specialized knowledge regarding the influences of their clients' ethnicity, culture, values, religious and health beliefs, and economic situations to understand their client's use of genetic information and services. In providing clinical services, social workers can obtain the socio-cultural knowledge through exploration with the client, starting with a family history, or health concern. The social worker will need to assess the meaning the client is placing on this concern. This process of cultural exploration is needed to assist in decision-making regarding the pursuit of genetic information and later the results of that decision on the individual, the family, the community and the wider social context.

There are many socio-cultural barriers to genetic services. Social workers should use and promote the use of appropriate language and literacy levels when discussing genetic information with clients and their families. When taking a genetic family history, they should be culturally sensitive and aware of language and underlying emotional content. The social worker should be alert to cultural factors in working with individuals and families regarding their understanding of genetic information and issues in genetic decision-making. As a client advocate, the social worker must address genetic privacy and confidentiality of genetic information with an awareness of possible cultural meaning and social stigma for an individual or a group.

It is observed that social workers may assist in overcoming cultural barriers to genetic services by using and promoting the use of appropriate language and literacy levels when communicating with clients and their families in regard to genetic information being culturally sensitive in obtaining a genetic family history being aware of cultural factors in working with individuals and families regarding the genetic decision-making process and in adapting to genetic information addressing genetic privacy and confidentiality of genetic information with an awareness of possible cultural meaning and social stigma for an individual or a group advocating for cultural competence in service delivery and throughout the health system.

Social workers shall contribute to, support, and be cognizant of the development of research-based and practice-relevant knowledge of the psychosocial, cultural, economic, and ethical implications of genetics on individuals, families and society. Much remains to be learned about how to promote the well-being of individuals, families and society in the context of the genetic revolution. Research is needed on how individuals and families react to learning about their genetic risk status, how they make decisions based on that knowledge, and how society can ensure that genetic information is used for the common good. Research can inform our understanding of how genetic information may differentially affect the diverse cultural and ethnic groups within our society, and how to be culturally sensitive to these differences. The *Code of Ethics* states that social workers should "contribute to the knowledge base" of the profession and "promote and facilitate evaluation and research to contribute to the development of knowledge". Moreover, the Code states that "when generally recognized standards do not exist with respect to an emerging area of practice, social workers should...take responsible steps including appropriate education, research to ensure the competence of their work and to protect clients from harm".

Social work's "person-in-environment" perspective can make a unique contribution to the understanding of the impact of genetic information on our society. Social workers are ideally suited to observe the impact of genetic information on individuals, families, and society; draw preliminary generalizations; and form theories that may be tested in research studies to enhance social work practice. They can initiate surveys among client populations, and document potential problems created by genetic testing, such as discrimination in insurance and employment.

Social work research must be guided by basic ethical and cultural principles, as defined by the *Code of Ethics of the National Association of Social Workers*. Promotion of the well-being of the client is the primary responsibility of the social worker. Informed consent, the equitable selection of subjects, privacy and confidentiality, the right to withdraw from studies, and avoidance of harm are among the standards that are essential for ethical research studies. The consequences of research must be considered, and appropriate institutional review boards consulted in the early stages of project development. Social workers must also keep current with emerging research by other professionals, and should collaborate in multi-disciplinary research with other interested professions, such as medicine, nursing, genetic counseling, psychology, and law.

Social workers shall safeguard the privacy and confidentiality of genetic information of their clients and advocate for and with clients when appropriate to ensure fair social policies and access to quality genetic services. Social workers are keenly aware of the importance of maintaining their clients' privacy with regard to genetic information, as well as the potential for discrimination based on that information and the need for social advocacy and social action to better empower clients and communities.

To protect clients, social workers must be aware that there are limitations to the confidentiality of genetic test information. Insurance companies, employers, the criminal justice system, and other government agencies have enormous financial incentives to gain access to people's genetic information. Federal and state policies may not adequately protect people from the use of genetic tests for purposes of discrimination in underwriting and employment. Of particular concern to social workers is the potential for labeling individuals and withholding services from those with genetic conditions.

The right to confidentiality extends to both the decision whether to be tested and the decision of who is allowed access to the test results. Social workers should inform clients about the possible disclosure of confidential information and the potential consequences before the disclosure is made.

As public policy is developed to define access and funding for genetic services, social workers must be active participants to the process. Social workers should also keep current with federal and state legislation pertaining to genetics and encourage their clients to do the same.

# 9

# Community Health

## Community Health

The term "community health" refers to the health status of a defined group of people, or community, and the actions and conditions that protect and improve the health of the community. Those individuals who make up a community live in a somewhat localized area under the same general regulations, norms, values, and organizations. For example, the health status of the people living in a particular town, and the actions taken to protect and improve the health of these residents, would constitute community health. In the past, most individuals could be identified with a community in either a geographical or an organizational sense. Today, however, with expanding global economies, rapid transportation, and instant communication, communities alone no longer have the resources to control or look after all the needs of their residents or constituents. Thus the term "population health" has emerged. Population health differs from community health only in the scope of people it might address. People who are not organized or have no identity as a group or locality may constitute a population, but not necessarily a community. Women over fifty, adolescents, adults twenty-five to forty-four years of age, seniors living in public housing, prisoners, and blue-collar workers are all examples of populations. As noted in these examples, a population could be a segment of a community, a category of people in several communities of a region, or workers in various industries. The health status of these populations and the actions and conditions needed to protect and improve the health of a population constitute population health.

The actions and conditions that protect and improve community or population health can be organized into three areas: health promotion, health protection, and health services. This breakdown emphasizes the collaborative efforts of various public and private sectors in relation to community health.

Health promotion may be defined as any combination of educational and social efforts designed to help people take greater control of and improve their health. Health protection and health services differ from health promotion in the nature or timing of the actions taken. Health protection and services include the implementing of laws, rules, or policies approved in a community as a result of health promotion or legislation. An example of health protection would be a law to restrict the sale of hand guns, while an example of health services would be a policy offering free flu shots for the elderly by a local health department. Both of these actions could be the result of health promotion efforts.

### Factors that Affect Community and Population Health

There are four categories of factors that affect the health of a community or population. Because these factors will vary in separate communities, the health status of individual communities will be different. The factors that are included in each category, and an example of each factor, are noted here.

1. Physical factors—geography (parasitic diseases), environment (availability of natural resources), community size (overcrowding), and industrial development (pollution).
2. Social and cultural factors—beliefs, traditions, and prejudices (smoking in public places, availability of

ethnic foods, racial disparities), economy (employee health care benefits), politics (government participation), religion (beliefs about medical treatment), social norms (drinking on a college campus), and socioeconomic status (number of people below poverty level).

3. Community organization—available health agencies (local health department, voluntary health agencies), and the ability to organize to problem solve (lobby city council).
4. Individual behavior—personal behavior health-enhancing behaviors like exercising, getting immunized, and recycling wastes;

**Three Tools of Community Health Practice**

Much of the work of community health revolves around three basic tools: epidemiology, community organizing, and health education. Judith Mausner and Shira Kramer have defined epidemiology as the study of the distribution and determinants of diseases and injuries in human populations. Such data are recorded as number of cases or as rates number per 1,000 or 100,000. Epidemiological data are to community health workers as biological measurements are to a physician. Epidemiology has sometimes been referred to as population medicine. Herbert Rubin and Irene Rubin have defined community organizing as bringing people together to combat shared problems and increase their say about decisions that affect their lives. For example, communities may organize to help control violence in a neighborhood. Health education involves health promotion and disease prevention (HP/DP) programming, a process by which a variety of interventions are planned, implemented, and evaluated for the purpose of improving or maintaining the health of a community or population. A smoking cessation program for a company's employees, a stress management class for church members, or a community-wide safety belt campaign are examples of HP/DP programming.

## COMMUNITY AND POPULATION HEALTH THROUGH THE LIFE SPAN

In community health practice, it is common to study populations by age group and by circumstance because of the health problems that are common to each group. These groupings include mothers, infants less than one year old, and children (ages 1–14); adolescents and young adults (ages 15–24); adults (ages 25–64); and older adults or seniors (65 years and older).

Maternal, infant, and child (MIC) health encompasses the health of women of childbearing age from prepregnancy through pregnancy, labor, delivery, and the postpartum period, and the health of a child prior to birth through adolescence. MIC health statistical data are regarded as important indicators of the status of community and population health. Unplanned pregnancies, lack of prenatal care, maternal drug use, low immunization rates, high rates of infectious diseases, and lack of access to health care for this population indicate a poor community health infrastructure. Early intervention with educational programs and preventive medical services for women, infants, and children can enhance health in later years and reduce the necessity to provide more costly medical and/or social assistance later in their life.

Maternal health issues include family planning, early and continuous prenatal care, and abortion. Family planning is defined as the process of determining and achieving a preferred number and spacing of children. Also a part of family planning and MIC is appropriate prenatal care, which includes health education, risk assessment, and medical services that begin before the pregnancy and continue through birth. Prenatal care can reduce the chances of a low-birthweight infant, and the poor health outcomes and costs associated with it. A controversial way of dealing with unintended or unwanted pregnancies is with abortion.

Infant and child health is the result of parent health behavior during pregnancy, prenatal care, and the care provided after birth. Critical concerns of infant and childhood morbidity and mortality include proper immunization, unintentional injuries, and child abuse and neglect.

The health of the adolescent and young adult population sets the stage for the rest of adult life. This is a period during which most people complete their physical growth, marry and start families, begin a career, and enjoy increased freedom and decision-making. It is also a time in life in which many beliefs, attitudes, and behaviors are adopted and consolidated. Health issues that are particularly associated with this population are unintended injuries; use and abuse of alcohol, tobacco, and drugs; and sexual risk taking. There are no easy, simple, or immediate solutions to reducing or eliminating these problems. However, in communities where interventions have been successful, they have been comprehensive and communitywide in scope and sustained over long periods of time.

The adult population represents about half of the world population. The health problems associated with this population can often be traced to the consequences of poor socioeconomic conditions and poor health behavior during earlier years. To assist community health workers, this population has been subdivided into two groups: ages twenty-five to forty-four and ages forty-five to sixty-four. For the younger of these two subgroups, unintentional injuries, HIV human immunodeficiency virus infection, and cancer are the leading causes of death. For the older group, noncommunicable health problems dominate the list of killers, headed by cancer and heart disease, which account for almost two-thirds of all deaths. For most individuals, however, these years of life are the healthiest. The key to community health interventions for this population has been to stress the quality of life gained by good health, rather than merely the added years of life.

The senior population of the India has grown steadily over the years, and will continue to grow well into the twenty-first century. The growth in this population will create new economic, social, and health concerns, especially as the baby boomers reach their senior years. From a community and population health perspective, greater attention will need to be placed on the increased demands for affordable housing, accessible transportation, personal care created by functional limitations, and all segments of health care including adult day care and respite care. Though many communities have suitable interventions in place to deal with the issues of seniors including meal services like congregate meals at senior centers, and Meals-on-Wheels, the demands will increase in all communities.

## HEALTH PROMOTION

The three strategies by which community health practice is carried out are health promotion, health protection, and the provision of health services and other resources.

As noted earlier, health promotion includes educational, social, and environmental supports for individual, organizational, and community action. It seeks to activate local organizations and groups or individuals to make changes in behavior lifestyle, self-care, mutual aid, participation in community or political action or in rules or policies that influence health. Community health promotion lies in the areas in which the spheres of health action.

Two areas in which communities employ health promotion strategies are mental and social health, and recreation and fitness. Though both of these health concerns seem to be problems of individuals, a health concern becomes a community or population health concern when it is amenable to amelioration through the collective actions noted above. Action to deal with these concerns begins with a community assessment, which should identify the factors that influence the health of the subpopulations and the needs of these populations. In the case of mental and social health, the need will surface at the three levels of prevention: primary prevention measures that forestall the onset of illness, secondary prevention measures that lead to an early diagnosis and prompt treatment, and tertiary prevention measures aimed at rehabilitation following significant pathogenesis.

Primary prevention activities for mental and social health could include personal stress management strategies such as exercise and meditation, or school and workplace educational classes to enhance the mental health of students and workers. A secondary prevention strategy could include the staffing of a crisis hot line by local organizations such a health department or mental health center. Tertiary prevention might take the form of the local medical and mental health specialists and health care facilities providing individual and group counseling, or inpatient psychiatric treatment and rehabilitation. All of these prevention strategies can contribute to a communitywide effort to improve the mental and social health of the community or population. During and after the implementation of the strategies, appropriate evaluation will indicate which strategies work and which need to be discontinued or reworked.

As with mental and social health promotion, community recreation and fitness needs should be derived via community assessment. The community or population enhances the quality of life and provides alternatives to the use of drugs and alcohol as leisure pursuits by having organized recreational programs that meet the social, creative, aesthetic, communicative, learning, and physical needs of its members. Such programs can provide a variety of benefits that can contribute to the mental, social, and physical health of the community, and can be provided or supported by schools, workplaces, public and private recreation and fitness organizations, commercial and semipublic recreation, and commercial entertainment. As with all health-promotion programming, appropriate evaluation helps to monitor progress, appropriate implementation of plans, and outcomes achieved.

## HEALTH PROTECTION

Community and population health protection revolve around environmental health and safety. Community health personnel work to identify environmental risks and problems so they can take the necessary actions to protect the community or population. Such protective measures include the control of unintentional and intentional injuries; the control of vectors; the assurance that the air, water, and food are safe to consume; the proper disposal of wastes; and the safety of residential, occupational, and other environments. These protective measures are often the result of educational programs, including self-defense classes; policy development, such as the Safe Drinking Water Act or the Clean Air Act; environmental changes, such as restricting access to dangerous areas; and community planning, as in the case of preparing for natural disasters or upgrading water purification systems.

## HEALTH SERVICES AND OTHER RESOURCES

The organization and deployment of the services and resources necessary to plan, implement, and evaluate community and population health strategies constitutes the third general strategy in community and population health. Today's communities differ from those of the past in several ways. Even though community members are better educated, more mobile, and more independent than in the past, communities are less autonomous and more dependent on those outside the community for support. The organizations that can assist communities and populations are classified into governmental, quasi-governmental, and nongovernmental groups. Such organizations can also be classified by the different levels world, national, state province, and local at which they operate.

Governmental health agencies are funded primarily by tax managed by government officials, and have specific responsibilities that are outlined by the governmental bodies that oversee them. Governmental health agencies include: the World Health Organization (WHO), the Department of Health and Human Services, the various state health departments, and the over three thousand local health departments throughout the country. It is at the local level that direct health services and resources reach people.

Quasi-governmental health organizations have some official responsibilities, but they also operate in part like voluntary health organizations. They may receive some government funding, yet they operate independently of government supervision. An example of such a community health organization is the Red Cross (ARC).

Nongovernmental health agencies are funded primarily by private donations or, in some cases, by membership dues. The thousands of these organizations all have one thing in common:. They arose because there was an unmet need for them. Included in this group are voluntary health agencies; professional health organizations and associations; philanthropic foundations; and service, social, and religious organizations.

Voluntary health organizations are usually founded by one or more concerned citizens who felt that a specific health need was not being met by existing government agencies. Voluntary health agencies share three basic objectives: to raise money from various sources for research, to provide education, and to provide services to afflicted individuals and families.

Professional health organizations and associations are comprised of health professionals. Their mission is to promote high standards of professional practice, thereby improving the health of the community. These organizations are funded primarily by membership dues. Examples include the American Public Health Association, the British Medical Association, the Canadian Nurses Association, and the Society for Public Health Education.

Philanthropic foundations have made significant contributions to community and population health throughout the world. These foundations support community health by funding programs or research on the prevention, control, and treatment of many diseases, and by providing services to deal with other health problems.

Service, social, and religious organizations have also played a part in community and population health by raising money and funding health-related programs. For example, the Lions Clubs has worked to help prevent blindness.

The health services and resources provided through the organizations discussed above are focused at the community level. However, a significant portion of the resources are aimed at personal health care.

## Health Promotion and Education

The scope of health promotion is determined as much by expected health outcomes as by methods and forms. From its purpose to enable people to gain greater control over the determinants of their health, "health promotion" can be defined as "any combination of educational and environmental supports for actions and conditions of living conducive to health". The actions or behaviors in question may be those of individuals, groups, or communities; or of policymakers, employers, teachers, or others in organizations whose actions or practices control or influence the determinants of health. When the determinants are ones over which individuals can exert personal control, this control ideally resides with the individual. But with some aspects of complex lifestyle issues, especially those that affect the health of others e.g., drunk driving, public smoking, the control that people exercise must be through collective decisions and actions. Such strategies are reflected in the social policy targets of health promotion, which may call for aggressive and even coercive measures to regulate the behavior of those individuals, corporations, and government officials whose actions influence the health of others.

Health education aims primarily at learning experiences and the voluntary actions people can take, individually or collectively, for their own health, the health of others, or the common good of the community. Defining health education as "any combination of learning experiences designed to facilitate voluntary actions conducive to health". It emphasizes the importance of multiple determinants of behavior. It also suggests an appropriate matching of determinants with multiple learning experiences or educational interventions. Health education is a systematically planned activity, and can thus be distinguished from incidental learning experiences. Further, this construction of health education draws attention to voluntary behavioral actions taken by an individual, group, or community with the full understanding and acceptance of the purposes of the action—either to achieve an intended health effect or to build capacity for health.

Health education can be seen as enveloped by health promotion, with its aim of complementary social and political actions that can achieve the necessary organizational, economic, and other supports that enable the conversion of individual actions into health enhancements and quality-of-life gains. In essence, the task for health promotion, beyond health education, is how to make more healthful choices easier choices. The commitment to an educational approach to health promotion is part practical necessity, part political expediency, and part philosophical commitment to provide for informed consent and voluntary change before attempting to change social structures and ecologies.

That policy, organizational, economic, regulatory, and environmental interventions are necessary to accomplish the original intent of health education is not to disaffirm health education as the primary means for democratic social and behavioral change. Health education provides the consciousness-raising, concern-arousing, and action-stimulating impetus for the public involvement and commitment to social reform essential to its success in a democracy. Without health education, health promotion would be a manipulative social-engineering enterprise. Health education of the public keeps the social change component of health promotion accountable to the public it serves. Without the policy supports for social change, on the other hand, health education is often powerless to help people reach their health goals, even with effective individual efforts.

The evolution of health policy and programs for health promotion and education has reflected a shared responsibility among institutions, groups, and individuals that have an influence on health. From era to era, the balance of responsibility has swung like a pendulum between a heavy reliance on government and its institutions for environmental and policy change and a heavy reliance on individuals and families to change behaviors. Ideological attempts to shift the responsibility more exclusively from one side to the other have met with a seemingly inexorable cycle of political swings. The reality of program planning and execution is that both sides must be engaged.

Health promotion, encompassing health education, has achieved a shift in the locus of initiatives for health and control over its determinants from medical institutions and health professionals to individuals, families, schools, and worksites. This has occurred in a context of growing community, social, and technological support for shared responsibility for health. Health promotion has expanded rapidly, with notable provisions for institutional supports for employee participation. Schools increasingly emphasize organizational and social factors in programs for the modification or development of diet and the prevention of substance abuse. In many communities, an emphasis is given to concerns about the environment and about housing and other conditions of living that shape lifestyles, health, and quality of life. All of this calls for greater collaboration among sectors, organizations, and individuals.

Achieving an optimum blend of responsibility appropriate to the local context and the health issue of concern requires more participatory and socially responsive strategies than have prevailed in past eras. Responsive strategies call for individuals, families, professionals, private organizations, governments, and local and national agencies to decide case by case how to divide and share responsibility for each health issue. Whatever, the need or objective, participants must assess its urgency, causes, variability, distribution, and the extent to which people want and are able to influence its determinants. Those directly affected should have a voice in negotiating this division of responsibility. Providing opportunities for all voices to be heard derives from the principle of participation central to learning theory and effective community organization. It also affirms a linkage to the philosophical and ethical basis of the professional commitment to supporting voluntary rather than coercive change where possible.

## THE COMMUNITY AND HEALTH PROMOTION

The most appropriate "center of gravity" for health promotion is the community. Community health promotion requires the participation of local leadership and social networks to facilitate the transmission and uptake of interventions for the overall population, as well as environmental changes e.g., legislating or enforcing policies to support individual and organizational interventions to achieve social change. State and national governments can formulate policies, provide guidance, allocate funding, and generate data for health promotion purposes; and individuals can govern their behavior and control the determinants of their own health— up to a point—and they should be allowed to do so. Decisions on priorities and strategies for social change affecting the more complicated lifestyle issues are best made collectively, however, close to the homes and workplaces of those affected. This principle assures the relevance and appropriateness of the programs to the people affected, and it offers the best opportunity for people to be actively engaged in the planning process. It also reflects the evidence that has accumulated on the value of participation in learning and behavior— that people are more committed to initiating and upholding changes they helped to design or adapt to their own purposes and circumstances.

A "community" may be a town or county in sparsely populated areas; or it may be a neighborhood, worksite, or school in more populous metropolitan areas. It can also apply to groups of people not sharing a specific geographic association, but sharing social, cultural, political, or economic interests that link them together. Community represents, ideally, a level of collective decision-making appropriate to the urgency and magnitude of a health-related issue, the cost and complexity of the solutions implied, the local culture and traditions of shared decision-making, and the sensitivity and consequences of the actions required of people after the decision is made.

Ensuring the active participation of the people intended to benefit from a proposed program is an essential principle of health promotion. Community or citizen participation is a social process by which members of particular groups with shared needs in a community setting actively pursue identification of those needs and make decisions and establish mechanisms to meet the needs identified. Small group processes such as meetings, coalitions, and committee structures offer avenues for participation, set into motion by effective community organization or organizational development.

The principle of participation, critical at the local level, is of no less importance at the national and state levels. When policies and priorities set at one level depend on individuals or institutions at another, those responsible for planning health interventions need to make every effort to solicit active participation, input, and endorsement from that second level. Without such collaboration, the cooperation and support needed from the second level may not appear. Participation in this form requires acts of courtesy and respect, the time needed to foster dialogue, and, ultimately, trust.

Failure to engender cooperation is a major over-sight, as it can yield a threat to any proposed program. In contrast, consulting and reconciling differences through consensus decision-making fosters trust and enables collaboration.

## THE ECOLOGICAL APPROACH

Ecological approaches in health promotion view health as a product of the interdependence between the individual and subsystems of the ecosystem e.g., family, community, culture, and the physical and social environment. To promote health, an ecosystem must offer economic and social conditions conducive to health and healthful lifestyles. These environments must also provide information and life skills that enable individuals to engage in healthful behaviors. Finally, healthful options among goods and services must be available. In an ecological context, all such elements are viewed as determinants of health. They also provide support in helping individuals modify their behaviors and reduce their exposure to risk factors.

The ecological view of behavior holds that the functioning of an organism is mediated by behavior-environment interactions. This concept of reciprocal determinism suggests that the environment controls or sets limits on behaviors that occur in it, and that changing environmental variables result in the modification of behaviors. The inference is that health promotion can achieve its best results by way of individuals, groups, and organizations exercising control over their environment. The reciprocal side of this equation, however, holds that the behavior of individuals, groups, and organizations also influences their environments. This leads to the credo that health promotion seeks to enable the empowerment of people by allowing them greater control over the determinants of their health, whether these are behavioral or environmental. In taking greater control themselves, rather than depending on health professionals to exercise the control for them, people should be better able to adjust their behavior to changing environmental conditions, or to adjust their environments to changing behaviors.

Reflecting its accent on the multiple interdependencies of the elements making up a social web, an ecological approach suggests the need for interventions directed at several levels within a community and at multiple sectors of a social system e.g., health, education, welfare, commerce, and transportation. The specification and application of such a sweeping, holistic conceptual framework challenges the capabilities and time of practitioners. The specificity with which ecological guidelines can identify the particular levels and sectors in need of attention is inherently constrained by the infinite variety of interactions that can apply in each idiosyncratic organization, community, or other social system. As the effectiveness of any health promotion strategy depends on its appropriate fit with the people involved, the health issue of concern, and the environment in which it is to be applied, any practical application of the ecological approach must target specific levels and sectors of a complex system. A realistic strategy, therefore is to intervene where one can, with reasonable certainty, match actions with needs and where one can be accountable for unexpected side effects. Careful, systematic planning and practice are essential.

## EMPOWERMENT

Empowerment can exist at four levels: (1) the personal level, by gaining control and influence in daily life and in community participation; (2) the small-group level, through the shared experience, analysis, and influence of small groups on their own efforts; (3) the organizational level, through capacity building by influencing decision-making processes; and (4) the community level, by gaining and utilizing resources and strategies to enhance community control. Empowerment has been defined as "a process by which individuals gain mastery over their own lives and democratic participation in the life of their community". A more detailed definition highlights empowerment as "a social—action process that promotes participation of people, organizations, and communities towards the goals of increased individual and community control, political efficacy, improved quality of community life, and social justice". Participation is central to these definitions, not only as an outcome of empowerment but also as a means by which individuals can organize, assess resources, and plan strategies to achieve collective goals.

Empowerment is a multidimensional construct, implying individual change and change in the social setting itself. True environmental change is distinct from environmental support for behavioral interventions, with structural modification of the environment necessary to support empowerment as an outcome for community interventions. While some individually aimed actions may be sufficiently empowering for some individuals to engage in healthful behavior, others will enter or remain in the "at risk" population because collective action has not been achieved in addressing the broader, social forces that created the problem initially.

Understanding empowerment requires clarifying the counterpoint from which it evolves, widely conceived as a sense of powerlessness. For either individuals or groups, powerlessness accompanies marginalization. Central to powerlessness and marginalization are societal arrangements of power and property, related patterns of production and consumption, and the impact of social experiences as reflected by population patterns of health, disease, and well-being. Powerlessness concerns the expectancy that people, individually or collectively, cannot determine the outcomes that they seek. Health promotion aims to facilitate empowerment by enabling people to take greater control over the behavioral or environmental determinants of health.

It is sometimes helpful to distinguish individual empowerment from community empowerment, but movement away from a position of powerlessness nearly always occurs in the context of community. This interdependence is consistent with conceptions of individual and collective efficacy, whereby increases in self-belief and self-esteem enable people, individually and collectively, to take control of their environment. Low socio-political control, even among those who have high levels of control in other dimensions, may limit the effectiveness of health interventions. Individualistic approaches that do not provide meaningful opportunities to support new habits will yield few changes. The *status quo* of public policy often implies, however, that responsibility for health resides not with government or social structures, but with those individuals or groups suffering particular problems. Thus, health issues can be seen as problems of certain groups, rather than of the systemic determinants of conditions of living. The reality is that both individual and environmental factors must be addressed jointly to facilitate individual and community empowerment together with health and quality-of-life gains.

## PUBLIC HEALTH STRATEGIES FOR HEALTH PROMOTION AND EDUCATION

Programs for health promotion and education apply integrated strategies appropriate to the local context. Most community programs to change health-related behavior are to some degree ecological, that is, they seek to influence the social norms, cultural values, and economic and environmental conditions that affect health behavior at the community level. Such programs usually focus on any combination of the following actions: (1) interventions to promote health and prevent the development of disease primary prevention; (2) screening for early detection and treatment of previously unrecognized cases of disease secondary prevention; and (3) activities to help persons with known or established disease to more successfully manage their disorder tertiary prevention.

There are two alternative, but complementary strategies by which actions directed at the social and behavioral determinants of health are undertaken in the local context. The "community intervention" approach seeks to effect change in the social determinants of health and disease in order to reduce the prevalence of unhealthful behaviors or increase the prevalence of positive health outcomes. The "high-risk," or "intervention-in-a-community," approach aims to identify people at greatest risk for disease, often in a specific community site, and to intervene selectively.

These two approaches compete for policy and fiscal support. They are sometimes combined, however, with the high-risk approach invoked in the service of a community intervention approach. A combination strategy might use interventions such as self-help materials, health education, workplace policy change, and health legislation. Settings for implementation could be practitioner-based as well as community-wide, extending further into the arena of state and national determinants of community health. Methods of intervention delivery could range from health professionals interacting with individuals and groups to centralized planning and the actions of community agencies, consultants, and legislators, as well as mass media initiatives. The scope of programs would vary with the time accorded to achieving change, and with the strength of institutional and political commitment.

Community programs ideally target health-related behaviors not simply as isolated acts under the conscious control of the individual, but as socially conditioned, culturally embedded, and economically impelled forms of living that reflect unconscious behaviors that often have health consequences or risks. Such a complex of related practices and behavioral patterns in a person or group, maintained with a consistency over-time, constitutes a "lifestyle." Lifestyle is a composite expression of the social and cultural circumstances that condition and constrain behavior, as well as the consciously chosen personal behavior of individuals.

## PROS AND CONS OF COMMUNITY INTERVENTIONS

Compelling reasons exist for undertaking community interventions for primary prevention. Only by changing risk factor distributions in the middle of the curve for an entire population—not by focusing on the upper reaches of the risk distribution—can communities expect to see their overall morbidity and mortality reduced significantly. Ecological actions for lifestyle change require the cooperation of various community sectors and people with sway over social policy and norms. Given such cooperation, a community intervention has an advantage over a high-risk intervention as it links education with structural modification of the environment. This increases the likelihood of successful behavioral change and reaches more people with a wider range of risk levels or propensities. As norms change and as supply industries e.g., food stores and restaurants adapt to a new pattern, the maintenance of changes no longer requires a high level of individual effort. A high-risk approach does not offer the potential for normative change, because it targets only a small percentage of the population at risk, and the causes of presenting cases e.g., behavior are not necessarily the causes of incidence in populations e.g., social, political, and economic factors.

There is also an economic and political case for community interventions. This perspective maintains that mass prevention is an "investment" that produces a dividend of reduced morbidity and mortality; produces an informed electorate and a consumer demand through education; and that yields a broader spin-off of secondary benefits for community stakeholders in terms of costs averted, quality of life, and productivity. An informed electorate spurs political change, and consumer demand achieves commercial advantages. A reduced burden on medical care systems, and a reduction of costs associated with absenteeism and reduced productivity and achievement, benefits a wider range of stakeholders. Community interventions have greater potential than high-risk approaches to achieve these political and economic benefits. The mainstreaming, rather than marginalization, of health problems e.g., substance abuse gives them greater political support and the programs greater momentum.

The drawbacks of community interventions in primary prevention are the greater complexity and duration of programs and policies addressing lifestyle and health-related behaviors and conditions of living. It can be difficult to activate a community sufficiently to enable individual and collective change through the development and implementation of broad and meaningful intervention strategies. Inadequate implementation and low levels of penetration explain the limited success of many community interventions. Underlying these explanations are specific causes, including: (1) the appropriateness of the theoretical foundation on which a program is based; (2) the level to which theory is integrated with local logic and cultural concepts of health and disease; (3) the extent to which a community is truly active in planning and implementing interventions; and (4) whether interventions vary across several different levels of implementation e.g., individual, small group, organizational, and community. Also important is the continuation of a program: Too few programs allow for a sufficient duration of exposure to achieve sustainable changes and outcomes.

Allowing for diffusion and utilization of interventions to shift risk factor distributions for entire communities requires more time than for projects targeting change only in high-risk groups. On the other hand, high-risk groups often require greater levels of exposure than the community in general, as more intensive and sustained outreach strategies are required to reach the last cohorts in the diffusion of knowledge and risk-reduction practices. In either case, the potential for realizing benefits depends on time for interventions to become established and achieve momentum, and program implementation should continue over the duration of a social intervention. Time is required to integrate program components, to achieve synergy among components, and to increase the potential for diffusion throughout the community. Time is also needed for feedback on the comprehensiveness of information diffusion channels in order to ensure that a knowledge—behavior gap is not created or exacerbated among subgroups in a community. This requires intensity of effort combined with appropriate adaptation at all phases of the program process—which, in turn, requires iterative appraisal of the processes of intervention delivery.

Given the cost and effort involved, community interventions have been criticized on the basis of perceived inefficiency or lesser effectiveness, relative to the high-risk approach and its greater efficacy by selective high-risk screening and intervention. Fueling this criticism is the reality that most communitywide efforts have yielded only modest gains attributable to the program, while the high-risk approach achieves more palpable benefits of prevention at the level of the individual. Weak motivation based on health rewards, however, is often replaced in community interventions with stronger motivators for individuals of the social rewards of enhanced self-esteem and social approval. Furthermore, for diseases with multiple determinants, the community intervention approach could be highly robust. If communities can realize a normative effect in reducing disease risk factors, the cost-effectiveness and efficiency greater reach of community interventions could surpass the greater efficacy of the high-risk approach for prevention. For instance, interventions targeting healthful behaviors and the reduction of environmental risks for chronic disease are likely to reduce morbidity and mortality from other diseases also influenced by the same lifestyle and environmental conditions.

In their capacity to shift norms, the evidence thus far suggests that some community interventions have, in their application, compromised what programs need in order to work in specific communities. A main pitfall of appropriate adaptation stems from the insistence of various advocates of community-based models that practitioners must distance themselves from anything that is not communitywide. Some of the theoretical and definitional literature on community strategies has implied or insisted that "community-based" must be synonymous with "communitywide." This leads to shunning the inclusion of prevention activities based in organizations or institutions. While it is expressed sometimes as a mere preference for mass media and centralized planning approaches to community programs, in its extreme forms it takes on an avoidance, if not hostility, to programs or activities that serve people at the one-to-one level, those that deal with high risk groups, and those that treat disease rather than restricting their focus to people who are well and who seek primary prevention measures.

Life is not so dichotomous for individuals who must anticipate a life course of progression in risk factors, in presymptomatic disease, and in diagnosed chronic disease. Nor are the individuals living at these various stages of progression living in isolation from each other. The organizations and institutions in which people at various stages on the spectrum of health and disease are living, working, and playing share mutual dependencies on each other. These considerations make a more comprehensive, spectrum-inclusive approach to health promotion and disease prevention, detection, control, and management more sensible and efficient.

The expectation that social norms will respond over the short term to intensive media and policy initiatives at the community level is overly ambitious. Most social norms are institution—bound as much as they are the product of broader mass media messages and images. Without the inward involvement of institutions and organizations in changing their own norms rather than just outwardly cooperating in community-wide efforts, the occupants employees, students, residents, customers of those institutions will continue to follow norms dictated by their organizational surrounding.

# 10

# Community Health Workers

The term "community health" refers to the health status of a defined group of people, or community, and the actions and conditions that protect and improve the health of the community. Those individuals who make up a community live in a somewhat localized area under the same general regulations, norms, values, and organizations. For example, the health status of the people living in a particular town, and the actions taken to protect and improve the health of these residents, would constitute community health. In the past, most individuals could be identified with a community in either a geographical or an organizational sense. Today, however with expanding global economies, rapid transportation, and instant communication, communities alone no longer have the resources to control or look after all the needs of their residents or constituents. Thus the term "population health" has emerged. Population health differs from community health only in the scope of people it might address. People who are not organized or have no identity as a group or locality may constitute a population, but not necessarily a community. Women over fifty, adolescents, adults twenty-five to forty-four years of age, seniors living in public housing, prisoners, and blue-collar workers are all examples of populations. As noted in these examples, a population could be a segment of a community, a category of people in several communities of a region, or workers in various industries. The health status of these populations and the actions and conditions needed to protect and improve the health of a population constitute population health.

The actions and conditions that protect and improve community or population health can be organized into three areas: health promotion, health protection, and health services. This breakdown emphasizes the collaborative efforts of various public and private sectors in relation to community health. It shows the interaction of the various public and private sectors that constitute the practice of community health.

Health promotion may be defined as any combination of educational and social efforts designed to help people take greater control of and improve their health. Health protection and health services differ from health promotion in the nature or timing of the actions taken. Health protection and services include the implementing of laws, rules, or policies approved in a community as a result of health promotion or legislation. An example of health protection would be a law to restrict the sale of hand guns, while an example of health services would be a policy offering free flu shots for the elderly by a local health department. Both of these actions could be the result of health promotion efforts such as a letter writing campaign or members of a community lobbying their board of health.

## Factors that Affect Community and Population Health

There are four categories of factors that affect the health of a community or population. Because these factors will vary in separate communities, the health status of individual communities will be different. The factors that are included in each category, and an example of each factor, are noted here.

1. Physical factors—geography (parasitic diseases), environment (availability of natural resources), community size (overcrowding), and industrial development (pollution).

2. Social and cultural factors—beliefs, traditions, and prejudices (smoking in public places, availability of ethnic foods, racial disparities), economy (employee health care benefits), politics (government participation), religion (beliefs about medical treatment), social norms (drinking on a college campus), and socioeconomic status (number of people below poverty level).
3. Community organization—available health agencies (local health department, voluntary health agencies), and the ability to organize to problem solve (lobby city council).
4. Individual behavior—personal behavior (health-enhancing behaviors like exercising, getting immunized, and recycling wastes; see.

## Three Tools of Community Health Practice

Much of the work of community health revolves around three basic tools: epidemiology, community organizing, and health education. Though each of these is discussed in greater length elsewhere in the encyclopedia, they are mentioned here to emphasize their importance to community and population practice. Judith Mausner and Shira Kramer have defined *epidemiology* as the study of the distribution and determinants of diseases and injuries in human populations. Such data are recorded as number of cases or as rates (number per 1,000 or 100,000). Epidemiological data are to community health workers as biological measurements are to a physician. Epidemiology has sometimes been referred to as population medicine. Herbert Rubin and Irene Rubin have defined *community organizing* as bringing people together to combat shared problems and increase their say about decisions that affect their lives. For example, communities may organize to help control violence in a neighborhood. *Health education* involves health promotion and disease prevention (HP/DP) programming, a process by which a variety of interventions are planned, implemented, and evaluated for the purpose of improving or maintaining the health of a community or population. A smoking cessation program for a company's employees, a stress management class for church members, or a community-wide safety belt campaign are examples of HP/DP programming.

## COMMUNITY AND POPULATION HEALTH THROUGH THE LIFE SPAN

In community health practice, it is common to study populations by age group and by circumstance because of the health problems that are common to each group. These groupings include mothers, infants (less than one year old), and children (ages 1–14); adolescents and young adults (ages 15–24); adults (ages 25–64); and older adults or seniors (65 years and older).

Maternal, infant, and child (MIC) health encompasses the health of women of childbearing age from prepregnancy through pregnancy, labor, delivery, and the postpartum period, and the health of a child prior to birth through adolescence. Maternal, infant, and child health statistical data are regarded as important indicators of the status of community and population health. Unplanned pregnancies, lack of prenatal care, maternal drug use, low immunization rates, high rates of infectious diseases, and lack of access to health care for this population indicate a poor community health infrastructure. Early intervention with educational programs and preventive medical services for women, infants, and children can enhance health in later years and reduce the necessity to provide more costly medical and/or social assistance later in their life.

Maternal health issues include family planning, early and continuous prenatal care, and abortion. Family planning is defined as the process of determining and achieving a preferred number and spacing of children. Infant and child health is the result of parent health behavior during pregnancy, prenatal care, and the care provided after birth. Critical concerns of infant and childhood morbidity and mortality include proper immunization, unintentional injuries, and child abuse and neglect.

The health of the adolescent and young adult population sets the stage for the rest of adult life. This is a period during which most people complete their physical growth, marry and start families, begin a career, and enjoy increased freedom and decision-making. It is also a time in life in which many beliefs, attitudes, and behaviors are adopted and consolidated. Health issues that are particularly associated with this population are unintended injuries; use and abuse of alcohol, tobacco, and drugs; and sexual risk taking. There are no easy, simple, or immediate solutions to reducing or eliminating these problems. However, in communities where interventions have been successful, they have been comprehensive and communitywide in scope and sustained over long periods of time.

The adult population represents about half of the population. The health problems associated with this population can often be traced to the consequences of poor socioeconomic conditions and poor health behavior during earlier years. To assist community health workers, this population has been subdivided into two groups: ages twenty-five to forty-four and ages forty-five to sixty-four. For the younger of these two subgroups, unintentional injuries, HIV (human immunodeficiency virus) infection, and cancer are the leading causes of death. For the older group, noncommunicable health problems dominate the list of killers, headed by cancer and heart disease, which account for almost two-thirds of all deaths. For most individuals, however, these years of life are the healthiest. The key to community health interventions for this population has been to stress the quality of life gained by good health, rather than merely the added years of life.

## HEALTH PROMOTION

The three strategies by which community health practice is carried out are health promotion, health protection, and the provision of health services and other resources. It presents a representation of these strategies, their processes, their objectives, and anticipated benefits for a community or population.

As noted earlier, health promotion includes educational, social, and environmental supports for individual, organizational, and community action. It seeks to activate local organizations and groups or individuals to make changes in behavior (lifestyle, selfcare, mutual aid, participation in community or political action) or in rules or policies that influence health. Community health promotion lies in the areas in which the spheres of health action, as shown in, overlap.

Two areas in which communities employ health promotion strategies are mental and social health, and recreation and fitness. Though both of these health concerns seem to be problems of individuals, a health concern becomes a community or population health concern when it is amenable to amelioration through the collective actions noted above. Action to deal with these concerns begins with a community assessment, which should identify the factors that influence the health of the subpopulations and the needs of these populations. In the case of mental and social health, the need will surface at the three levels of prevention: *primary prevention* (measures that forestall the onset of illness), *secondary prevention* (measures that lead to an early diagnosis and prompt treatment), and *tertiary prevention* (measures aimed at rehabilitation following significant pathogenesis).

Primary prevention activities for mental and social health could include personal stress management strategies such as exercise and meditation, or school and workplace educational classes to enhance the mental health of students and workers. A secondary prevention strategy could include the staffing of a crisis hot line by local organizations such a health department or mental health center. Tertiary prevention might take the form of the local medical and mental health specialists and health care facilities providing individual and group counseling, or inpatient psychiatric treatment and rehabilitation. All of these prevention strategies can contribute to a communitywide effort to improve the mental and social health of the community or population. During and after the implementation of the strategies, appropriate evaluation will indicate which strategies work and which need to be discontinued or reworked.

As with mental and social health promotion, community recreation and fitness needs should be derived via community assessment. The community or population enhances the quality of life and provides alternatives to the use of drugs and alcohol as leisure pursuits by having organized recreational programs that meet the social, creative, aesthetic, communicative, learning, and physical needs of its members. Such programs can provide a variety of benefits that can contribute to the mental, social, and physical health of the community, and can be provided or supported by schools, workplaces, public and private recreation and fitness organizations, commercial and semipublic recreation, and commercial entertainment. As with all health-promotion programming, appropriate evaluation helps to monitor progress, appropriate implementation of plans, and outcomes achieved.

## HEALTH PROTECTION

Community and population health protection revolve around environmental health and safety. Community health personnel work to identify environmental risks and problems so they can take the necessary actions to protect the community or population. Such protective measures include the control of unintentional and intentional injuries; the control of vectors; the assurance that the air, water, and food are safe to consume; the proper disposal of wastes; and the safety of residential, occupational, and other environments. These protective measures are often the result of educational programs, including self-defense classes; policy development, such as the Safe Drinking Water Act or the Clean Air Act; environmental changes, such as restricting access to dangerous areas; and community planning, as in the case of preparing for natural disasters or upgrading water purification systems.

## HEALTH SERVICES AND OTHER RESOURCES

The organization and deployment of the services and resources necessary to plan, implement, and evaluate community and population health strategies constitutes the third general strategy in community and population health. Today's communities differ from those of the past in several ways. Even though community members are better educated, more mobile, and more independent than in the past, communities are less autonomous and more dependent on those outside the community for support. The organizations that can assist communities and populations are classified into governmental, quasi-governmental, and nongovernmental groups. Such organizations can also be classified by the different levels (world, national, state/ province, and local) at which they operate.

**Community Mental Health Services** (CMHS) support or treat people with mental disorders (mental illness or mental health difficulties) in a domiciliary setting, rather than being admitted to a psychiatric hospital (asylum). Community services include supported housing with full or partial supervision (including halfway houses), psychiatric wards of general hospitals (including partial hospitalization), local primary care medical services, day centers or clubhouses and self-help groups for mental health. They may be provided by government organizations and mental health professionals, including specialized teams providing services across a geographical area, such as assertive community treatment and early psychosis teams. They may also be provided by private or charitable organizations. They may be based on peer support and the consumer/survivor movement.

The World Health Organization states that community mental health services are more accessible and effective, lessen social exclusion, and are likely to have less possibilities for the neglect and violations of human rights that were often encountered in mental hospitals. However, WHO notes that in many countries, the closing of mental hospitals has not been accompanied by the development of community services, leaving a service vacuum with far too many not receiving any care.

New legal powers have developed in some countries, such as the United States, to supervise and ensure compliance with treatment of individuals living in the community, known as outpatient commitment or assisted outpatient treatment or community treatment orders.

## History

The 19th to mid-20th century saw a large expansion of the number and size of asylums in Western countries. Originally based on principles of moral treatment, they were often situated in rural areas or on the outskirts of cities. Following human rights and financial concerns, a deinstitutionalization movement led to the closing down of many asylums. Community services known in the UK as Care in the Community were meant to take their place, but were often were poorly funded, uncoordinated and unable to meet complex needs. Homelessness and prison were the result for many. Expectations that community care would lead to fuller social integration were not achieved, with many remaining without employment, having limited social contacts and often living in sheltered environments that still lead to institutionalization. Services in the community sometimes provided a new ghetto, where service users meet each other but have little contact with the rest of the community. It has been said that instead of "community psychiatry", reforms established a "psychiatric community".

In recent years, many countries have expanded their health systems by training community health workers (CHWs) on a large scale. These community health workers are either paid or voluntary workers. They are part of government or national programs, and differ from community health workers trained in small scale, often non-government projects influenced by charismatic leaders and funded externally. The success of small, well-managed projects is evident in the literature and there is ample evidence that community health workers in small scale well managed projects can be effective.

Hówever, it is much less clear about the large scale national CHW programs being effective and making a difference in peoples' lives. Voices have been raised questioning, among other things, meeting people's needs, the quality of their work, the amount of work they do, attrition rates, the precedence curative or facility work takes over preventive or community work, etc.

What is the evidence of community health workers in South Asia? There is no documentation yet at the regional level on this specific matter. In this backdrop, we looks at national, large scale programs in five countries, viz., Bangladesh, Bhutan, India, Nepal and Sri Lanka and reviews the existing policies, practices and lessons learned within the overall context of primary health care in these countries, hoping that it will help the community health practitioners, program managers or policymakers of the countries region to adapt, replicate and/or scale up the best evidences and learn from the mistakes.

## Community Health Workers Definitions

Since the role of the community health worker was re-emphasized during the Alma Àta Conference in 1978, there have been several variations and definitions of this term. Globally, they are called by a variety of names including Health Auxiliaries, Barefoot Doctors, Health Agents, Health Promoters, Family Welfare Educators, Health Volunteers, Village Health Workers, Community Health Aides, Community Health Volunteers and Community Health Workers. With the varying demands and differing levels of health within countries, regions, districts, and villages, each community has its own version of the community health worker.

According to WHO, " Community health workers are men and women chosen by the community, and trained to deal with the health problems of individuals and the community, and to work in close relationship with the health services. They should have had a level of primary education that enables to read, write and do simple mathematical calculations". Witmer *et al* (1995) define community health workers as community members who work almost exclusively in community settings and who serve as connectors between health care consumer's and providers to promote health among groups that have traditionally lacked access to adequate care. By identifying community problems, developing innovative solutions, and translating them into practice, community health workers can respond creatively to local needs.

Walt (1989) provides the following definition of community health workers: ...generally local inhabitants given a limited amount of training to provide specific basic health and nutrition services to the mothers of their surrounding communities. They are expected to remain in their home village or neighborhood and usually only work part-time as health workers. They may be volunteers or receive a salary. They are generally not, however, civil servants or professional employees of Ministry of Health.

## Alternative Titles for Community Health Workers

| | |
|---|---|
| Shasthyo Sebikas | Bangladesh |
| Village Health Worker | Bhutan |
| Village Health Guide | India |
| Female Community Health Volunteer | Nepal |
| Community Health Worker | Sri Lanka |

In addition to the various definitions that are applied to the CHW, there are also many different titles that are used.

## Country Experiences

A review of the published literature on CHW reveals that there is a large body of papers and reports describing many small scale locally initiated projects by NGOs, specifically designed field experiments and official pilot projects. In these reports one can find many variations on CHW selection, training, incentives, management, etc. In contrast, there are very few papers and reports available documenting large scale national programs. While scientific studies of impact are rarer, there are evidences that suggest dramatic improvements can be achieved with well-designed and run community-based health volunteer programs.

## Bangladesh

In Bangladesh, the government has provided a few essential services and encouraged NGOs to work with communities through a large array of approaches to provide responsive health and development initiatives. Hence, there is not one standard model of community health program forced by government but rather a proliferation of efforts by nongovernmental organizations, most with a firm base in the community. The experiences of NGOs range from national house to house education efforts by BRAC, one of the largest national nongovernmental organizations in Bangladesh, with their unsalaried community health workers called Shastho Shebikas, teaching every woman how to prepare oral rehydration solution to treat diarrhea to the efforts of World Vision/Bangladesh with community partners; experience of the Local Initiatives Program and the Jiggasha approach with community collaborators or, ICDDR/B to empower the communities to take full control of their health with the help of community health workers. The BRAC health program addresses the health and nutritional status of women and children in Bangladesh and covers 35 million people with approximately 25,140 Shastho Shebikas (SSs). The concept of SS was first introduced in 1977 through a small scale integrated health development program in five sub-districts. Subsequently the approach was found to be successful and expanded into another 21 sub-districts in 1992 and then to 330 sub-districts by 1999. As the BRAC experience with SS at national scale provides compelling evidence that local-level community health workers can effectively provide health services to the entire local population, this paper primarily highlights on BRAC's experiences with the SS.

## Selection of Shastho Shebikas

The SSs are members of the BRAC village organizations, that consist of women from the poorest communities and which are aimed at improving their socioeconomic conditions. In the beginning of the program, five women form a group and about ten such groups constitute a village organization in each community. These village organization members suggest names of prospective SS during the village organization meetings. Based on these recommendations, the final selection of SS is done at BRAC's regional office. Selection of SS is based on the following criterion: female, socially acceptable, age 25 to 35 years, married, youngest child's age above five years, eager to do work, preferably educated, not living near a local health care facility or big bazaar. They are not paid a salary but they retain a small profit from the sale of drugs prescribed for common illnesses.

## Role of Shastho Shebikas

The breadth of the health activities of SS in community based health care is quite extensive, especially considering that SS are illiterate or, at best semi-literate and unsalaried. The SSs give health education, motivation, and mobilization regarding the five components of Essential Health Care Program which consists of water and sanitation, immunization, health and nutrition education, family planning and basic curative services. Each SS facilitates 150-300 households for their health care needs and also to link them up with BRAC's multidimensional development interventions. They sell medicine, contraceptives, sanitary latrines, tubewells, and vegetable seeds. They diagnose, treat, and provide health education on diarrhea, dysentery, fever, common cold, anemia, worm infection, gastric ulcer, allergic reaction, scabies, and ringworm infection.

The SSs go on follow-up visits in the afternoons and encourage pregnant women to utilize government facilities. Furthermore, the SSs are involved in attending their daily household chores, village organizations related income-generating activities, establishing liaison with government health workers, and preparing and submitting monthly progress reports. Total monthly working days for each SS are 15.

## Training

The SSs are given foundation or basic training on essential health care, which lasts for 21 days, at 4 days per week at the regional office. Then refresher training is given for one day every month for two years.

## Incentives/motivation

According to Khan *et al* (1998), there are various motivational factors for becoming a SS e.g. to do some work for children, to earn a profitable income, to have access to medicine, to make people aware about contraception and immunization, to learn about health and hygiene of her own children and neighbors. Additionally, the SSs think that if she or anyone in the village became ill there would be an advantage in knowing all this health information and to earn name and fame if she gave treatments for such illnesses. For making the SS economically self-dependent, BRAC supplied credit to the SS so that they could undertake small income-generating activities such as poultry raising.

## Monitoring/follow Up

BRAC's program organizers (POs) provide supportive supervision and technical advice to SSs. Each PO supervises 25-30 SSs and visits each SS two to three times per month. The PO also visits 25% households served by SS as part of routine monitoring.

## Replication/Scaling Up

Lovell *et al* (1993) note that BRAC has been able to scale-up its health programs (e.g. nation-wide, single purpose oral rehydration teaching program reaching 13 million households, Child Survival Program assisting government in immunization covering a third of a the country) through replication of best practices. After the development stage at one place (i.e. at Sulla), where the idea was tested, changed, retested and tried again, it was replicated later in many other areas. A strong monitoring and evaluation program made it possible to identify weaknesses that could be corrected before scaling up to the next level.

Analysis of BRAC's experience suggests that several factors are essential for successful scaling-up. Primarily, they are related to qualified, experienced and dedicated human resources to support the program; effective management systems (including monitoring and evaluation systems) and capabilities in the organization; learning environment (generating ideas from interaction with the field and encouraging learning in and between all levels of the organization) and adequate financial support.

## Sustainability

Khan *et al* (1998) reported that the drop out rate for SS ranged from 31 percent to 44 percent. Some dropped out after only a few months and there were others who did so after a few years of service. There were multiple reasons for discontinuing the work: lack of time due to more time spent looking after little children and doing household chores, not much profit earned from selling medicine, more profit earned from other activities, too much effort spent for too little profit, could not find enough customers to sell medicine to, target set by office too high to be achieved, unwillingness to do this work without a salary, people buying medicine on credit purchase basis, people reluctant to buy medicine because of their perception that BRAC got the medicine free, availability of cheaper medicine at the local bazaar, preference for buying medicine from local shops, family members disliked the work, socially unacceptable for a woman to do this work, etc.

BRAC has learned that progress cannot be made on health issues without the full involvement and leadership of women. It has also proved that, once empowered, the poorest illiterate women can become leaders in health improvements. By developing strong, better educated and empowered village groups, capable of utilizing and making demands on government health services, a higher quality of preventive health measures will be practiced in the community (Lovell *et al*, 1993)

## Constraints

The major challenge is that could the BRAC model be adopted by the government at national level. As successful implementation of the voluntary program needs intensive monitoring and supervision, would it be easy for the government to institutionalize an intensive monitoring system similar to that of BRAC and to integrate volunteering into the formal health program.

## Bhutan

Royal Government of Bhutan, Ministry of Health initiated the Village Health Worker (VHW) program in 1979 with the training of first batch of volunteers at Thimpu. The basic philosophy of VHW program in Bhutan was to establish a link between the community and the health services. The concept of Primary Health Care (PHC) is disseminated to the community through this group of volunteers, including improvement of basic hygiene and sanitation, prevention of vaccine preventable diseases and other preventive and promotive aspects of health.

The VHW program has two main objectives (Government of Bhutan, MOHE): to increase people's access to health care services thus, enhancing the health coverage in the country and to improve health and hygiene practices of the people in the communities through dissemination of health information and provision of simple treatment and first aid.

## Selection of Village Health Workers

The communities select the VHW following a set of criteria which are as follows (Government of Bhutan, MOHE):

A Village Health Worker must be: confident, trusted and popular in the community, living permanently in the community and not frequently absent, a good example in terms of personal hygiene, health care and community participation, healthy and physically able to fulfill the role of VHW, sufficiently confident to attend the training and willing to be a VHW for at least one year.

While selecting, priority should be given to the villages which are more than one hour walking distance from the nearest health centre. One Village Health Worker covers more than one village if the villages are small and close by approximately 20-30 households.

## Role of VHWs

The Village Health Workers are not an integral extension of the national health system, but a complimentary force to support the activities of the health system for the enhancement of health of the people. The role of a Village Health Worker is to spend a fraction of his time carrying out health related activities in his own community. It is not envisaged that a single Village Health Worker cover a large population, nor is the VHW expected to spend all his time for this; he is only a part-time volunteer.

The Village Health Workers are supposed to be primarily the link between the community and the health system. They are expected to be able to provide health education towards better health care, including family planning, provide simple first aid treatment for emergencies and minor illnesses, notification of the outbreak of any epidemics in the community, recognizing danger signs and symptoms of serious and chronic patients, playing an important role in out-reach clinics and expanded program of immunization and referral to the nearest health centre. They are also expected to participate in any development activities in the community, for example electricity and water programs.

## Training

Although the Village Health Worker Scheme in Bhutan had been initiated by 1979, the beginning of training of such workers in most of the districts began only by mid '80s. By 1994, more than 1,000 Village Health Workers were trained throughout Bhutan. They were given an initial training of 12 working days followed by yearly refresher training of five days' duration.

The basic training consists of ten modules covering the basics of preventive health (e.g. child health, nutrition, safer motherhood, family planning and sexual health), identification and treatment of minor illnesses, attending to injuries and guiding people to take timely action during sickness and other health needs.

## Incentives

As Village Health Workers do not constitute a regular cadre and the services offered are voluntary, the Village Health Worker s do not receive any kind of financial benefit from the government, except during the training period when each VHW would receive a daily stipend at par with other sectors Government of Bhutan, MOHE. The Village Health Worker s work in the community because they have been trusted and trained to care for the community and it gives them recognition for their service. Some Village Health Workers see this recognition as a way of getting higher level community and block leadership.

In Bhutan, it is a traditional practice to offer something to traditional and religious practitioners. The Gewog Yargay Tschogchung GYT or Block Development Committee decides upon a system of remunerative compensation for the time, effort and services rendered by the Village Health Workers. Some communities have devised the ways of exempting them from contributing labor to local development work. However, such an offer or contribution would be purely voluntary and should be acceptable to the Village Health Worker.

The other motive that drives the Village Health Worker s to continue is the central Buddhist tenet of service for the sake of improving ones "karma". Many Village Health Workers tell that although they receive nothing for their service now, they feel that the good that they have done will certainly help shape a better "karma" for the next life. There is also a general attitude in Bhutan that responsibility delegated in some way has to be fulfilled. However, with modernization and increasing wants for this life, it is a debatable point and for how long can such a sentiment be sustained.

## Monitoring

According to the Ministry of Health and Education Strategy Paper, the Village Health Workers' activities would be regularly supervised and routinely monitored by the respective GYTs (Block Development Committee) and basic health unit (BHU) staff. VHWs would maintain simple records of the activities undertaken and submit reports to the BHU. The BHU staff would submit the reports of VHWs activities to District Health Supervisory Officers, who in turn would submit to the national program manager. The National Program Manager would be responsible for overall planning, implementation and evaluation of the VHW program and monitor all activities carried out by different Dzongkhags in the country.

## With Doctors Scarce, Bhutanese Turn to Village Health Workers

Though Village Health Worker s do not provide routine checkups and immunizations, they do assist the mobile health units that make frequent visits to villages. They also provide health, hygiene and nutrition information that helps alleviate respiratory infections, poor nutrition, anemia and inadequate maternal health care — major causes of death and disease. Kencho Tshering, like other Village Health Workers, knows a lot about prevention. Sitting behind his crude wooden desk, he dispenses advice about everything from safe water and household hygiene to birth spacing. His clients listen respectfully and nod their heads in solemn agreement. Surrounding them are brightly colored wall posters illustrating the diseases of childhood, the importance of immunizing children, nutrition tips and ways to keep toilets clean. But watching over the health of so many people is a huge added responsibility for a man whose primary occupation is farming...

Mr. Tshering's age has a lot to do with the respect he receives in his traditional society, where advanced years are correlated with wisdom. Like many Village Health Workers, Mr. Tshering has no formal education, yet he wields the authority of a professor, and a popular one at that. Though his services and government supplied drugs are free, his clients nevertheless heap him with small, thoughtful gifts. When he falls ill, they help with cooking and fieldwork. And when he walks through the village, the men quickly put out their cigarettes in deference to his anti-smoking campaign.

Although, the government has follow-up guidelines, refresher training was found to vary as were supervisory practices. Most often Village Health Worker s meet at the outreach sites or come to the BHUs for monthly meetings.

## Replication

Village health workers have been recognized as a positive force in the community at all levels, including the National Assembly. The 2003 Annual Health Conference, which was attended by Village Health Workers, recommended sustaining and scaling up the VHW program. There is a great demand for Village Health Worker training from those communities which do not have Village Health Workers, either, because no-one was trained before or, to replace the dropouts. However, as the program is totally dependent on donors, even maintaining the network of close to 1,300 Village Health Workers is becoming a challenge. In this situation, the only feasible option is to find ways of keeping the Village Health Workers working and to continue refresher-training program to maintain their knowledge and skills and this is the direction the VHW program has opted for.

## Sustainability

There is no direct input from the Government into the Village Health Worker Program except the supervision and support given to the Village Health Worker s through the decentralized health system. There is a very high attrition rate and there is no specific mechanism in place to prevent or decrease the high attrition rate. Except UNICEF, there has been a gradual reduction of support for Village Health Workers from development partners. The probable reason is that they are being perceived as "just another pair of hands" in providing health services. Without a very specific support from the Government or community and a shift in strategy, it may be very difficult to sustain the existing VHW network.

## Constraints

In 1993/94, UNICEF supported a study of the VHW program implemented by the Health Division, Ministry of Health and Education (MOHE). The evaluation had identified a number of problems related to selection of Village Health Workers (uniform selection criteria and process), time needed to perform their functions, supervision (no opportunity for on the job training or any form of supervision), 'career' advancement (no scope), compensation and sustainability. In order to respond to some of these issues, Health Division, MOHE developed a strategy paper for strengthening of Village Health Worker Program in Bhutan where the selection criteria, incentives, supervision and monitoring system, training and retraining arrangements and roles and functions of Village Health Workers were clearly laid out.

It was observed that the five year attrition rate for VHW in Bhutan was 50 to 55%. Individual districts had attrition rates ranging from 21% to 63%. The most common reasons given for the high attrition was that the work interfered with their personal work (70%), family pressure (12%), too hard job (9%) and there was nothing to be gained from it (6%). Given the Bhutanese nature of being indirect, it would not be surprising if the majority left as there was no remuneration and career prospect as a VHW, but did not want to put it so plainly. Given the high attrition rate and increasing need for Village Health Workers, priority attention needs to be given to problems related to this program. In some areas the situation has improved and attrition rates have decreased as a result of Village Health Workers being released from volunteer service in the community as a form of compensation. Still the issues needing clarification include the policy for recruiting replacements for Village Health Workers who resign.

## India

Following reports of successful experiments in the non-governmental sector with the community health workers, the Indian government introduced a CHW Scheme across the country in 1977 envisaging "provision of health services at the doorsteps of villager". However, the names of the worker and the scheme changed over-time—from CHW in 1977 to Community Health Volunteer in 1980 and Village Health Guides in 1981.

The Village Health Guide (VHG) Scheme was made 100% centrally sponsored under the Family Welfare Program until April 2002. In 2000-01, a very high level review committee was established to study in details the entire scheme. The review committee looked at the work done by CHWs, their abilities and honorarium and sustainability issues. Based on this study recommendation, the government of India communicated to the state governments that the national government's funding will be discontinued starting April 2002 and the states were asked to run the scheme on their own, if they could mobilize the resources. However, with this change in financing arrangements, it is reported that no states are currently running the VHG scheme.

Based on the available written documents and personal communication, this paper highlights on India's experiences and lessons learned on VHGs up to April 2002. Maru (1983) summarized the following as the objectives of Village Health Guide Scheme based on the various official pronouncements: To provide basic curative, preventive and promotive health care at the door-steps of the people, To involve rural people in the provision, monitoring and control of basic health services, to place "people's health in people's hand" and To create a resource person trusted by the local population who could provide a link between primary health centre and the local community.

The scheme included training of one community health volunteer for every village community comprising of 1000 population. As of 2000, about 323,000 VHGs were working throughout India, under the Government of India sponsored scheme.

## Selection of Village Health Guides

The community used to select one of its own members as the community health volunteer or the VHW. The most common procedure adopted for selection of VHGs was that Village Panchayats, village self-government councils recommended two or three names to the primary health centre and a final decision made by a committee consisting of Medical Officer, Block Development Officer and the elected chairperson of the Block Panchayat Committee. Although the selection was to be made in an open meeting of the total village council, in practice, most often, only a few important village leaders were involved in the selection.

As the men were the main targets of the family planning program in the 1970s and early 1980s, males were selected as VHGs. However, after 1986, realizing the importance and neglect of domiciliary maternal and child health services and fresh attention given to women as the main target for family planning, the policy was changed and attempts were made to phase out male workers and recruit females in their place. But the organized male CHWs brought political pressure and legal procedures initiated against their removal, paralyzing the scheme in most states. Until the end of the program, about 80% of the VHGs were male. The national directives had laid out a few standards concerning the VHG profile: he was to live in the village, have minimal schooling and be willing to devote two to three hours a day to community health activities. He had to be acceptable to all the groups forming the community, and was not to be a member of any political organization. The selection procedure gave the primary health centre personnel the responsibility of enforcing the standards.

## Roles of Village Health Guides

The VHG was expected to know the health needs of the community and provide basic health services: minor treatments, preventive measures, including education and liaison with specialized health institutions. He/she would receive a manual of instructions and a 'health kit' for his/her works as well as a small supply of medicine for first treatments. If the action required was beyond his/her skill or resources, he/she would draw on the resources of the formal health structure and in the process render it more responsive to community needs.

The VHG was expected to educate the village population about health problems, such as family planning or public sanitation and personal hygiene, which might not be perceived by the community members as their felt needs. AVHG used to be a change agent as well as a representative of the community.

## Training

After the VHG was identified and approved by the selection committee, he/she used to undergo through a three-months training in simple and basic health care at the primary health centre. During the training period, the community health volunteer used to receive from the government, a monthly stipend of Rs. 200. After the training, the VHG used to spend 2-3 hours a day for health work in his community

## Incentives

The government used to provide an honorarium of Rs 50 per month plus basic medicines worth Rs. 50 and both of these were disbursed to VHGs through the primary health centre (Maru 1983). Although, the government made it clear at the outset that the VHGs were volunteers and accountable to the communities they came from and served, communities viewed them as government employees because they were 'paid' a small monthly stipend. The health system personnel also perceived the CHWs as government employees and therefore, assigned them additional tasks. Providing the stipend for each VHG was a sizeable recurring expense for the government. Therefore, in 1981, the central government had decided to reduce its contribution from 100 to 50 per cent of the costs of the scheme and asked the State Government to meet the remainder. But, this led to several states backing out of the program. Later, following the conviction that women should be employed as VHGs, the central government decided to fund the scheme fully once again.

All this led to employment considerations becoming more important to VHGs than social service and ultimately they were demanding for higher remuneration. As a result, by 2001, there were at least 23 cases in various courts all over India demanding for raising the honorarium but all the cases failed as the court took a decision that being a volunteer scheme it did not stand well against the demand for increasing honorarium.

## Monitoring

The routine functions and activities of the VHG were supervised and controlled by the community. As he/she was not a government employee, there was no direct line relationship with the primary health centre staff. The local community could decide to change the CHV if he/she did not perform well after the training. But, in such cases, the community was expected to bear the cost of training the second VHG.

## Replication

There is no plan of reviving the VHG scheme by Government of India

## Sustainability

Because of the failure of taking ownership of the program by the state governments and discontinuation of financial support from the central government, the VHG scheme ultimately came to an end after 25 years of running. There is a great lesson to be learned from this case about whether the honorarium to be given or not to CHWs if it can not be sustained as well as the importance of involvement and buy-in of the local governments (state governments in this case) and community support, from the very beginning of the program.

## Constraints

Village Health Guides in India had encountered a number of difficulties stemming from inadequate support from their communities and the health system alike. One of the main issues enveloping the VHGs was their 'medicalization'. Trained for three months, they focused on providing curative services, to the neglect of preventive and promotive tasks. This was due in large part to their orientation to curative care during their initial training which was conducted by Primary Health Centre Doctors and Health Supervisors, who were themselves not instructed appropriately in how to train basic health workers. The VHGs began to perceive themselves as village medical practitioners, often even demanding further training for this purpose. While village communities concurred because their perceived need was for curative services, they usually viewed the VHGs as "third class doctors", and bypassed their services, whenever possible. At the same time, India's powerful medical lobby, the Indian Medical Association, opposed the scheme on the grounds that these workers would indulge in quackery, inflicting inferior or even dangerous care on underserved and unsuspecting villagers. Poor role definition led to other difficulties in the scheme. VHGs were seen as extensions of the health system, especially to undertake family planning motivation and sanitation tasks.

## Nepal

In Nepal, there are many forms of volunteer service and types of volunteers, including religious service volunteerism. Community members consider traditional birth attendants, female ward members (political leaders), functional users group and committee members to be volunteers. In addition, there are many volunteer programs supported by national and international NGOs for health and family planning programs. In the late 1970s, the Government of Nepal launched its first National Community Health Volunteer Program. During the last 25 years, the volunteer program has evolved, changed and expanded into the current national Female Community Health Volunteer (FCHV) program, with more than 48,550 trained volunteers in all 75 districts throughout the country. Since the implementation of the National FCHV Program in 1988, the context in which Female Community Health Volunteers have been involved in community health improvement has witnessed significant changes. The roles and responsibilities have continually evolved, the variety of different health programs utilizing community-based approaches has increased and Village Development Committees have begun to take local responsibility for the management of Sub Health Posts in accordance with the Local Self-Governance Act.

## Selection of Female Community Health Volunteers

The official criteria for selection of Female Community Health Volunteers state that in each ward (an administrative division with approx. 500 inhabitants) of Village Development Committees (lowest geo-political unit), one FCHV will be selected by local mothers' group. According to the national strategy, criteria for the selection of Female Community Health Volunteers are as follows.

"The Female Community Health Volunteer must be a local resident, willing and capable to work as volunteer, at least 20 years old and literate. If literate woman is not available illiterate women meeting other criteria may be selected. But such illiterate women should be willing to attend literacy classes. Preference will be given to those involved in social works/health activities and married women with one or two children, and those who have completed primary education" In recent years, some districts have implemented a population-based system, which varies depending on the population density: one volunteer for 400 population in the Terai, 250 in the hills and 150 in the mountains. However, this official criterion for selecting the FCHVs is currently being reviewed by the Family Health Division, Ministry of Health.

In a study on the concept of volunteerism many community people observed favoritism in the selection of Female Community Health Volunteers. The overall impression was that selection occurs through informal networks and, therefore, the process was in the hands of local elites. The majority of Female Community Health Volunteers were described as being selected or appointed by Village Development Committee members, political leaders, local elites or health workers and many appointed volunteers were related to local leaders and health workers. Several community members complained about excluding women who were poorer and from "lower" castes and ethnic groups in the selection process. The exceptions were in those areas where NGOs have taken an active role in the formation of mothers' groups and adequate attention given in the process for selecting government supported FCHVs. People who were active, educated, and with some connections were viewed as having the best chance of being selected. Most often Female Community Health Volunteers were not selected by the mothers' groups and in fact, it was reported that mothers' groups were often formed after the FCHV was selected.

## Role of Female Community Health Volunteers

Female Community Health Volunteers played an important, multifaced role related to family planning, maternal and neonatal health, child health and select infectious diseases such as diarrhea, acute respiratory infections at the community level. They promoted the utilization of available health services and the adoption of preventive health practices among community members. They were recognized as health educators and promoters, community mobilisers, referral agents and community-based service providers.

The FCHV was expected to conduct mothers' groups meetings to discuss and teach health messages from her manual as well as use other opportunities to meet the mothers in groups or individually to discuss health messages and advise them for applying good maternal and child health and family planning practices.

The study on the concept of volunteerism noted that many community members and even some Village Development Committee officials were unaware of the responsibilities of FCHVs. The activities most frequently and consistently identified by the community members were those associated with national programs (e.g. Vitamin A distribution and polio campaigns). The national Vitamin A program (supported by the Nepal Technical Assistance Group) provided training and active supervision, clearly defined job responsibilities and training allowances for vitamin A. In addition, participation was required for only a few days twice yearly, rather than throughout the year, as were other FCHV responsibilities. Volunteers were described as being best able to carry out such clearly defined, concrete tasks, rather than activities such as health education.

However, community members expressed a preference for volunteers to provide treatment and distribute medicines, rather than health education. In the study on the concept of volunteerism, volunteers also said that they wanted to be trained to distribute medicines. Acute respiratory infection (ARI) program provided another good example of the community's positive assessment of the FCHV's role in distribution of cotrimoxazole. In the ARI program, volunteers had concrete tasks, were given good training and were closely supervised and monitored. In a study conducted in 1997 by Child Health Division, Ministry of Health Nepal on Assessment of ARI Strengthening Program, it was found that FCHVs were acceptable care providers to mothers, because they were easily accessible and gave good advice. They were also seen as affordable and they gave good medicines. Especially, poor people and those living in remote areas greatly benefited from their services and for times when other care providers were not available like at night times. In the study on the concept of volunteerism, many volunteers and community members referred to the increasing burden of work and time commitment expected of volunteers. At central level, the people interviewed expressed concern that an increased burden could overwhelm volunteers and undermine their performance and the program.

## Training

Training has been identified as the most important component of the FCHV program. The National Health and Training Centre developed the national guidelines for an initial training of 15 days, followed by refresher training for two days every 6 months. Usually, the initial training was organized in the nearest health facilities (health post or sub-health post) by Health Assistants, Assistant Nurse Midwives and Auxiliary Health Workers under the direction of the District Health Office. The initial training for FCHVs were focused on family health care with emphasis on motivation and health education in relation to immunization, diarrhea control, nutrition, hygiene, acute respiratory infection, maternal health and family planning. The training was primarily knowledge-oriented and not skills-oriented, except the specific training on integrated management of childhood illnesses (IMCI), community-based acute respiratory infection and control of diarrhoeal diseases, and vitamin A deficiency disorders.

The study on concept of volunteerism noted that FCHVs were not given training on interpersonal communication, how to provide counseling, how to conduct meetings, or how to teach and present information – even though these activities were essential for performing many of the responsibilities assigned to FCHVs. The study also revealed that training was not regular in all areas and where it was more frequent, volunteers reported that it had become repetitive and ritualistic, with rote teaching methods most often used by local health workers. Some volunteers attended many different types of training sessions provided by government and other organizations — the many types of training did not appear to be coordinated or prioritized. However, volunteers said that they liked training, and many expressed an interest in learning new things and they needed refresher training to be able to teach people in the community.

## Incentives

Compensation or remuneration of CHVs continues to be an issue of intense debate in Nepal. The debate intensified in 1988 when the FCHV program was established and volunteers were given Rs. 100 per month. Provision of this allowance could not be sustained and was discontinued after the first year, but is still remembered and discussed. The issue became complicated by the fact that there were several types of community-based health workers who were called volunteers and received payment from NGOs, but volunteers with the national health volunteer program did not receive a salary or financial compensation except for a daily allowance during training sessions.

Although volunteerism was described as being free service, there was a consensus among most of the people concerned (e.g. central and district officials, health workers, NGOs staff, community members and leaders) that FCHVs need to be remunerated or receive regular incentives. These could be in the form of financial allowances or non-monetary benefits such as bicycles, radios, saris, etc. Such benefits were considered to have a positive influence on the family's willingness to give permission for women to serve as volunteers; improve the volunteer's status in the community; provide compensation for the time taken from household and agricultural responsibilities; and be an incentive for long-term service.

In addition to remuneration and incentives, community recognition and public appreciation for the contribution of volunteers in the form of awards, certificates, ceremonies, etc., was desired especially by volunteers. This recognition was identified by volunteers as an important factor in their own sense of satisfaction and motivation to continue as a volunteer.

## Monitoring

Village Health Workers were the primary contact and Village Health Workers were the primary contact and responsible government health cadres for supervision of Female Community Health Volunteers. However, the study on the concept of volunteerism noted that supervision was not found to take place in many areas and in others it was irregular and informal, except for the national health programs, e.g. vitamin A, polio immunization days, which were reported to provide regular supervision and some allowances for these activities.

The study report noted that most interactions with FCHVs took place at outreach clinics (ORCs) and often FCHV participation in ORCs was not regular and in some areas, the ORCs themselves were held irregularly. In addition, these meetings were brief and did not serve as a forum for guidance or problem solving. The health workers were not found to be providing much support for the volunteers. According to the study, refresher training was described as the major form of supervision and for many these training sessions were the only events when they received supervision. It was also noted that supervision was difficult because FCHVs did not have a clear job description and were not paid. Questions were raised about the appropriateness of supervising volunteers. Contrastingly, some NGO supported volunteer programs, such as Family Planning Association of Nepal paid volunteers for specific tasks and targets, and provided supervision on the basis of their ability to carry out these responsibilities.

## Replication

The Female Community Health Volunteer Program has already been expanded to all 75 districts in the country. There is a plan for phased replacement of those who are now quite aged and of those who are inactive. The FCHVs' original role has been modified a great deal to include diagnosing, treating or referring cases of pneumonia, involvement in national immunization days, Vit. A distribution, etc. As the IMCI strategy is implemented in more and more districts, demands on the FCHVs are increasing. FCHV program has also been expanded to select municipalities.

## Sustainability

Through orientations and review meetings, efforts were made to generate support from local government bodies and from communities in organising mother's group meetings, replenishing FCHV medicine supplies, disseminating information and providing incentives for FCHVs, etc. At present, 47 (out of 75) districts have established a district level endowment fund for supporting FCHV activities. This Fund needs to be activated and transferred into Village Development Committee (VDC) level endowment fund. There is a lot of interest and encouragement to the VDCs to sustain the FCHV program. Approximately 400 VDCs of 18 districts have already established endowment funds.

## Constraints

As noted above, among rural villagers there is a greater interest in curative services rather than health education. This was also reflected in an anthropological survey conducted in Nepal by Stone (1986). She concluded that in the villages she visited there was a social pressure to move the health workers away from the health education role and toward a community 'doctor' role. This pressure came from both the community people and the health workers themselves. CHVs reported frustration that, contrary to the expectation of their fellow villagers, they were not really able to treat illnesses. When asked directly how the program could be improved, CHVs unanimously asked that they be given more medical training and more drugs.

## Sri Lanka

In Sri Lanka, the involvement of school teachers and village/community leaders in voluntary work can be traced as far back as 1915, to the Rockfeller Foundation sponsored campaign for control of hookworm infestation. During the malaria epidemic of 1934/35, extensive involvement of voluntary workers was a special feature of the government's malaria control program while the non-government organizations began involving volunteers from the 1950s.

The main growth of the volunteer program, however was from the mid 1970s. Service organizations such as the Family Planning Association started to train volunteers in the 1970s, expanding from 60 in 1973 to 40,000 in 1987. Many other non-government agencies (e.g. Oxfam, Save the Children (UK and US), SIDA and JOICFP, a Japanese organization) also supported small volunteer programs. The largest trainer of volunteers within the government, however is the Health Education Bureau, part of the Public Health Division of the Ministry of Health. From 1976 onwards, the Health Education Bureau developed its volunteer program and trained 100,000 volunteers (Walt *et al* 1989). However, opinions differ on the current number of volunteers working regularly, with one conservative estimate being 15,000.

**Selection of Community Health Workers**

Although all countries have had standard criteria for selecting CHWs that included involvement of community members in the selection process, most often the volunteers were appointed by local elites, political leaders and health workers and were related to these people. Given this situation and the fact that the ethnic minorities or marginalized and poorer groups in the community get excluded from the selection process, equitable involvement of community members in selecting CHWs and using their services appears to be critical to successful CHW programs.

Though the criteria for selecting CHWs could vary depending upon the local and national context, based on the successful examples, the generic selection criteria could include the following: selection by the community members equitably, married female (so the CHW would not leave the community) of 20 to 35 years from the same community, socially acceptable, preferably literate (so that they can record health information and use written materials), demonstrated involvement in and willing to work for the community. The evidence from India shows that involvement of local government in selecting CHWs and their buy-in from the beginning of the program is extremely important for having success.

## Roles

Evidence shows that Community Health Workers can be extremely effective to work as a complimentary force promoting utilization of available health services and the link between the community and the health system. However, with regards to their roles, whether the CHWs should have a single or multiple focus, maintaining a delicate balance between the curative and preventive role seems to be of critical importance. The evidence from Nepal and Bangladesh shows that prevention is extremely hard to sell while curative care (treatment of ARI and other minor health problems) is generally more welcomed and appreciated by the community members.

Additionally, Community Health Workers are best able to carry out clearly defined, concrete tasks over a short and specific time period such as national health campaigns (vitamin A distribution, polio campaigns, etc) rather than carrying out broad-based activities such as health education. One should also take into consideration that increased burden of work and excessive time commitment for multiple tasks could overwhelm volunteers and in turn, negatively affect their performance and the program.

## Training

All the countries reviewed had provisions of basic foundation training that ranged from five days to three months, and refresher training (one to five days) in regular intervals. Most often, the basic training focused on preventive health, health education and first aid. It would be a formal lecture based and knowledge-oriented training rather than the one which is skills-oriented and community specific or contextual.

The review of the community health workers literature revealed a strong need for the training in interpersonal communication and counseling skills, including methods of adult participatory learning. It also noted that continuous training is found to be an essential prerequisite for an effective CHW program and an important factor in retaining their motivation level.

## Incentives/Motivation

Except India, all countries reviewed did not pay salaries or provide any kind of monetary incentives to community health workers, because the governments did not consider the salaries to be sustainable. Although Nepal started with a provision of small allowance per month (less than $ 2), it was discontinued after the first year as this could not be sustained. However, they were paid nominal allowances during the training period in all countries.

Contrarily, countries are encouraging communities and local governments for providing them either monetary or, non-monetary incentives such as bicycles, radios or community recognition and public appreciation for the contribution of volunteers in the form of awards, certificates, etc. And, some communities have even set up special funds for supporting the community health workers (e.g. Nepal).

Ideally speaking, it is said that service to the community as the primary motivation factor for volunteering. However, it is reported that training stipend, earning an income through selling medicines and possibility of future employment opportunities are the motivational factors for many community health workers. But, evidence has shown that monetary incentives often bring a host of problems: money may not be enough, may not be paid regularly or may stop altogether (e.g. Nepal and India). Hence, non-monetary incentives are critical to the success of any CHW programs. Additionally, the role of community health workers that required them to deliver curative services rather than just promoting utilization of available health services seems to greatly increase their motivation level.

## Monitoring

Although community members express some appreciation of the work of Community health workers and some satisfaction with their services, often community support is largely passive. Monitoring and follow up of CHW is seldom done by communities. It largely depends upon the initiative and interest of the government health workers at periphery level, who receive no incentives for supervising the volunteers. Hence, in reality, the interactions with community health workers usually take place at the out-reach clinics or refresher training which are held irregularly.

The evidence from the field shows that regularity of supportive supervision and appropriate refresher training helps to sustain the interest and motivation of community health workers to do their assigned tasks (e.g. Bangladesh and Nepal). Similarly, frequent interactions of community members and community health workers are also critically important in affecting their motivation levels.

## Replication

In most of the reviewed countries, the CHW approach has "gone to scale" based on the results, real and perceived, of the small scale pilot projects. These pilot projects had demonstrated that with intensive support, community health workers can provide effective interventions of adequate quality, coverage and equity to achieve significant reductions in mortality and associated improvements in health status. Particularly, analysis of Bangladesh's experience suggests that several factors are essential for successful scaling-up. They are qualified, experienced and dedicated human resource base to support the program, effective management systems including monitoring and evaluation systems, learning environment (encouraging learning from interaction with the field) and adequate financial support.

## Sustainability

A basic lesson from this review is that community health workers must be adequately supported and such adequate support requires more resources from the government or communities than what are spent now on CHW programs. Community health workers cannot be seen as a marginal addition to existing services funded by limited one-time special expenditures. Evidence from Bangladesh suggests that the level of institutional support in training and retraining, program management and supportive supervision by health workers greatly determine the sustainability of the CHW scheme. By developing strong, better educated and empowered women and village groups, sustainable improvements can be achieved and a higher quality of preventive health measures will be practiced in the community.

## Constraints

The major issues identified are related to selection of CHWs (community involvement, uniform selection criteria and process), time commitment and workload, communities' preference for curative services, remuneration/ incentives (continuity, source, uniformity), prospect for career advancement and high attrition rates, etc.

The evidence shows that from the very beginning stage of the program, clarity on community role, selection criteria, community health workers role, mechanisms for compensating community health workers time involvement and incentives, together with adherence to these basic principles helps to enhance the effectiveness of the CHW program.

**Overview of Competencies**

*A. Client Interviewing/Intake*

1. Begin the Interview
2. Discuss Policy and Procedures
3. Practice Communication Techniques
4. Assess Client Needs

*B. Client Orientation*

1. Discuss Agency Services
2. Explain Agency Policy and Procedures

*C. Coordinating Client Care*

1. Keep a Client File
2. Develop a Plan of Care
3. Track Clients

*D. Document and Report Client Information*

1. Document Client Information
2. Report Client Information

*E. Provide Referral Services*

1. Give Referrals
2. Maintain Referrals

*F. Provide Health Information*

1. Provide Client with Health Information
2. Assist in Health Service Planning and Development

*G. Community Health Education*

1. Planning, Implementation and Evaluation
2. Working in Groups
3. Community Outreach
4. Community Organizing

*A. Client Interviewing/Intake*

## I. Beginning the Interview

Preview client information

Introduce self to the client

Welcome the client/establish rapport

Establish a comfortable and quiet interviewing environment

Identify and address language barriers

Explain the purpose and process of the interview

### *Discuss Policy and Procedures*

Explain confidentiality policy and exceptions

Advise clients of legal rights/immigrant policy

Obtain a signed release/waiver from client

Assist client in filling out forms and paperwork

### *Practice Communication Techniques*

Use appropriate eye contact and body language

Use plain language instead of jargon

Use open-ended questions

Use active listening skills

Verify what you heard to the client

Obtain a translator, if needed

### *Client Needs Assessment*

Determine, evaluate and prioritize needs with the client

Clarify client needs and concerns by paraphrasing

Determine client eligibility for services

Seek consultation from supervisor, if needed

Inform client about what will happen next

## II. Client Orientation

### *Discuss Agency Services*

Explain services the agency offers

Explain agency schedule of services (i.e., specific clinic days)

Inform client about what to expect during agency visits

Give the client agency resources, handouts and pamphlets

Explain managed care and utilization of the system in non-technical language

Explain roles of health team members

### *Explain Agency Policies and Procedures*

Take client on a tour of the agency

Explain appointment protocol: cancellation policy, hours, after hours

Explain caregiver team approach

Explain emergency procedures

## III. Coordinating Client Care

### *Keep a Client File*

Set up a client file using agency format

Document client history/information/progress

Give the client agency resources, handouts and pamphlets

Follow established agency legal guidelines

Conduct case presentations in staff meetings

Store client files securely

***Develop a Plan of Care***

Create a treatment plan with the client

Discharge client upon termination

***Track Clients***

Make and keep appointments with clients

Make follow up contact with the client based on agency policy

Review treatment to date

Visit client at other sites: home, shelter, hospital, jail

Refer client to other services

**Document and Report Client Information**

***Document Client Information***

Explain to the client what you are documenting

Explain how the information will be used

Record client history

Write general notes for self

Follow established charting protocols: date, sign, initial

***Report Client Information***

Review cases with supervisors

Give case presentations

Write reports

Explain reporting protocols

## IV. Provide Referral Services

### *Give Referrals*

Explain the purpose and procedures of referrals

Explain referrals and how they will benefit the client

Explain detailed information about the referral agency

Identify and address possible client barriers to accessing referrals

Call referral agency to advocate for client access and track access

### *Maintain Referrals*

Develop and maintain a community resource/referral book

Establish and maintain contact with referral agencies and key contacts

Assess and evaluate referral information

## V. Provide Health Information

### *Provide Client with Health Information*

Provide health advising: routine/low-risk situations

Perform health presentations and demonstrations

Distribute informational handouts and pamphlets

Identify myths and misconceptions

Discuss effective ways to address myths and misconceptions

Assist client with personal issues: goal setting, empowerment

***Assist in Health Service Planning and Development***

Develop or obtain literacy-appropriate educational materials

Demonstrate general knowledge about health issues

**VI. Community Health Education**

Planning, Implementation and Evaluation

Conduct needs assessments

Participate in program planning, implementation and evaluation

Administer pre-and post-test evaluations

Determine target populations

Stay current with health issues and statistics

***Working in Groups***

Plan and give presentations

Facilitate and participate in group process

***Community Outreach***

Participate in the outreach process

Plan and participate in health workshops/fairs

Distribute educational materials

Work on crisis hotlines

***Community Organizing***

Initiate and participate in community events/health fairs

Recruit and work with volunteers

Act as a liaison between community leaders and members

Use the media for community announcements

Build and organize networks

Develop written materials for community

### *Performance Based Education for Community Health Workers*

A three-day training session for health workers who do street outreach, counseling and partner notification in sexually transmitted diseases in a major city. A series of doctors lecture to the health workers, showing slides of patients with STDs, and presenting on diagnosis and treatment. They reel off facts and figures which the health workers are supposed to memorize for their pre-and post-tests. The doctors drone on and by the end of each day the health workers' eyes are glazed over and they are completely frustrated.

### What's wrong?

1. The doctors are teaching what they were taught, not what the health workers need to know how to do. The content of the training is determined by "experts," not by people who really do the work on the ground in the community. The people who are teaching have never done what the health workers need to know how to do.
2. Learning is evaluated by regurgitation of facts, not by the mastery of skills in a real-life situation. This kind of pencil-and-paper evaluation favors people with more formal education, not necessarily people with knowledge of the community who are most effective in the field.
3. The health workers get an informal certificate of completion, but not college credits that contribute to raises, career mobility or educational advancement. No matter how much they know, how high their

skill level, or how much responsibility they take, they are too often ghettoized in a dead-end job.

4. Every topical specialty—for example, sexually transmitted disease, or nutrition, or perinatal—designs its own training program. None of these programs recognize the trainings put on by other programs, so that health workers find it hard to advance no matter how many trainings they attend. However, when our project compared job descriptions across specialties, we found that many process skills—for example client interviewing or health advising -- are common to Community health workers no matter what their topical focus.

## Competencies of Community Health Works

The seven competencies are client interviewing/intake; client orientation; care coordination or case management; documenting and reporting; providing referrals; providing health information; and community health education or outreach/organizing. With the input of veteran community health workers and supervisors, each competency is broken down into subcompetencies, and each one is described in detail: What does it look like when this competency is done well or poorly? In this way each person in the program knows she is learning what is critical, and that she has mastered the competency well enough for use in a real life situation. On the first day a learner comes to class, she or he receives this roadmap of what they are to learn and what criteria will be used to evaluate mastery? The curriculum addresses the knowledge, skills, and attitudes that a health worker needs to be successful. Potential employers know that graduates of the Certificate program are capable of consistent performance.

Community health workers need to master not only technical information, but also be able to serve as a voice of the community in the political process that has such a big effect on community health.

## Recruitment

### Based in the Community

While there are often few physicians and nurses in resource-poor settings, a large number of underemployed or unemployed persons are frequently available. CHWs are always recruited from the communities they support. Recommendations are sought from respected members of the community such as village elders, spiritual leaders, nurses and teachers. Some programs have organized community meetings to find CHWs, while others have advertised through local newspapers and radio announcements. Religious groups, schools, and other community-based organizations providing outreach activities are also good places to find potential community health workers. Patients are another source as they are able to serve themselves and to recommend people in their village who are trustworthy and caring.

## Selection of Communication Health Works

### Requirements

- The community health workers must be an adult (usually over 18 years of age) and preferably literate.
- Since the community health workers is in daily contact with patients in their homes, he or she should live in or close to the community served; having lived in the community for a specific number of years is often required.
- The community health workers should have a background that is similar to the background of the patients so that they feel comfortable sharing their concerns. This also enables the CHW to have first-hand knowledge of the problems and obstacles

patients face every day. In some cases, community health workers are themselves HIV positive or former TB patients. They frequently know someone who has HIV or TB in their community.

- Motivation and character are critical requirements. A CHW must be a trustworthy and respected member of the community with a strong desire to help the needy and a strong sense of empathy with those who are vulnerable and sick. A CHW's work is not only focused on improving health status, but also on social justice and solidarity with the community, through working to support affected individuals and households and reduce social isolation.

## Interviewing Community Health Workers Candidates

The clinical team usually interviews people who wish to become CHWs to see if they meet the above requirements. Team members that may be involved in the interview process include doctors, nurses, social workers or program managers. The candidate may be asked to take a basic literacy test. He/she may also be called upon to read a medication label or write his/her name, to distinguish medications by color and size and to count the number of pills in a month's supply. In some programs, preference is given to candidates who are extremely poor and could, therefore particularly use the additional income and skills-training. Given the specific vulnerabilities of women in the HIV epidemic, women may be preferred.

## Pairing a Patient with a Community Health Workers

Community health workers are chiefly selected by patients themselves. In the case of an established program, a patient may already know a CHW in his community, and may even have been referred to the health center by him/

her. If the patient does not know any community health workers, or doesn't feel comfortable with the one(s) he/she knows, then the clinical team suggests a possible candidate from those CHWs who live in the vicinity of the patient.

## Roles and Functions

Community health workers serve as counselors, educators, treatment supervisors, and advocates experienced in identifying the needs of their communities. They:

Provide home-based care, provide psychosocial support to patients undergoing treatment, act as the link between the patient and the health center carry out active case finding and educate the community on a variety of health topics

## Provide Home-Based Care

At PIH programs, community health workers provide the bulk of daily care to patients, especially in supporting those who have chronic illnesses such as HIV and TB. Community health workers are responsible for administering all outpatient TB- and HIV-related medications. They directly observe the ingestion of pills at the same time once or twice a day in the patient's home and record the patient's adherence. By working to ensure that patients adhere to medications, Community health workers fulfill an essential function in optimizing patients' clinical outcomes and preventing or delaying the emergence of drug-resistant disease. CHWs also routinely visit HIV-positive patients who are not receiving ART to assess their ongoing needs and those of the family.

Community health workers explain the importance of adherence to medication and work with the patient to identify and address obstacles to adherence. Through their daily visits, Community health worker teach patients how to manage complex drug treatments and cope with possible side effects. Community health workers ensure that they safely store the medications they provide to patients, keep them away from children, away from sunlight, in a dry place and in the same container in which they come from the health center. The community health workers are also responsible for ensuring that drugs are taken with the appropriate food and drink if required, and that any allergic reactions or side effects to medicines are quickly identified and reported to the health center.

CHWs are also a vital link between the health center and pregnant women in the community. CHWs stress the importance of prenatal and postnatal care and encourage pregnant women to visit the health center for check-ups, undergo HIV testing, and deliver at the health center. In the case of a home delivery, they encourage women to bring their babies to the health center as soon as possible after the birth.

### Provide Psychosocial Support to Patients Undergoing Treatment

As the primary contact with the patient and the patient's family through daily visits, Community health workers see first-hand the stresses that affect a patient's health status and adherence to treatment and health status. Through their own experience as members of the same community, and their knowledge, commitment, and ability to access to other resources, CHWs can support the patient and his/her family in important non-medical ways during treatment and beyond.

Community health workers respect the **privacy and confidentiality** of the patient. When the patient and the community health worker start working together, they establish ways to respond to questions about their relationship. Some patients may prefer to describe the community health worker as a friend or a cousin. Following the wishes of the patient and keeping information about him/her confidential are crucial for building trust.

Community health workers provide emotional and practical support to patients by helping reduce their sense of isolation and by encouraging them to discuss their illness with their families. They alert the staff at the health center if the patient's mental, social, or economic state is precarious.

### Act as the Link between the Patient and the Health Center

Community Health Workers are the eyes and ears of the clinical team in the community. CHWs also accompany their patients to the health center, sometimes assisting with arranging transportation, child care, or other logistics.

At the same time, they advocate for the patient by assessing, monitoring, and attending to patients' need for food, housing, safe water, education, or financial assistance. They notify the clinical staff and the social worker at the health center when these non-medical problems impact patients' adherence, treatment or overall health.

### Carry Out Active Casefinding

As community health workers are living and working in the community, they may be able to proactively identify sick or otherwise needy people, especially family members or other close contacts of patients. They may recognize opportunistic infections or TB symptoms and encourage these people to undergo testing and treatment at the health center; CHWs should pay particular attention to groups at particular risk for TB: children, people living with HIV/AIDS, and malnourished people. CHWs may also identify social and economic obstacles that impact on health, such as problems with children's schooling, or housing or economic hardship, and help to obtain support for these social needs.

### Educate the Community on a Variety of Health Topics

CHWs provide accurate information about chronic diseases such as HIV/AIDS and TB, explain how to prevent them, encourage community members to undergo testing, and correct people's misunderstandings or myths. They also encourage community members to accept and provide support to people living with HIV/AIDS, especially orphans. Beyond AIDS and TB, CHWs formally and informally educate the community on a wide array of health center activities and health topics, ranging from vaccination campaigns to hygiene and sanitation.

## Payment

### Community Health Workers should be Paid for their Efforts

Community Health Workers should be paid for their efforts. CHWs are trained to carry out essential care, often under very difficult circumstances. Furthermore, CHWs' role in identifying patients in need of care and in ensuring adherence to treatment results in significant short- and long-term cost savings through earlier initiation of treatment and by preventing or delaying the emergence of drug resistant-disease. They should not be asked to volunteer their services in settings of great poverty. Rather, their efforts should be fairly compensated. Salarying CHWs in settings with high unemployment and overall poverty helps jump-start economic activity in addition to being a critical recognition of the vital services they provide.

### How the Payment is Calculated?

In determining how much to pay CHWs, it is important to keep in mind local pay scales for public sector employees, from schoolteachers to staff at health facilities. When a new CHW program is established in an area where community health workers already exist, the payment for both groups should be harmonized as much as possible.

## Training

### Organization

Before they begin supporting patients, CHWs receive an orientation from the clinical staff at the health center as well as participate in a rigorous training program.

The number of participants varies according to need; 25 participants or fewer is ideal. All participants are provided with meals and a stipend. Trainers and facilitators are drawn from the staff at the health centers and should have experience in training or education to ensure that they are knowledgeable about and competent in participatory-based learning and training methods suited to low-literate adult learners.

Regardless of the specific content areas covered, the primary objective of CHW training is consistent: to instill a sense of solidarity and social justice in supporting patients, households and the community. Specific goals include: Providing correct information about treatment, prevention, and risk factors for HIV, TB, malaria, and other infectious diseases. Defining the roles and responsibilities of CHWs. Helping CHWs recognize and reduce stigma and discrimination in their communities. Developing CHWs' competence in active casefinding for diseases and social needs. Helping CHWs improve their skills related to effective communication and psychosocial support and Directing CHWs to additional resources or people at the health center and in the community who can guide or assist their work.

### Training Principles

Based upon adult learning principles, the CHW training curriculum presented here incorporates a variety of participatory approaches to teaching and learning that build upon the existing knowledge, skills, and experiences of the participants, including: Large-and small-group activities and discussions, Role plays, Case studies, Brainstorming, Panel discussions and Peer teaching.

**Continuing Education**

After the initial program, CHWs participate in ongoing monthly education sessions for one year and beyond, with additional training in areas such as nutrition, malaria, pediatric HIV/AIDS, diarrheal disease, family planning, active casefinding, worms and parasites, chronic disease, first aid, the role of traditional healers, and oral hygiene. Trainings are led by health center staff or other available teachers.

**Shadowing a CHW**

After completing his/her initial training, the new CHW joins a veteran CHW in conducting patient visits. This provides a practical, hands-on learning experience and helps the new CHW develop a support network of fellow CHWs.

**Supervision**

Historically, CHWs have been directly supervised by clinical staff, usually a doctor or nurse involved in the care of HIV or TB patients. As our programs have grown, we have increasingly recognized a need for more formal supervision structures that take advantage of the experience and skills of more senior CHWs. Recently, we have introduced the role of Accompagnateur Leader at several of the program sites.

**CHW Leaders**

Most often, the leader is an existing CHW who has been chosen based on the high quality of his/her work, leadership qualities and standing in the community. The length of time the CHW has been working as an accompagnateur and his/her level of education are also factors.

## Roles and Responsibilities

The primary responsibility of the CHW leader is to ensure that the CHWs are visiting their patients daily, administering medications correctly, and vigilantly monitoring patient health. The leader also helps the clinical team by answering patients' questions, joining the team on patient visits, and identifying problems between CHWs and patients.

Another point of supervision is at the pharmacy, which CHWs visit regularly to pick up medications for their patients. Pharmacy logs and interactions with the pharmacist are important points of supervision. The CHW leader and other members of the health center identify problems between CHWs and patients through unannounced visits to patients' homes. When a conflict does arise, the CHW is called to the health center to discuss the situation. CHW leaders meet regularly with health center staff to exchange information and discuss common issues. CHWs meet monthly with health center staff for ongoing training and to discuss any problems or concerns.

## Implementation

## Begin with Community

Establishing services in a community begins with an informal (and ongoing) process of surveys and meetings with the local population to find out their specific needs and desires.

## Organizational structure

The CHW represents the health center to the community and is an integral part of the medical team, interacting continually with the rest of the staff. It is important that he/she knows the different staff roles and responsibilities in order to direct medical and non-medical issues to the appropriate person.

## The Number of Community Health Workers

The CHW—to-patient ratio varies from site to site depending on how many CHWs can be recruited or how many CHWs already exist, population density, the logistical demands of the area's topography, and the types of patients being supported.

## Work Schedule

After the initial training, the CHW meets with those patients he/she will support who are undergoing or about to start ARV or TB treatment. The CHW can be chosen by the patient, or, with the patient's agreement, the CHW may be assigned to a patient depending on where he/she lives.

Ideally, CHW-patient pairings remain stable over the course of treatment/care. While the schedule of visits varies according to the population and geographic spread of the community and their specific health needs, there is a common set of visits that occurs in all the programs.

## At the Patient's Home

- Once a patient begins AIDS or TB treatment, the CHW visits the patient's home once a day to administer medications. The CHW should watch the patient take his/her medication. If the patient is having trouble with ART, the CHW visits twice a day to observe both doses.
- CHWs meet with the members of the health center team when the team makes home visits to patients, or when the CHW leader makes unannounced visits to meet with patients and monitor the work of the CHWs.

## At the Health Center

The CHW accompanies his/her AIDS patients for a consultation with clinical staff two weeks after ART initiation. In some programs, each AIDS patient is assigned to a group based on the starting date of treatment. Each group is assigned a specific day of the week for visits to the health center, thus allowing for coordinated care and monitoring of patient cohorts. Additional visits when: A patient is ill and needs to be seen by clinical staff. A CHW identifies a person in the community who shows symptoms of HIV, TB, or other illness. A CHW is assigned to a new patient. The staff at the health center asks to meet with the CHW. Twice a month If supervising TB patients, visit the health center to collect TB medicines. Once a month visit the health center to collect ART if supervising AIDS patients. Collect salary. Attend ongoing training and education sessions, CHW meetings, and meetings with health center staff. In some programs: Accompany HIV and TB patients for their monthly consultations. Accompany pregnant women enrolled in the PMTCT program for their monthly consultations and accompany HIV-positive mothers and their newborns for biweekly consultations.

In early drafts of the ANC health plan, CBHWs were seen as an important resource for PHC because of their potential to play a significant role in expanding and improving health services, provided they received effective support and ongoing training. They were viewed as catalysts for community development, who could mobilise people around issues such as the need for clean water, sanitation, waste disposal, safe playgrounds and parks. Further, they could empower people with health knowledge and encourage their participation in health issues such as nutrition, family planning and HIV/ AIDS. It was envisaged that they would form an integral part of the decentralised health services, and be compensated, either by the government, or the local community, according to their level of skills. This implied that they were to have career structure and pathways for promotion within the health system.

After the democratic transition in 1994, the hope that this idea would be implemented was initially in limbo.

The official policy watered down their role by stating that although CBHWs' programmes would be encouraged where they were integrated into local services, there would be no national programme.

In 1995, a national task force funded by the Health Systems Trust produced a report *"Assessing the Feasibility of Greater State Support to Community Based Health Programmes"* (CBHP) which recommended that a phased CBHP model be considered for implementation by the national government. In the first phase, it recommended that financial, political, structural and other support be given by the government to existing programmes in order to strengthen them.

## Community Baser Health Works

### *Advocates with experience in working with CBHWs value them because they:*

Are excellent health promoters who also play an important role in prevention, treatment, rehabilitation and palliation enhance community participation provide the District Health System (DHS) with a link to communities and a means of getting feedback. In a sense this allows DoH staff to feel the pulse of the people, helping them understand, for example, why people do or don't use certain services; what people know and why they are not accepting responsibility for certain issues. Unearth sensitive social problems such as child or woman abuse and reach people with physical disabilities who can otherwise only access the service with difficulty. Similarly, mental disease, which was previously felt to be a shame on the family – children once hidden or even chained, are now identified and referred for help. Bring all the stakeholders who need to collaborate into one forum. In this way a CBHWs' programme acts as a core integrative process around which all vertical programmes and diverse services can rally and provide a mechanism for socioeconomic development undertaken by a variety of other sectors.

### *Current Challenges for Current CBHWs' Programmes*

During the process of gathering material for this article, certain critical issues emerged repeatedly and provide a useful framework for analysis and suggest how improvements could be incorporated into future policy and programmes. Common challenges for CBHWs programmes are:

The fragmented roles of many different kinds of community based health workers – different and often competitive CBHWs provide DOTS support, HIV/AIDS, sex education, nutrition, IMCI, first aid, home-based care, etc. often without reference to each other or to 'generalist' CBHWs. They often lack the skills necessary to deal with even simple issues outside their range of narrow specialisation and this can lead to conflict. Many projects, in their urgency to implement vertical programmes, often introduce their own cadres of CBHWs only to find out later that this was not the best course of action. The large variation in incentives and payments for similar types of work. This has been responsible for confusion and conflict. Some 'volunteer' incentives are as low as Rs 250 per month, whereas other paid CHWs get about Rs. 600 per month. The excessive amount of days per week that unpaid workers or partially paid CBHWs are often expected to work. This has blurred the boundaries of 'voluntarism' and sometimes over-extended the resources of very poor people.

The disconcerting range in the amount and quality of training offered to different groups. This is not due to the justifiable need to adapt to local circumstance. Rather it is due to a lack of cooperative working. Curricula vary widely. Teaching materials that have already been produced are not being adequately disseminated, used and adapted. There is a continual re-invention of the wheel. Existing materials do not always seem to be consulted before new materials are developed. The inconsistent support and supervision given to different groups as is evident in many programmes

Monitoring of programmes is weak and evaluation results are sparse. This continues to be a problem, although there is an increasing amount of information on programmes that have been evaluated. Regrettably many of these evaluations reach a limited audience.

Transport constraints are a major obstacle even for those programmes where there are paid CBHWs. Many successful projects have required CHFs to have their own vehicles prior to being employed. Alternatively some are subsidised so that they can own their vehicles, and receive a transport allowance for their travel. Inadequate linkages with the district health system and a lack of involvement in intersectoral activity. Many districts do not understand the critical role of CBHWs' contribution to the success of their programmes. Poor integration with the work of community-based professionals, CBOs, NGOs, faith-based organisations (FBOs), funders, local and provincial government in different sectors. Functional District and Health Forums, which coordinate the activities of all stakeholders in the district, are absolutely essential and require strong government support. Without such forums, even the excellent work of a few NGOs or the government itself, flounders in the long term and the potential for developing conflict between different groups of CBHWs is great if vertical programmes do not agree on working together jointly at community level.

## Remuneration Issues

The question of who pays CBHWs is an important one from the point of view of the CBHW's accountability to the community. Ideally, salaries should be paid by the community-based NGO and not directly by the formal health services. The district health authority could pay the NGO or community structure responsible for the CHWs, according to the contractual agreement. Donor funding should be supplementary and used for testing innovations prior to widespread adoption. The principal funder should be the state given that the CBHWs is one components of the district health system budget.

The feasibility of national or provincial salary structures, standardised according to level of training and years of service should also be considered. There are various options for funding. The best option, given that government resources are restricted, is to promote public-private partnerships between the provincial Departments of Health and local private or overseas funding organisations who together can achieve more that what is possible from government sources alone.

### *Community Relationships and the Sustainability of CBHWs' Programmes*

Ignoring important lessons such as the need to pay CBHWs and not create conflicting roles is illustrated by the following case study of emerging conflict between a group of CHWs and home based volunteers. This type of situation has arisen in many different communities and is likely to occur, whenever the circumstances create these conditions.

### *Management of CBHWs' Programmes*

Various studiese have shown that the training of many health professionals such as doctors and nurses does not adequately prepare them for work in a community setting. In addition, the reported universal shortage of doctors, nurses, and other health personnel has been exacerbated recently by emigration of many professions from South Africa. As a result it has proved difficult to bring about transformation even within clinical settings where systems can be more easily managed within an environment that health professions understand. Community Based programmes which are poorly understood have therefore been almost entirely neglected.

Despite the difficulties, there is considerable agreement that CBHWs have a role to play in improving the health of communities and fill the gap in areas which existing health personnel cannot reach. In these areas CBHWs have a vital role and to do this, they need to be formally recognised as members of the district health team. The first crucial step requires the acknowledgement and recognition of CBHWs as an essential part of the district health team from the highest level in terms of both policy and committed funding.

### *Supervision Procedures and Structures of Accountability*

A simple practical system would be for each district health authority which receives funds from the provincial department of health, to contract one or more NGOs to provide specific sets of health, welfare and development outputs to be undertaken by CBHWs working within a defined population. In this way district health authorities retain responsibility for the services, while recognising that these specific services are best delivered by NGOs using CBHWs supported by CBOs and FBOs. Examples of services that could be contracted include DOTS services, HIV pre-and post-test counselling, HBC, care of orphans and vulnerable children, health promotion, rehabilitation work and potentially even antiretroviral treatment supervision. Some of the tasks would be undertaken by full-time paid CBHWs, while other tasks might be undertaken by part-time workers or volunteers, receiving remuneration or acknowledgement appropriate to the amount of time they contribute.

### Training of CBHWs

In general training should be a continuous, community-based, problemoriented, experiential education process. Apart from an initial orientation course and short specific course(s) the training should be undertaken where CBHWs

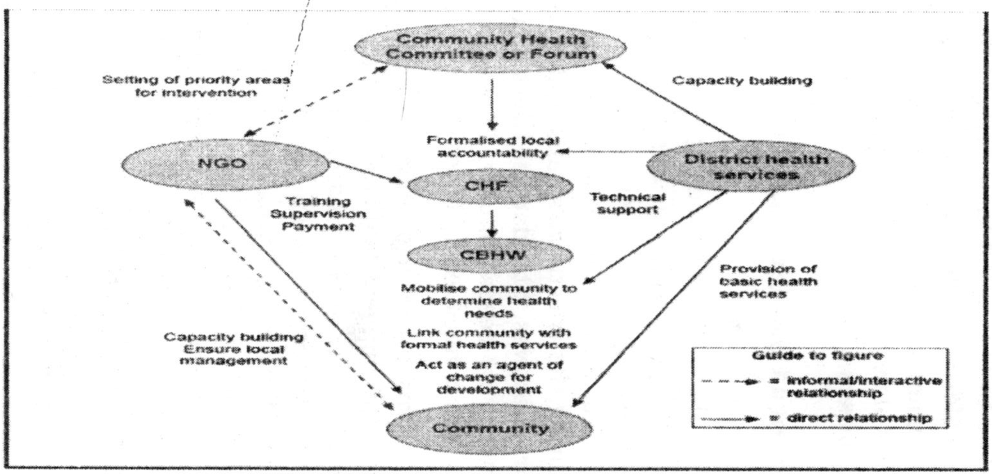


**Fig. 10.1:** Model for CHW supervision, support and accountability in the District Health System.

operate. The curriculum should be comprehensive, task oriented and outcomes based. Usually the training should start with an intensive course and then continue gradually over a few years with the CBHWs functioning during this time, gradually extending their range of their work as they become more competent. Most training programmes are not currently accredited by an approved educational institution, and this deprives CBHWs of recognition, which would enable them to develop their careers.

## New Tasks and Roles in a Complex, Changing Environment

Apart from CBHWs, the community and organisational support structures also require training. These include health professionals who require reorientation to the CBHWs scope of practice, as well as project managers responsible for monitoring the effectiveness and ability of CBHWs to meet their objectives. Standardised recording and reporting instruments are needed in order to evaluate progress and several projects have examples of these.

Figure 10.2: An approach to integrating the work of CBHWs in an HIV/AIDS environment could take on the role of coordinating and supporting community based support for sick adults and vulnerable children, including orphans. The model tries to incorporate the complex situation that exists at the moment where there are both full-time generalist CBHWs working in the same communities as a wide variety of more specialist volunteer cadres.

Primarily CBHWs would support caregivers in households, supplemented when necessary by volunteers from neighbourhood care groups, community or faith-based organisations. Organisational development would be undertaken to enhance the functioning of such groups. Other community groups who sew, garden, teach literacy, undertake para-legal work, etc. are all important in providing holistic care. In certain countries, where voluntary work is undertaken, credit is given to volunteers through the allocation of 'points', to which can be allocated certain benefits in respect of training, etc. Although less valuable than money, such schemes could at least document and acknowledge the large amount of time that some individuals volunteer.

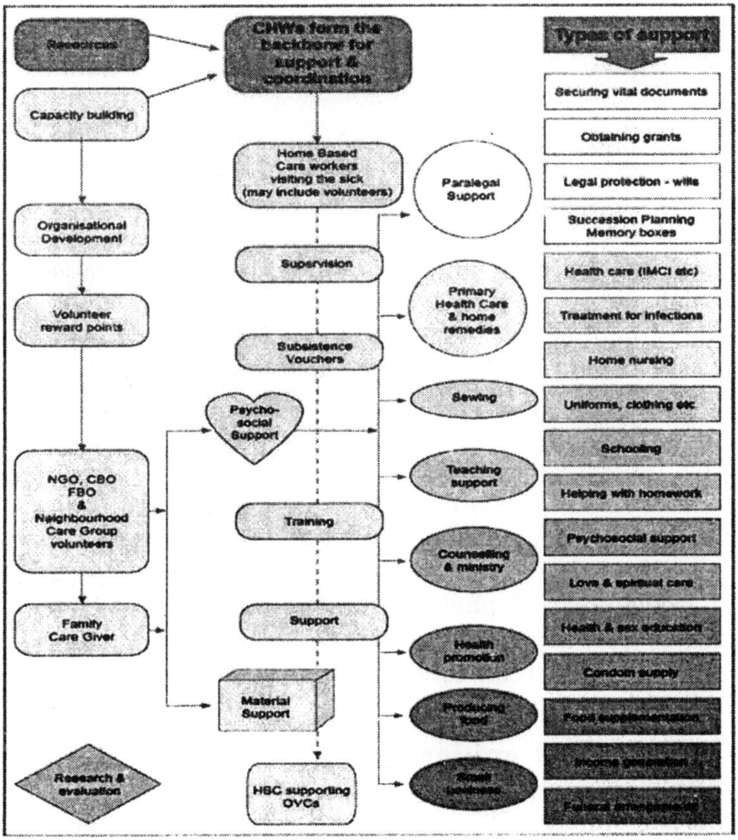


**Fig. 10.2:** Presents a comprehensive community based care model showing how CBHWs, adequately supported with resources and training.

# 11

# Social Epidemiology

Social epidemiology is defined as "The branch of epidemiology that studies the social distribution and social determinants of health," that is, "both specific features of, and pathways by which, societal conditions affect health." Social epidemiology may focus on individual-level measures, or on emergent social properties that have no correlate at the individual level; simultaneous analysis at both levels may be warranted. Use of such multilevel models also known as hierarchical and mixed effects models has grown in recent years, but as for all observational epidemiology, this approach suffers from theoretical and practical concerns. Social epidemiology overlaps with fields in the social sciences, most notably medical sociology and medical geography. However, these latter fields often use health and disease in order to explain specifically social phenomenon such as the growth of lay health advocacy movements, while social epidemiologists generally use social concepts in order to explain patterns of health in the population.

In **social epidemiology**, to speak of theory is simultaneously to speak of society and biology. It is, to speak of embodiment. At issue is how we literally incorporate, biologically, the world around us, a world in which we simultaneously are but one biological species among many—and one whose labour and ideas literally have transformed the face of this earth. To conceptualize and elucidate the myriad **social** and biological processes resulting in embodiment and its manifestation in populations' epidemiological profiles, we need theory. This is because theory helps us structure our ideas, so as to explain causal connections between specified phenomena within and across specified domains by using interrelated sets of ideas whose plausibility can be tested by human action and thought. Grappling with notions of causation, in turn, raises not only complex philosophical issues but also, in the case of **social epidemiology**, issues of accountability and agency: simply invoking abstract notions of 'society' and disembodied 'genes' will not suffice. Instead, the central question becomes: who and what is responsible for population patterns of health, disease, and well-being, as manifested in present, past and changing **social** inequalities in health?

Not surprisingly, theorizing about **social** inequalities in health runs deep. One reason is that it is fairly obvious that population patterns of good and bad health mirror population distributions of deprivation and privilege. Comments to this effect can be found in the Hippocratic corpus and in early texts of ancient Chinese medicine. Shared observations of disparities in health, however, do not necessarily translate to common understandings of cause; it is for this reason theory is key. Consider only centuries of debate in the US over the poor health of black Americans. In the 1830s and 1840s, contrary schools of thought ask: is it because blacks are intrinsically inferior to whites?— the majority view, or because they are enslaved?—as argued by Dr James McCune Smith (1811–65) and Dr James S Rock (1825–1866), two of the country's first credentialled African American physicians. In contemporary parlance, the questions become: do the causes lie in bad genes? bad behaviours? or accumulations of bad living and working conditions born of egregious **social** policies, past and present? The fundamental tension, then and now, is between theories that seek causes of **social** inequalities in health in innate *versus* imposed, or individual *versus* societal, characteristics.

Yet, despite the key role of theory, explicit or implicit, in shaping what it is we see—or do not see, what we deem knowable—or irrelevant, and what we consider feasible—or insoluble, literature articulating the theoretical frameworks informing research and debates in **social epidemiology**—and **epidemiology** more broadly—is sparse.

## 'Social Epidemiology' Gains a Name

Building on holistic models of health developed between World War I and World War II and on the '**social** medicine' framework forged during the 1940s, it is in the mid-20th century that **social epidemiology** gains its name-as-such. The term apparently first appears in the title of an article published by Alfred Yankauer in the *American Sociological Review* in 1950: 'The relationship of fetal and infant mortality to residential segregation: an inquiry into **social epidemiology**', a topic as timely now as it was then; Yankauer later becomes editor of the *American Journal of Public Health*. The term then reappears in the introduction to one of the first books pulling together the behavioural and medical sciences, edited by E Gartly Jaco, published in 1958, *Patients, Physicians, and Illness: Sourcebook in Behavioral Science and Medicine,* and is included in the title of Jaco's next book, *The Social Epidemiology of Mental Disorders; A Psychiatric Survey of Texas*, published in 1960. By 1969, enough familiarity with the field exists that Leo G Reeder presents a major address to the American Sociological Association called '**Social epidemiology**: an appraisal'. Defining '**social epidemiology**' as the 'study of the role of **social** factors in the aetiology of disease', he asserts that '**social epidemiology** ... seeks to extend the scope of investigation to include variables and concepts drawn from a theory'—in effect, calling for a marriage of sociological frameworks to epidemiological inquiry.

Soon thereafter, the phrase '**social epidemiology**' catches on in the epidemiological literature. Articles appear with such titles as: 'Contributions of **social epidemiology** to the study of medical care systems', published by S

Leonard Syme in 1971, and **Social epidemiology** and the prevention of cancer', published by Saxon Graham *et al.* in 1972. By the end of the century, the first textbook is published with the title *Social Epidemiology*, co-edited by Lisa Berkman and Ichiro Kawachi. Despite these gains, it is nevertheless sobering to realize that among the slightly over 432 000 articles indexed in Medline by the keyword **epidemiology** between 1966 and 2000, only 4% also employ the keyword '**social**', and—as Reeder surely would be sorry to learn—fewer than 0.1% are additionally indexed by the term 'theory'. Clearly, there is room for improvement—and reflection.

## Current Theoretical Trends in Social Epidemiology

Contemporary **social epidemiology**, however, is not without its theories. The three main theories explicitly invoked by practising **Social** epidemiologists are: (1) **psychosocial**, (2) **social** production of disease and/or political economy of health, and (3) **ecosocial** theory and related multilevel frameworks. All seek to elucidate principles capable of explaining **social** inequalities in health, and all represent what we would term theories of *disease distribution,* which presume but cannot be reduced to mechanism-oriented theories of *disease causation*. Where they differ is in their respective emphasis on different aspects of **social** and biological conditions in shaping population health, how they integrate **social** and biological explanations, and thus their recommendations for action.

## Psychosocial Theory

First, **psychosocial** theory As is typically the case with scientific theories, its genesis can be traced to problems prior paradigms could not explain, in this case, why it is that not all people exposed to germs become infected and not all infected people develop disease. One response, first articulated in the 1920s and refined in the 1950s as epidemiologists increasingly study cancer and cardiovascular disease, is to expand the aetiological framework from simply 'agent' to 'host-agent-environment'. Despite conceptual expansion, several restrictive assumptions still pervade the new framework's very language. 'Agency', for example, remains located in the 'agent'—typically an exogenous entity that acts upon a designated 'host'; terminology alone renders it inhospitable to conceive of the 'host' having 'agency'! 'Environment', moreover, serves as a catch—all category, with no distinctions offered between the natural world, of which we humans are a part and can transform, and **social** institutions and practices which we, as humans, create and for which we can hold each other accountable. Gaining complexity without an explicit accounting of **social** agency, the model becomes increasingly diffuse and, by 1960, the spiderless 'web of causation' is born.

The importance of the 'host-agent-environment' model for **psychosocial epidemiology** is evidenced by the title of one of the field's still-defining papers: John Cassel's (1921–76) final opus, 'The contribution of the **social** environment to host resistance'. Published in the *American Journal of* ***Epidemiology*** in 1976, the year of Cassel's death, this article expands upon frameworks elaborated in the 1940s and 1950s linking vulnerability to disease to both physical and psychological stress. Positing that in 'modern' societies exposure to pathogenic agents is ubiquitous, Cassel argues that to explain disease distribution we must, therefore investigate factors affecting susceptibility:

The question facing epidemiological inquiry then is, are there categories or classes of environmental factors that are capable of changing human resistance in important ways and making subsets of people more or less susceptible to these ubiquitous agents in our environment? To Cassel, in prosperous nations, relevant modifying factors are unlikely to include 'nutritional status, fatigue, overwork, or the like'. More promising candidates lie in what he calls the '**social** environment', comprised of **psychosocial** factors generated by human interaction. Cassel's central hypothesis is that the '**social** environment' alters host susceptibility by affecting neuroendocrine function. His list of relevant **psychosocial** factors includes: dominance hierarchies, **social** disorganization and rapid **social** change, marginal status in society, including **social** isolation, bereavement, and, acting as a buffer to all of the above, the '**psychosocial** asset' of '**social** support'. In Cassel's view, these **psychosocial** factors, considered together, explain the puzzle of why particular **social** groups are disproportionately burdened by otherwise markedly distinct diseases, e.g. tuberculosis, schizophrenia and suicide. Shifting attention from 'specific aetiology' to 'generalized susceptibility'—while acknowledging that what disease a person gets is dependent on prior exposures—Cassel ultimately concludes that, in his own words, the most 'feasible' and promising interventions to reduce disease will be 'to improve and strengthen the **social** supports rather than reduce the exposure to stressors'.

Following Cassel's article, research in **psychosocial epidemiology** blossoms. Between 1966 and 1974, the keywords 'psycho**social**' and '**epidemiology**' together index only 40 articles in Medline; between 1995 and 1999 alone, the number jumps to nearly 1200. Indicating new ideas are 'in the air', new polysyllabic terms emerge—such as psychoneuroendocrinology, psychoneuroimmunology and biopsycho **social**—whose proliferating prefixes hint some important concepts have yet to be tabbed down. Fortunately, newer additions gaining currency are appreciably shorter. One is 'allostasis', introduced as an alternative to 'homeostasis' in 1988 by Peter Sterling and Joseph Eyer to describe systems that achieve balance through change. Its successor, 'allostatic load', is then introduced by Bruce McEwen to describe 'wear-and-tear from chronic over—activity or underactivity' of systems 'that protect the body by responding to internal and external stress', including 'the autonomic nervous system, the hypothalamic-pituitary-adrenal axis, and cardiovascular, metabolic, and immune systems'. One new implication is that psychosocial stressors can be directly pathogenic, rather than alter only susceptibility. And, consonant with the emerging lifecourse perspective—which holds that health status at any given age reflects not only contemporary conditions but prior living circumstances, *in utero* onwards' allostatic load' draws attention to long-term effects of both chronic and acute stressors. Other new work extends Cassel's insights to focus on 'social capital' and 'social cohesion', which—although defined differently by diverse schools—are construed and contested as population-level psychosocial assets which shape population health by influencing norms and strengthening bonds of 'civil society'.

In nutshell, then, a psychosocial framework directs attention to endogenous biological responses to human interactions. Its focus is on responses to 'stress' and on stressed people in need of psychosocial resources. Comparatively less attention, theoretically and empirically, is accorded to: (1) who and what generates psychosocial insults and buffers, and (2) how their distribution—along with that of ubiquitous or non-ubiquitous pathogenic physical, chemical, or biological agents—is shaped by social, political and economic policies. Time also takes a back seat, in that except for reference to periods of rapid social change, the question of whether changing levels of stress are sufficient to explain secular trends in disease and death receives little attention. It is as if, paraphrasing Aaron Antonovsky's (1923–94) penultimate lament, the study of why some people swim well and others drown when tossed into a river displaces study of who is tossing whom into the current—and what else might be in the water. To ask the latter questions, however, brings us to other schools of thought.

## Social Production of Disease or Political Economy of Health

A second theoretical framework accordingly introduces agency to the 'upstream-downstream' metaphors increasingly invoked in **social epidemiology** today. Hearkening back to **social** analyses of health of the 1830s and 1840s, as well as 1930s and 1940s, this school of thought—emerging in the politically turbulent 1960s and 1970s—focuses on what it terms the '**social** production of disease' and 'political economy of health'. Articles appear with such titles as: 'A case for refocusing upstream: the political economy of illness', 'the **social** production of disease and illness', and—recalling the trend's Marxist origins and its advocacy of 'materialist' analyses of health, even: 'Hypertension in American society: an introduction to historical materialist **epidemiology**'. These and kindred papers are published, however in journals unlikely to be on the regular browsing list of most epidemiologists—for example, the International Journal of Health Services, founded in 1971 by Vicente Navarro and Review of Radical Political Economics. By 1979, the trend's broad theoretical contours are encapsulated in two books: The Political Economy of Health, by Lesley Doyal, a British health policy analyst, and Epidemiologia Economia Medicinay Politica, by Jamie Breilh, an Ecuadorian epidemiologist.

Arising in part as critique of proliferating blame-the-victim 'lifestyle' theories, which emphasize individuals' responsibility to 'choose' so called 'healthy lifestyles' and to cope better with 'stress', these new analyses explicitly address economic and political determinants of health and disease, including structural barriers to people living healthy lives. At issue are priorities of capital accumulation and their enforcement by the state, so that the few can stay rich or become richer while the many are poor—whether referring to nations or to classes within a specified country. Recast in this manner, determinants of health are analysed in relation to who benefits from specific policies and practices, at whose cost. Core questions include: how does prioritizing capital accumulation over human need affect health, as evinced through injurious work-place organization and exposure to occupational hazards, inadequate pay scales, profligate pollution, and rampant commodification of virtually every human activity, need, and desire? What, too, is the public health impact of state policies enforcing these priorities?—whether by regulation or de-regulation of corporations, the real estate industry, and interest rates; or by enactment or repeal or enforcement or neglect of tax codes, trade agreements, labour laws, and environmental laws; or by absolute and relative levels of spending on **social** programmes *versus* prisons and the military; or by diplomatic relations with, economic domination of, and even invasion of countries abroad? The underlying hypothesis is that economic and political institutions and decisions that create, enforce, and perpetuate economic and **social** privilege and inequality are root— or 'fundamental' —causes of **social** inequalities in health. Revisiting issues of agency and accountability, theoretical analyses examine interdependence of institutional and interpersonal manifestations of unjust power relations; resources to counter these adverse conditions are reframed, no longer 'buffers' but rather strategies for community not just individual 'empowerment' and **social** change.

Within this trend, initial conceptual and empirical analyses chiefly focus on class inequalities in health within and between countries. Related contemporary questions include: what are the health impacts of rising income inequality, of structural adjustment programmes imposed by the International Monetary Fund and the World Bank, of neoliberal economic policies favouring dismantling of the welfare state, or of free-trade agreements imposed by the World Trade Organization? Other analyses address **social** inequalities involving race/ethnicity, gender and sexuality, as they play out within and across socioeconomic position, within and across diverse societies. Relevant questions include: what are the health consequences of experiencing economic and non-economic forms of racial discrimination?—or of men dominating and abusing women?—or of civilians and soldiers verbally or physically queer-bashing lesbian, gay, and transgendered people? Recently emerging environmental justice movements likewise bring critical attention to corporate decisions and government complicity in transferring toxic waste to poor countries and to poor regions within wealthy countries, especially poor communities of colour. The call for action premised on this framework is thus, minimally, for 'healthy public policies', especially redistributive polices to reduce poverty and income inequality, if not for 'wider campaigns for sustainable development, political freedom, and economic and **social** justice'.

Four implications for action accordingly flow from a **social** production of disease/political economy of health perspective. One is that strategies for improving population health require a vision of **social** justice, backed up by active organizing to change unjust **social** and economic policies and norms. Another is that absent concerns about **social** equity, economic growth and public health interventions may end up aggravating, not ameliorating, **social** inequalities in health if the economic growth exacerbates economic inequality and if the public health interventions are more accessible and acceptable to affluent individuals. A third is that greater familiarity with the emerging field of health and human rights—supplemented by analyses of who gains from neglecting or violating these rights—is likely to improve the real-world efficacy of **social** epidemiologists' work, by providing a systematic framework for delineating governmental accountability to promote and protect health, premised, in the first instance, upon the 1948 Universal Declaration of Human Rights and its recognition of the indivisibility and interdependence of civil, political, economic, **social** and cultural rights. And fourth, **social** epidemiologists must be key actors in ensuring viability of the vital public health activity of monitoring **social** inequalities in health, for without such work—which is our particular job to do—it is impossible to gauge progress and setbacks in reducing **social** inequalities in health.

Yet, despite its invaluable contributions to identifying **social** determinants of population health, a **social** production of disease/political economy of health perspective affords few principles for investigating *what* these determinants are determining. Biology is opaque. Focusing on relative risks across specified **social** groups, these analyses rely chiefly on critical appraisals of population distributions of known risk and protective factors, most of which ironically are individual-level characteristics identified by conventional epidemiological research. In the case of breast cancer, for example, analyses might focus on **social** determinants of a variety of reproductive risk factors e.g. age at menarche, use of oral contraceptives, age at and number of pregnancies, but would be as constrained as conventional analyses in explaining the portion of cases not attributable to these factors. Nor does an emphasis on 'fundamental **social** causes' offer principles for thinking through, systematically, *whether*—and if so, *which*—specific public health and policy interventions are needed to curtail **social** inequalities in health, above and beyond securing adequate living standards and reducing economic inequality. In the background is Thomas McKeown's (1914–88) famous argument that 19th century declines in infectious disease mortality in the UK and US are due chiefly to improved nutrition, not medical interventions. Yet, as Simon Szreter and other public health historians have convincingly demonstrated, McKeown is only half right: although medical care *per se* can claim little credit for declines in incidence or mortality before World War II, economic growth alone did not improve health. Rather, specific public health policies, e.g. those aimed at cleaning the water and eliminating bovine tuberculosis, were also of fundamental importance. Stated another way, both improved living standards and non-economic interventions albeit with economic costs and consequences matter. Moving from an 'either/or' to a 'both/ and' logic requires multilevel frameworks integrating **social** and biological reasoning and history, and it is to such new theoretical efforts in **social**

**epidemiology**—building on prior ideas infused into '**social** medicine' in the 1940s.

## Ecosocial Theory and Related Multilevel Dynamic Perspectives

Perhaps one sign of the ferment in contemporary **social** epidemiological thought is the fact that pictorial depictions of newer frameworks to explain current and shifting patterns of disease distribution refuse to stay in a single plane. Instead, unlike prior images—whether of a triangle connecting 'host', 'agent' and 'environment', or a 'chain of causes' arrayed along a scale of biological organization, from 'society' to 'molecular and submolecular particles', or a spiderless two-dimensional 'web of causation', or a 'causal pie' sans cook,—the new mental pictures are both multidimensional and dynamic. The terminology, too, is changed, as each invokes literal—and not just metaphorical—notions of ecology, situating humans as one notable species among many cohabiting, evolving on, and altering our dynamic planet. They are explained have.

1. **'ecosocial' theory**, a term was introduced in 1994, with its visual fractal metaphor of an evolving bush of life intertwined at every scale, micro to macro, with the scaffolding of society that different core **social** groups daily reinforce or seek to alter;
2. **'eco-epidemiology'** proposed by Mervyn Susser in 1996, with its image of 'Chinese boxes', referring to nested 'interactive systems', each with its localized structures and relationships; and
3. the **'social-ecological systems perspective'** invoked by Anthony McMichael in 1999, depicting a cube, representing the 'present/past', whose three axes extend from individual-to-population, proximate-to-distal, static/modular to life course and which is projected forward, to 'future'.

Their goal is not a totalizing theory to explain everything and, therefore nothing, but rather to generate a set of integral and testable principles useful for guiding specific inquiry and action, much as evolutionary theory biological disciplines ranging from paleontology to molecular biology. And, specifically in the case of **ecosocial** theory, its fractal image deliberately fosters analysis of current and changing population patterns of health, disease and well-being in relation to *each* level of biological, ecological and **social** organization e.g. cell, organ, organism/ individual, family, community, population, society and ecosystem as manifested at *each* and every scale, whether relatively small and fast e.g. enzyme catalysis or relatively large and slow e.g. infection and renewal of the pool of susceptibles for a specified infectious disease.

That each of these frameworks explicitly incorporates the prefix 'eco' or term 'ecological' in its name is revealing. Ecology, after all, is a science devoted to study of evolving interactions between living organisms and inanimate matter and energy over time and space. Core to an ecological approach are concerns with:

1. *scale*: referring to quantifiable dimensions of observed spatiotemporal phenomenon, whether measured in nanoseconds or millennia, microns or kilometres;
2. *level of organization*: theorized and inferred, in relation to specified nested hierarchies, from individual to population to ecosystem;
3. *dynamic states*: reflecting combined interplay of specified animate and inanimate 'inputs' and 'outputs', with recognition that operative processes and phenomena may be scale-dependent e.g. factors relevant to self-regulation of an organism's body temperature differ from those involved in self-regulation of the earth's global temperature;
4. *mathematical modelling*: employed to illuminate how groupings of organisms and processes work

together, using both idealized minimal and detailed synthetic models—both to render complexity intelligible and because large-scale experiments are rarely feasible;

5. *understanding unique phenomena in relation to general processes*: in the case of populations, for example, no two forests are ever identical, yet share important features and processes in common relevant to understanding their genesis, longevity, and degradation or decline.

Recognizing, however, the importance of **social**, political, and economic processes in shaping epidemiological profiles, two of the frameworks—'eco**social'** and '**social**-ecological systems perspective'—additionally explicitly indicate in their very names that ecological analysis is not intended to be a substitute or metaphor for **social** analysis. Rather, they distinguish ecological theory from the diverse **social** theories upon which they and the other **social** epidemiological frameworks rely. In doing so, these frame works part company with other theoretical perspectives that invoke 'ecology' as a metaphor, e.g. '**social** ecology' and 'human ecology', and which employ organic analogies that obscure accountability for **social** divisions and processes by reinterpreting them as 'natural' phenomena e.g. migration of populations to cities and gentrification recast as analogous to plant succession.

Nascent, these emerging ecologically inclined multi-level **social** epidemiological frameworks remain rather sketchy, the bare beginnings of a mental map. Much more elaboration is required; calling the question can perhaps spur the needed work. Concomitantly, explicit applications to aetiologic inquiry and to interventions are only just underway. From an eco **social** perspective, however, it is possible to formulate several constructs that can begin to serve as a mental checklist for epidemiological research. Focused on the guiding question of 'who and what drives current and changing patterns of **social** inequalities in health', the **ecosocial** approach but not necessarily the other multilevel frameworks fully embraces a **social** production of disease perspective while aiming to bring in a comparably rich biological and ecological analysis. Relevant **ecosocial** constructs thus minimally include:

1. embodiment, a concept referring to how we literally incorporate, biologically, the material and **social** world in which we live, from conception to death; a corollary is that no aspect of our biology can be understood absent knowledge of history and individual and societal ways of living.
2. pathways of embodiment, structured simultaneously by: (a) societal arrangements of power and property and contingent patterns of production, consumption, and reproduction, and (b) constraints and possibilities of our biology, as shaped by our species' evolutionary history, our ecological context, and individual histories, that is, trajectories of biological and **social** development;
3. cumulative interplay between exposure, susceptibility and resistance, expressed in pathways of embodiment, with each factor and its distribution conceptualized at multiple levels (individual, neighbourhood, regional or political jurisdiction, national, inter—or *supra*-national) and in multiple domains (e.g. home, work, school, other public settings), in relation to relevant ecological niches, and manifested in processes at multiple scales of time and space;
4. accountability and agency, expressed in pathways of and knowledge about embodiment, in relation to institutions in terms of government, business and public sector, households and individuals, and also to accountability and agency of epidemiologists and other scientists for theories used and ignored to

> explain **social** inequalities in health; a corollary is that, given likely complementary causal explanations at different scales and levels, epidemiological studies should explicitly name and consider the benefits and limitations of their particular scale and level of analysis.

With these constructs at hand, we can begin to elucidate population patterns of health, disease and well-being as biological expressions of **social** relations, and can likewise begin to see how **social** relations influence our most basic understandings of biology and our **social** constructions of disease—thereby potentially generating new knowledge and new grounds for action.

Consider, as one example, the phenomenon of pregnancy in relation to risk of cancer. Let us start with breast cancer. As is wellknown, pregnancy decreases risk of breast cancer over the lifetime if it occurs early, but thereafter increases risk, especially after age 35. This phenomenon is often invoked to explain, in part, why incidence of breast cancer increases with affluence and why the rate has climbed during the 20th century over and above increases due to earlier age at menarche, since more educated women tend to have children later in life and educational level of women, especially in industrialized societies, has generally been on the rise. Notably, all three **social** epidemiological frameworks—**psychosocial, social** production of disease, and **ecosocial**—would highlight how **social** conditions, including women's **social** status, available birth control technology and access to abortion, affect age at first pregnancy. An eco **social** approach, however, would raise questions beyond **social** determinants of age at first pregnancy to inquire how pregnancy itself is conceptualized in relation to risk of breast cancer. Constructs of 'embodiment', 'pathways of embodiment', and the 'dynamic and cumulative interplay between exposure, susceptibility and resistance' would require analysing pregnancy in relation to developmental biology of the breast especially maturation of lobules and ducts and also altered rates of apoptosis as well as its effects on the endocrine system synthesis of hormones within the breast plus alteration in magnitude and frequency of hormonal fluctuations and cardiovascular system increased vascularization of the breast. A concern with 'accountability and agency', as well as scale and level, would additionally challenge gender-biased views positing reproductive hormones as primary determinants of women's health. The net result would be to *reconceptualize* pregnancy not simply as an 'exposure' but also as a biological process capable of altering susceptibility to exogenous carcinogens. This is the thinking, in part, behind new aetiologic research on environmental pollution and breast cancer; although 'answers' are not yet in as to causal relationships, at least the question is posed.

Similar fresh and integrative thinking motivates a recent novel study including men and women which asks if relationships between parity and cancer incidence are due to the biology of pregnancy or to other **social** factors 'that are influenced by or are influencing family size'. Tellingly, parity is *equally* associated among women and men with risk of three types of cancer: oral and pharyngeal reflecting greater use of tobacco and alcohol by childless men and women, a topic itself meriting investigation and malignant melanoma—for which the parity/ risk association had been previously interpreted only in hormonal terms, and only for women. For two sites, however, thyroid and Hodgkin's disease, parity is associated with incidence only among women. One implication of these findings is not to presume parity exerts effects solely by pregnancy—related biological processes; the other is to consider the **social** meaning of parity even when the biology of pregnancy is relevant. Simplistic divisions of the **social** and biological will not suffice. Consider, too, how an **ecosocial** perspective can contribute to unravelling the unexplained excess risk of hypertension among African Americans. Moving beyond eclectic, purely psychological, or purely economic sets of risk factors, the four **ecosocial** constructs can systematically be used to propose six discrete—yet entangled—multilevel pathways linking expressions of racial discrimination and their biological embodiment across the lifecourse. These are:

1. *economic and social deprivation*: for example, residential and occupational segregation lead to greater economic deprivation among African Americans and increased likelihood of living in neighbourhoods without good supermarkets; risk of hypertension is increased by cheap, high fat, high salt and low vegetable diets; also, economic deprivation increases risk of being born preterm, thereby harming development of kidneys and increasing likelihood of chronic salt retention;
2. *toxic substances and hazardous conditions*: residential segregation increases risk of exposure to lead paint in older houses and to soil contaminated by lead from car exhaust due to closer proximity of residences to streets or freeways; lead damages renal physiology, increasing risk of hypertension;
3. ***socially** inflicted trauma*: perceiving, recalling or anticipating interpersonal racial discrimination provokes fear and anger, triggering the 'flight-or-fight' response; chronic triggering of this pathway increases allostatic load, leading to sustained hypertension;
4. *targeted marketing of commodities*: targeted marketing of high—alcohol content beverages to black communities increases likelihood of harmful use of alcohol to reduce feelings of distress; excess alcohol consumption elevates risk of hypertension;

5. *inadequate health care*: poorer detection and clinical management of hypertension among African Americans increases risk of untreated and uncontrolled hypertension;
6. *resistance to racial oppression:* individual and community resources and **social** movements to counter racism and to enhance dignity, along with enactment and implementation of legislation to outlaw racial discrimination, reduces risk of hypertension among African Americans.

Embracing **social** determinants ignored by biomedical approaches, the **ecosocial** approach thus recasts alleged 'racial' differences in biology e.g., kidney function, blood pressure as mutable and embodied biological expressions of racism. Emphasizing accountability, it extends beyond **psychosocial** explanations focused on 'anger' and 'hostility' to the **social** phenomena—in this case, interpersonal and institutional discrimination—eliciting these responses, as mediated by material pathways. Highlighting dynamic and cumulative interplay between exposure, susceptibility and resistance, it advances beyond **social** production of disease analyses typically focused on racial/ethnic disparities in socioeconomic position among adults to highlight discrimination within class strata plus ongoing biological impact of economic deprivation in early life. Urging conceptual integration, it advocates coordinated research and action cognizant of the specified multiple pathways and geared to explaining current and changing rates of hypertension, premised on the view that our common humanity demands no less if we are to understand and rectify **social** inequalities in health. Thus, more than simply adding 'biology' to '**social**' analyses, or '**social** factors' to 'biological' analyses, the **ecosocial** framework begins to envision a more systematic integrated approach capable of generating new hypotheses, rather than simply reinterpreting factors identified by one approach, viz., biological in terms of another, viz., **social**. Suggesting much work remains to be done.

Scientific theories provide explanations for what can be systematically observed. They include exemplars—typical problem-solutions within a discipline—and they may also include qualitative principles, quantitative laws or rules, and sometimes the methods used to test them. Some theories are almost exclusively qualitative, while others are primarily quantitative, and some are a mix of concepts, methods and empirical generalizations, the latter leading to predictions—the hypotheses mentioned earlier—that are then tested in studies. Scientific theories are often contrasted with the "facts" that empirical studies produce as a way of testing those theories.

Theories of ethics, on the other hand, are typically qualitative and are used to illuminate our understanding of what we believe is right and good in the context of our professional practice. Theories of ethics and their accompanying methods also help guide the actions taken by those who practice a discipline. They are especially important for health-related disciplines, such as epidemiology, demography, medicine and nursing, wherein practitioners take actions that affect the health and well-being of others. The relationship of ethical theory to ethical decisions is not analogous to the relationship between scientific theory and empirical evidence. Although there is a growing interest in descriptive ethics, wherein investigators systematically describe what ethical positions individual patients, physicians, research participants, and others have on issues relevant to epidemiology and other health disciplines, contrasting ethical theory with these empirical results as way of testing theory is not typically undertaken.

Some specific examples of scientific and ethical theories relevant to epidemiology will be provided below, but first it will be important to define more carefully what is meant by the "practice" of epidemiology?

## The Practice of Epidemiology

The practice of epidemiology is characterized in terms of two closely connected activities: the scientific study of the determinants and distributions of disease and the application of the knowledge gained to prevent disease and improve the health of populations. Although this definition has changed over time and some debate exists about the extent to which epidemiologists should participate in public health advocacy, the practice of epidemiology covers a broad territory: doing scientific studies, communicating the results of those studies, and participating along with many other disciplines and institutions in public health interventions and policymaking.

## Two Types of Theory for the Practice of Epidemiology

Two major categories of theories are relevant to this practice: scientific theories and theories of ethics. Scientific theories provide explanations and predictions for epidemiologic studies of disease etiology and prevention. Scientific theories explain, in other words, why disease occurs and how it manifests itself in cells, tissues, individual organisms and in the diverse social groups populations that inhabit the globe. For example, theories of the healthy worker effect provide explanations for why comparison of disease rates between occupational populations and general populations have specific patterns. Causal theories of disease are centrally important to epidemiology. Over the years, they have featured miasma, germs, individual risk factors, and more recently, social determinants in the context of probabilistic and counterfactual models. Some have argued that scientific theories appropriate to epidemiology should be narrowly conceived as universal laws subject to strict falsification in line with a longstanding fascination by epidemiologists with Popperian philosophy. Others propose that theoretical development in epidemiology should include a much broader range of explanatory constructs incorporating biological and social determinants. We suspect that the latter approach may be the wiser one, although the testability of any causal theory is an important concern. Developing and testing scientific theories is consistent with a core value of the discipline: that the fundamental goal of the profession is to better understand why disease occurs and how public health can be improved through disease prevention and control efforts. Epidemiologists have a pragmatic bent, in other words, and will use, whatever intervention "works" from currently available theories, subject to ethical constraints.

Theories of ethics provide principles, warrants, and methods for acquiring and acting upon the knowledge gained in epidemiology's scientific pursuits. Theories of ethics guide epidemiologic practitioners in making good—justified—decisions about when and under what conditions public health interventions should be undertaken. Theories of ethics can also provide a strong foundation for guiding scientific practices; a good example is the role that virtue theory can play in the prevention of scientific misconduct. Theories comprised of mid-level bioethical principles— respect for persons, nonmaleficence, beneficence, and justice—are perhaps the most familiar to health professionals and are often used in the context of research ethics, the ethics of preventive interventions, and as foundations for professional ethics guidelines. Other theories of ethics—e.g. communitarian ethics—will likely become increasingly relevant to epidemiology as its relationship to public health is further developed.

### Is Epidemiology Atheoretical?

In light of the material presented above, a negative answer to the question "is epidemiology atheoretical?" may seem obvious, although a better crafted answer will emerge by carefully defining what is meant by "atheoretical?" Three candidate definitions follow:

1. devoid of theory none used in practice and none impacting on practice and none lurking behind the scenes
2. without a unique theory without a theory for epidemiology to call its own
3. practice largely unaffected by explicit applications of theory, tests of theories, or efforts to develop and apply theories

Epidemiology is not—cannot—be atheoretical in the first-two senses above. No one can deny the continued relevance of the germ theory of important diseases—AIDS, tuberculosis, hepatitis—and the closely—related models of infectious disease epidemics that have been used for nearly a hundred years with ever increasing precision. Epidemic theory *is* an essential theory for epidemiology. Nevertheless, epidemiology can legitimately be considered "atheoretical" in the third sense given above. Theory just does not matter much in contemporary literature and practice; this is especially true in what is often referred to as chronic disease epidemiology? If it were possible to survey the typical practitioner of epidemiology about the role of theory in their practice, it is suspected that most would respond with a puzzled shrug of the shoulders much more often than with a hearty retort along the lines of "Yes, theory is very important to my work!" Observing the discipline as it reveals itself in print and on podiums worldwide, one can easily get the impression that epidemiology is, as some have claimed, primarily an applied science, devoid of theory unless method and ethical issues count as theories. Scientific and ethical theories may lurk in the background, but do not play a prominent role in the design and analysis of scientific studies nor, for that matter, do they clearly affect the interpretation of evidence and the application of the knowledge gained to improve the public's health in current practice.

Theory, in other words, remains a low priority in contemporary epidemiology. True, there are some relatively recent threads of debate to the contrary for scientific theories, a tradition especially within behavioral and social epidemiology to study health related phenomena in terms of theoretical models, a growing interest in linking causal models with statistical analysis, and a complementary effort to bring theories of ethics to bear on the practice of epidemiology. And epidemiology has for at least fifty years promoted its methods to the point where one could argue that they constitute a "theory" although it is causal and statistical theory that form the foundation for epidemiologic methodology. But I cannot in good conscience argue that theory is a prominent concern in the daily lives of professional practitioners, including its university-based scholars.

**Theory Matters**

In conclusion, theory matters: both to define **social epidemiology** and to distinguish among trends within this field. These diverse frameworks encourage us to think critically and systematically about intimate and integral connections between our **social** and biological existence—and, especially in the case of **social** production of disease and eco**social** theory, to name explicitly who benefits from and is accountable for **social** inequalities in health. By focusing attention on under-theorized and under-researched conjoint **social** and biological determinants of disease distribution, these theories, even in nascent form, can potentially give new grounds for action—and underscore that theory, absent action, is an empty promise.

Ultimately, it remains to be seen whether any of the three theoretical frameworks discussed in this article—psycho**social, social** production of disease/political economy of health, and emerging **ecosocial** and other multilevel frameworks—are best suited for guiding **social** epidemiological research in the 21st century. If not these theories, however, other frameworks will need to be elaborated to enhance **social** epidemiologists' ability to analyse and provide evidence useful for addressing the myriad ways we both embody and transform the co-mingled **social** and biological world in which we live, love, work, play, fight, ail and die. To generate the data required to test and refine our theoretical frameworks, priority must thus be accorded to: (1) enhanced monitoring of **social** inequalities of health, so that data are available—cross-stratified—by class, gender, and race/ethnicity and any other **social** groups subject to economic and **social** deprivation and discrimination, to gauge progress and setbacks in reducing **social** inequalities in health, (2) funding interdisciplinary aetiologic research to identify conjoint **social** and biological determinants of disease at appropriate spatiotemporal scales and levels of organization, and (3) funding interventions based on the findings of this research—with the content of all three priority areas determined by coalitions including sectors of society most burdened by **social** inequalities in health.

# 12

# Bioethics in Medical Profession

During the past decade, biomedical ethics commonly called bioethics has become a popular topic for media coverage. This is largely due to increased complexity of caring for patients and the difficult decisions that new technologies demand. Examples include high-visibility issues like the completion of the human genome project, cloning, patenting of human tissue products, and transplants. However, doctors worry or should worry more often about less visible but more common issues such as ensuring patient self-determination and proper informed consent for medical procedures, end-of-life decision-making, research ethics, reproductive medicine, and managed care and related economic issues.

Students and physicians need education about ethical issues and laws. Despite the trendy nature of cloning and other hot issues, there are numerous ways in which the knowledge that practicing physicians have about medical ethics and law can have a more direct impact on the type and quality of care that the average patient receives. In order to provide medical care in an ethical and humane way, physicians need to be *better* educated about specific aspects of ethical medical practice and learn to think critically about the increasingly complex world of medical practice. Routine bioethics education for medical students and resident physicians, and continuing medical education for practicing doctors, are the best ways to accomplish this goal.

What skills and characteristics in physicians in addition to scientific expertise are necessary for them to practice good medicine? It is vital that physicians understand basic aspects of law and the legal system in order to practice good medicine. This means that knowledge of law has profound ethical implications for patient care and well-being. It could be noted that physicians know substantially less about medical law when they get such legal information from other physicians. This is not to suggest that all physicians are ignorant of relevant law but rather, that there is great variability among physicians in knowledge of law and ethics. Thus bioethicists, who are trained in specific aspects of medical law and who may themselves be physicians, are appropriate persons to supplement physicians' knowledge in this area. Other research has demonstrated that how people think about risk like the risk of malpractice lawsuits affects the way they react to it, creating ethical consequences. Because risk management is an issue that concerns most physicians, improving doctors' knowledge of medical law can help them better understands and estimate risks, as well as learns where they may be unconsciously overestimating certain risks in ways that have negative effects for patient care. Thus, law and ethics are inevitably intertwined in clinical medicine.

Knowledge of the health care delivery system is vital. Understanding social and institutional aspects of health care delivery is also vital. Doctors should know how hospitals and other medical institutions function and how different health care providers and administrators work together. These relationships include physicians' interactions with nurses, respiratory therapists, physical therapists, occupaticnal therapists, nurses' aides, and members of hospital administration in the areas of finance and risk management. Bioethicists can assist physicians-in-training to understand how such institutional relationships may function differently from those to which they are accustomed and help them assimilate to new institutional structures.

Good physician-role-models also play a significant part in this process.

Bioethicists can teach doctors and students about clinical ethics. Practical application of bioethics concepts is essential for the well-being of both patients and physicians. The integration of bioethics into clinical medicine through the practice of "clinical ethics" is a major part of many bioethicists' jobs. This usually occurs in at least two ways, first by educating physicians-in-training, and second, by conducting clinical ethics consultations, which have both an educational role and are designed to assist with a particular ethical problem in a clinical setting. In this setting, the bioethicist provides services that assist specific patients and their families, as well as health care providers. By modeling good clinical ethics practice, bioethicists can teach physicians ways to better perform these functions.

Physicians should be aware of current health policies and legislation. Understanding health policy and the legislative process is an important part of delivering good health care in the modern world. Some good examples of issues from the realm of health policy, of which physicians should be aware, include: state and central governmental regulation of health care financing; public health and health promotion efforts; legislative action on end-of-life decisions and pain control; pharmaceutical regulation; and the impact of emerging genetic testing and other biotechnology. Physicians having a strong interest in one or more of these issues may wish to become active in advocating a particular piece of legislation or other policy. Because many physicians do not ordinarily think in these terms, bioethicists can make them aware of ways that health care providers can become more active in the public policy process.

Bioethicists can also introduce physicians to medical humanities. Knowledge and experience of the humanities is a key element of caring for patients as persons. For example when physicians read poetry or fiction that explores aspects of human illness and suffering, it provides them with exposure to the human experience of health care that may become lost in the daily activities of technological medicine. The humanities can thus add to the richness of both patients' and physicians' experiences. Many bioethicists are trained in particular disciplines of the humanities, and some bioethicists have specific training in "medical humanities." Thus, the bioethicist is the ideal person to provide such background for aspiring physicians.

Physicians should be wary of conflict-of-interest situations. With academic medicine becoming ever more dependent on the private sector in health care, the ability to think critically about ethical issues and take appropriate action in response is a key element of academic physicians' work. A good example is the increasing impact of conflicts of interest. As research physicians increasingly have a direct financial interest in the outcome of their research, bioethicists can provide a sensitivity to the public perceptions that may emerge from such financial relationships. Critical thinking is the stock-in-trade of bioethicists and they can foster it in many ways with physicians.

## Role of Bioethicists

Bioethicists have the expertise to examine the complex issues facing the medical profession. Bioethicists are generally trained in philosophical ethics and law, as well as the social sciences and humanities. However, the level and type of training among individuals varies to a significant extent, so physicians seeking bioethics consultations should be aware of the particular type of expertise they need and search out a bioethicist with proper background when possible.

Bioethicists can provide a more objective and balanced view of complex ethical issues in health care settings. In other words, bioethicists can often provide an outside perspective on medical care. However, as bioethics practice becomes a more routine part of medicine there is a danger of bioethicists being co-opted by the system they are charged with improving. For this reason, bioethicists should be scrupulous in maintaining their objectivity where possible. Many bioethicists have extensive experience in analyzing and resolving actual dilemmas in clinical medicine. In fact, "clinical ethics" has become an unofficial sub-specialty of the field. Educational efforts specifically targeted to teach bioethics issues to physicians are effective. Recent research suggests that after a course in bioethics, physicians have a more subtle understanding of ethical issues and are better able to analyze relevant issues critically.

## Factors Converge in Bioethicists

Controlling a terminally ill patient's pain is a good example of treatment complexity. An excellent example of the importance of all these factors is the ongoing debate over control of severe pain in terminally ill patients. First, because of the risk of diversion of narcotic medications into illegal markets, there are strong legal restrictions placed on prescribing of these drugs. Fear of overly-zealous government enforcement of these laws may cause many physicians to err on the side of caution and prescribe lower doses of these medications than necessary to relieve patients' pain. Thus, regulations affecting pain relief medication can have unintended consequences of diminishing patients' ability to obtain legitimate relief. Improved legal knowledge among physicians may reduce fear and misunderstanding and may increase prescribing of appropriate levels of medication for pain relief.

However, knowledge of these unintended effects is also necessary among policymakers and legislators. The misnamed Pain Relief Promotion is but one example of how policy and medical care may collide in ways that have negative effects on patient care. This law was designed to override the physician-assisted suicide law currently in effect in Oregon and to prohibit other states from enacting similar laws. Expert bioethicists believe that if this law were to pass, palliative care could be compromised due to the fear of criminal prosecution of physicians. Thus, physicians concerned about being able to prescribe appropriate pain control for their dying patients should take an active role in the legislative and process to ensure that patients' interests are upheld. As part of this effort, physicians could be active in public education about the impact of such legislation as well as contacting legislators directly to voice the concerns of the health care community and make clear the possible unintended consequences.

Finally, but not least in importance, viewing cases through the lens of medical humanities can better enable physicians to understand their patients' experience of pain and alleviate suffering to the extent possible. Thus, legal, social, institutional, policy, and humanistic factors all play a role in such analysis.

**What are Barriers to Practices Bioethicists**

Bioethics education is under funded. The most critical barrier to achieving uniform bioethics education in the medical curriculum is financial constraints.

Bioethics curricula lack national standards. Another barrier to bioethics implementation throughout medical curricula is that there remains substantial variation in the quantity and quality of curriculum. Because the field is fairly new and remains underfunded, less effort has been expended in developing programs than in other aspects of medical education. However, the proliferation of graduate programs awarding Ph.Ds. in bioethics means there will soon be a good supply of well trained persons able to fill this gap.

Bioethics courses are often meager in content. Another barrier is giving bioethics lip service but not substance. Although accrediting organizations require institutions to address ethics issues to some extent, the compliance bar is set fairly low. Institutions with ethics programs that only satisfy the minimum requirement of accrediting agencies do not have adequate services to ensure ethical patient care. Physicians who are mentors and teachers must indicate to students and trainees that ethics is an crucial part of what they are learning. This message must permeate the educational environment. In all these efforts, however, the role of the bioethicist should be one of a colleague possessing specialized knowledge and skills, who is working with doctors, rather than an outside professional seeking to monitor physician behavior.

Patient care may suffer if physicians are not educated about bioethical issues. The most important implication of these barriers is for patient well-being. If young physicians are not taught the importance of bioethics issues for their clinical practice, patients may suffer needless pain, their legal rights of self-determination may be disregarded, and their experience of health care will be less than optimal. If this is to be avoided, bioethics must receive a higher priority in medical education in the future than it has occupied in the past.

It is noted that bioethics education should be mandatory for medical students and physicians. One way to convince medical institutions that bioethics is necessary may be to appeal to their bottom line. If having an excellent bioethics program in a medical school and affiliated teaching hospitals can reduce exposure to legal risks, then administrators may begin to view it as more important. Myra Christopher. has noted that when viewed in this light "good ethics is good business." If appealing to the benefit for suffering patients is insufficient to foster the development and continuation of good bioethics programs, approaching the issue from a legal perspective should provide ample alternative justification. Whichever, rationale is more persuasive, bioethics education should emerge as a permanent and routine part of medical education.

*"Men are neither angels nor devils; that makes morality both necessary and possible."* New technologies force us to make ethical choices. Scientists from the human genome project predict that we will determine the genetic causes of human disease long before treatments are available. Access to genetic and sequence maps will alter the face of clinical medicine in the twenty-first century. With the gap between our ability to diagnose and treat or cure genetic diseases ranging from five to twenty or more years, coupled with the high economic and social costs of disease, there is increasing pressure to explore genetic manipulation of somatic cells. How do we decide among current scientifically available options? How do we make those difficult ethical choices?

Young people are eager to debate ethical issues. Adolescents are passionately interested in ethical questions suggesting adolescence may be a critical period for including bioethics in science education. Knowledge arises when the mind interacts with content; an understanding of ethical issues develops as an evolving process around real-life situations. The question is what role should teachers play in the acquisition of this knowledge?

## How do we Make Ethical Choices?

Do we need to teach bioethics? Plato asked a form of this question more than two thousand years ago: Is ethics taught, inherited or passed on by some other mechanism? Does ethics need to be taught? Experts have studied how we learn ethical concepts and behavior and what roles nature and nurture play in the process (Figure 12.1). Their hypotheses don't always agree.

Some believe that ethics are learned by observation. *Hypothesis 1: Nature is more influential than nurture.* Can the mind actually build knowledge from sensory information? We instinctively know some things, although group interactions and environmental factors may modify this knowledge. For example, as an extension of the mother-infant bond, we learn kinship preferences, recognition of specific individuals, social communication, and long term infant care. Some scientific studies support this view. For example, neurologist Oliver Sacks befriended a young boy named Stephen, an autistic savant who was capable of memorizing complex scenery at a glance and retaining the information for long periods of time. From an early age he appeared to have little need for nurture — human or otherwise.

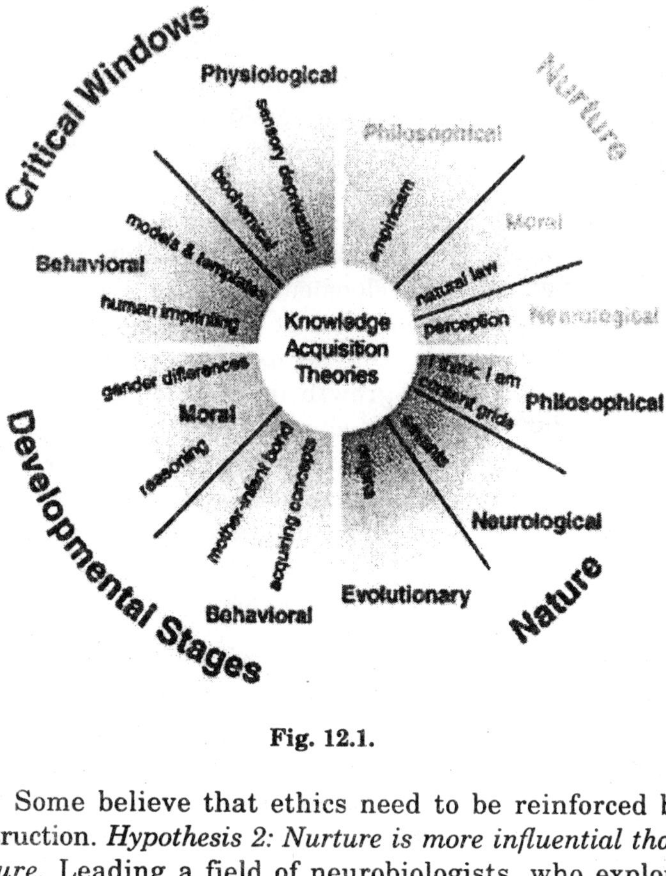


**Fig. 12.1.**

Some believe that ethics need to be reinforced by instruction. *Hypothesis 2: Nurture is more influential than nature.* Leading a field of neurobiologists, who explore how the human brain learns about the world, Nobel

Laureate Gerald Edelman hypothesizes that with repeated experiences, we develop and reinforce anatomically based concept maps. These concept maps subsequently modify how sensory information is processed and organized.

"Natural Law" ethics, which has been traced to the writings of Aristotle and Plato, states that decision-making principles can be discovered through careful reflection and by observing nature. The law of nature, rather than individual preferences, determines what actions are right? The human mind need only possess the capacity for reasoned thought and the ability to communicate.

Some believe that observation is balanced by instruction. *Hypothesis 3: Nature and nurture interact in sequential stages.* In a series of elegantly designed experiments, child psychologist Jean Piaget proposed that children pass through developmental stages where one stage builds on an earlier stage through assimilation and accommodation to the real world. Psychologist Lawrence Kohlberg strongly believed that moral development occurs in six stages. We grow from a point of self-interest to one of an increasingly larger circle of people. Our perspective changes with age and is comparable to growth in areas of psychological development. Educators should note that educational psychologist Carol Gilligan, Kolberg's student, criticizes his theory because it is based on studies of males and, therefore, contains a significant gender bias. Others have also criticized Kohlberg for placing a higher value on one form of moral reasoning over another.

Some believe there is a critical window of opportunity through which we learn bioethics.

*Hypothesis 4: Nurture interacts with nature at the critical window stage.* We appear primed to receive specific environmental stimuli that are most easily incorporated during windows of opportunity (i.e., critical windows). For example:

A familiar example of a critical developmental window is the medical condition known as "lazy eye." If the human brain fails to receive input from both eyes before about the age of five years, the information from the eye with very poor vision is permanently ignored even after corrective surgery or lenses. The acquisition of bird songs has also been extensively studied in the context of what is inherited and learned. For example doves, who have a species specific cooing rhythm, are unaffected by efforts to disrupt their learning. Their song likely has a genetic model that does not require a specific environmental stimulus .The sparrow, however, needs to acquire a template for its species-specific song sometime during its first four months of life. If no template is provided, the sparrow fails to produce a normal song even with subsequent adult song exposure.

Evolutionist Ernst Mayr observes, "Man is distinguished from all other animals by the openness of its behavioral program... so in human beings ethical norms and definite values are laid down in the open behavior program of an infant." He further states this is a very special type of learning akin to imprinting based on an innate capacity to acquire ethical beliefs.

## Observations to Science Education

Students need classroom opportunities to engage in discussions and practice conflict resolution. The acquisition of ethics and other forms of knowledge are dependent on exposure to content, properly timed experiences, and practice with reasoning skills. Since we acquire this knowledge from heritable and external sources, such as the classroom, students need an opportunity to: engage in discussions that allow them to examine their values practice resolving ethical conflicts in a real world context and science discoveries are occurring with unprecedented speed. Every day, we are faced with new ethical choices posed by these discoveries. The inclusion of bioethics in classroom curricula is more important than ever before. Bioethics is an excellent vehicle to generate interest and establish the relevancy of science content:

Bioethics instruction must assist students in distinguishing between fact and opinion. The ambiguities of ethical viewpoints challenge critical thinking abilities and promote the development of problem solving strategies. After students become interested in an ethical problem at the emotional level, they are motivated to discover the facts, better understand the problem, and come up with a reasoned solution and science topics are not void of personal or societal values and are open to subjective interpretation.

It is significant to hole that studying bioethics can help a student's self-discovery process.

- Bioethical decisions often come down to a question of values or determining priorities in competing values. Students need to understand the difference between fact, opinion, and values; and develop an ability to make rational decisions, while recognizing the role of subjective interpretation.

## EDICAL PROFESSIONALISM IN A PHYSICIAN CHARTER

Professionalism is the basis of medicine's contract with society. It demands placing the interests of patients above those of the physician, setting and maintaining standards of competence and integrity, and providing expert advice to society on matters of health. The principles and responsibilities of medical professionalism must be clearly understood by both the profession and society. Essential to this contract is public trust in physicians, which depends on the integrity of both individual physicians and the whole profession.

At present, the medical profession is confronted by an explosion of technology, changing market forces, problems in health care delivery, bioterrorism, and globalization. As a result, physicians find it increasingly difficult to meet their responsibilities to patients and society. In these circumstances, reaffirming the fundamental and universal principles and values of medical professionalism, which remain ideals to be pursued by all physicians, becomes all the more important. The medical profession everywhere is embedded in diverse cultures and national traditions, but its members share the role of the healer, which has roots extending back to Hippocrates. Indeed, the medical profession must contend with complicated political, legal, and market forces. Moreover, there are wide variations in medical delivery and practice through which any general principles may be expressed in both complex and subtle ways. Despite these differences, common themes emerge and form the basis of this charter in the form of three fundamental principles and as a set of definitive professional responsibilities.

Fundamental Principles Principle of primacy of patient welfare. The principle is based on a dedication to serving the interest of the patient. Altruism contributes to the trust that is central to the physician-patient relationship. Market forces, societal pressures, and administrative exigencies must not compromise this principle. Principle of patient autonomy. Physicians must have respect for patient autonomy. Physicians must be honest with their patients and empower them to make informed decisions about their treatment. Patients' decisions about their care must be paramount, as long as those decisions are in keeping with ethical practice and do not lead to demands for inappropriate care. Principle of social justice. The medical profession must promote justice in the health care system, including the fair distribution of health care resources. Physicians should work actively to eliminate discrimination in health care, whether based on race, gender, socioeconomic status, ethnicity, religion, or any other social category.

A Set of Professional Responsibilities Commitment to professional competence. Physicians must be committed to lifelong learning and be responsible for maintaining the medical knowledge and clinical and team skills necessary for the provision of quality care. More broadly, the profession as a whole must strive to see that all of its members are competent and must ensure that appropriate mechanisms are available for physicians to accomplish this goal.

Commitment to honesty with patients physicians must ensure that patients are completely and honestly informed before the patient has consented to treatment and after treatment has occurred. This expectation does not mean that patients should be involved in every minute decision about medical care; rather, they must be empowered to decide on the course of therapy. Physicians should also acknowledge that in health care, medical errors that injure patients do sometimes occur. Whenever, patients are injured as a consequence of medical care, patients should be informed promptly because failure to do so seriously compromises patient and societal trust. Reporting and analyzing medical mistakes provide the basis for appropriate prevention and improvement strategies and for appropriate compensation to injured parties. Commitment to patient confidentiality Earning the trust and confidence of patients requires that appropriate confidentiality safeguards be applied to disclosure of patient information. This commitment extends to discussions with persons acting on a patient's behalf when obtaining the patient's own consent is not feasible. Fulfilling the commitment to confidentiality is more pressing now than ever before, given the widespread use of electronic information systems for compiling patient data and an increasing availability of genetic information. Physicians recognize, however, that their commitment to patient confidentiality must occasionally yield to overriding considerations in the public interest for example, when patients endanger others.

Commitment to maintaining appropriate relations with patients given the inherent vulnerability and dependency of patients, certain relationships between physicians and patients must be avoided. In particular, physicians should never exploit patients for any sexual advantage, personal financial gain, or other private purpose.

## Commitment to Improving Quality of Care

Physicians must be dedicated to continuous improvement in the quality of health care. This commitment entails not only maintaining clinical competence but also working collaboratively with other professionals to reduce medical error, increase patient safety, minimize overuse of health care resources, and optimize the outcomes of care. Physicians must actively participate in the development of better measures of quality of care and the application of quality measures to assess routinely the performance of all individuals, institutions, and systems responsible for health care delivery. Physicians, both individually and through their professional associations, must take responsibility for assisting in the creation and implementation of mechanisms designed to encourage continuous improvement in the quality of care.

## Commitment to Improving Access to Care

Medical professionalism demands that the objective of all health care systems be the availability of a uniform and adequate standard of care. Physicians must individually and collectively strive to reduce barriers to equitable health care. Within each system, the physician should work to eliminate barriers to access based on education, laws, finances, geography, and social discrimination. A commitment to equity entails the promotion of public health and preventive medicine, as well as public advocacy on the part of each physician, without concern for the self-interest of the physician or the profession.

## Commitment to a Just Distribution of Finite Resources

While meeting the needs of individual patients, physicians are required to provide health care that is based on the wise and cost-effective management of limited clinical resources. They should be committed to working with other physicians, hospitals, and payers to develop guidelines for cost effective care. The physician's professional responsibility for appropriate allocation of resources requires scrupulous avoidance of superfluous tests and procedures. The provision of unnecessary services not only exposes one's patients to avoidable harm and expense but also diminishes the resources available for others.

## Commitment to Scientific Knowledge

Much of medicine's contract with society is based on the integrity and appropriate use of scientific knowledge and technology. Physicians have a duty to uphold scientific standards, to promote research, and to create new knowledge and ensure its appropriate use. The profession is responsible for the integrity of this knowledge, which is based on scientific evidence and physician experience. Commitment to maintaining trust by managing conflicts of interest Medical professionals and their organizations have many opportunities to compromise their professional responsibilities by pursuing private gain or personal advantage. Such compromises are especially threatening in the pursuit of personal or organizational interactions with for-profit industries, including medical equipment manufacturers, insurance companies, and pharmaceutical firms. Physicians have an obligation to recognize, disclose to the general public, and deal with conflicts of interest that arise in the course of their professional duties and activities. Relationships between industry and opinion leaders should be disclosed, especially when the latter determine the criteria for conducting and reporting clinical trials, writing editorials or therapeutic guidelines, or serving as editors of scientific journals.

Commitment to professional responsibilities as members of a profession, physicians are expected to work collaboratively to maximize patient care, be respectful of one another, and participate in the processes of self regulation, including remediation and discipline of members who have failed to meet professional standards. The profession should also define and organize the educational and standard-setting process for current and future members. Physicians have both individual and collective obligations to participate in these processes. These obligations include engaging in internal assessment and accepting external scrutiny of all aspects of their professional performance.

The practice of medicine in the modern era is beset with unprecedented challenges in virtually all cultures and societies. These challenges center on increasing disparities among the legitimate needs of patients, the available resources to meet those needs, the increasing dependence on market forces to transform health care systems, and the temptation for physicians to forsake their traditional commitment to the primacy of patients' interests. To maintain the fidelity of medicine's social contract during this turbulent time, we believe that physicians must reaffirm their active dedication to the principles of professionalism, which entails not only their personal commitment to the welfare of their patients but also collective efforts to improve the health care system for the welfare of society. This Charter on Medical Professionalism is intended to encourage such dedication and to promote an action agenda for the profession of medicine that is universal in scope and purpose.

How does one ensure that appropriate ethical values are being applied within hospitals? Effective hospital accreditation requires that ethical considerations are taken into account, for example with respect to physician integrity, conflicts of interest, research ethics and organ transplantation ethics. The following and the imperfect.

### Autonomy

Autonomy is a general indicator of health. Many diseases are characterised by loss of autonomy, in various manners. This makes autonomy an indicator for both personal well-being, and for the well-being of the profession. This has implications for the consideration of medical ethics: "is the aim of health care to do good, and benefit from it?" or "is the aim of health care to do good to others, and have them, and society, benefit from this?" It could be noted that ethics — by definition — tries to find a beneficial balance between the activities of the individual and its effects on a collective. By considering Autonomy as a gauge parameter for (self) health care, the medical and ethical perspective both benefit from the implied reference to Health.

### Beneficence

James Childress and Tom Beauchamp in Principle of Bioethics (1978) identify beneficence as one of the core values of health care ethics. Some scholars, such as Edmund Pellegrino, argue that beneficence is the only fundamental principle of medical ethics. They argue that healing should be the sole purpose of medicine, and that endeavors like cosmetic surgery, contraception and euthanasia fall beyond its purview.

### Non-Maleficence

In practice, however, many treatments carry some risk of harm. In some circumstances, e.g. in desperate situations where the outcome without treatment will be grave, risky treatments that stand a high chance of harming the patient will be justified, as the risk of not treating is also very likely to do harm. So the principle of non-maleficence is not absolute, and must be balanced against the principle of beneficence (doing good).

Some American physicians interpret this principle to exclude the practice of euthanasia, though not all concur.

Probably the most extreme example in recent history of the violation of the non-maleficence dictum was Dr. Jack Kevorkian, who was convicted of second-degree homicide in Michigan in 1998 after demonstrating active euthanasia on the TV news show, 60 Minutes.

In some countries euthanasia is accepted as standard medical practice. Legal regulations assign this to the medical profession. In such nations, the aim is to alleviate the suffering of patients from diseases known to be incurable by the methods known in that culture. In that sense, the "Primum no Nocere" is based on the realisation that the inability of the medical expert to offer help, creates a known great and ongoing suffering in the patient. "Not acting" in those cases is believed to be more damaging than actively relieving the suffering of the patient. Evidently the ability to offer help depends on the limitation of what the practitioner can do. These limitations are characteristic for each different form of healing, and the legal system of the specific culture. The aim to "not do harm" is still the same. It gives the medical practitioner a responsibility to help the patient, in the intentional and active relief of suffering, in those cases where no cure can be offered.

"Non-maleficence" is defined by its cultural context. Every culture has its own cultural collective definitions of 'good' and 'evil'. Their definitions depend on the degree to which the culture sets its cultural values apart from nature. In some cultures the terms "good" and "evil" are absent: for them these words lack meaning as their experience of nature does not set them apart from nature. Other cultures place the humans in interaction with nature, some even place humans in a position of dominance over nature. The religions are the main means of expression of these considerations. Depending on the cultural consensus conditioning expressed by its religious, political and legal social system the legal definition of Non-maleficence differs. Violation of non-maleficence is the subject of medical malpractice litigation. Regulations thereof differ, over-time, per nation.

**Double Effect**

Some interventions undertaken by physicians can create a positive outcome while also potentially doing harm. The combination of these two circumstances is known as the "double effect." The most applicable example of this phenomenon is the use of morphine in the dying patient. Such use of morphine can ease the pain and suffering of the patient, while simultaneously hastening the demise of the patient through suppression of the respiratory drive.

**Informed Consent**

Informed consent in ethics usually refers to the idea that a person must be fully-informed about and understand the potential benefits and risks of their choice of treatment. An uninformed person is at risk of mistakenly making a choice not reflective of his or her values or wishes. It does not specifically mean the process of obtaining consent, nor the specific legal requirements, which vary from place to place, for capacity to consent. Patients can elect to make their own medical decisions, or can delegate decision-making authority to another party. If the patient is incapacitated, laws around the world designate different processes for obtaining informed consent, typically by having a person appointed by the patient or their next-of-kin make decisions for them. The value of informed consent is closely related to the values of autonomy and truth telling.

**Confidentiality**

Confidentiality is commonly applied to conversations between doctors and patients. This concept is commonly known as patient-physician privilege. Legal protections prevent physicians from revealing their discussions with patients, even under oath in court. Confidentiality is also challenged in cases involving the diagnosis of a sexually transmitted disease in a patient who refuses to reveal the diagnosis to a spouse, and in the termination of a pregnancy in an underage patient, without the knowledge of the patient's parents. Traditionally, medical ethics has viewed the duty of confidentiality as a relatively non-negotiable tenet of medical practice. More recently, critics like Jacob Appel have argued for a more nuanced approach to the duty that acknowledges the need for flexibility in many cases.

## Criticisms of Orthodox Medical Ethics

It has been argued that mainstream medical ethics is biased by the assumption of a framework in which individuals are not simply free to contract with one another to provide, whatever medical treatment is demanded, subject to the ability to pay. Because a high proportion of medical care is typically provided via the welfare state, and because there are legal restrictions on what treatment may be provided and by whom, an automatic divergence may exist between the wishes of patients and the preferences of medical practitioners and other parties. Tassano has questioned the idea that Beneficence might in some cases have priority over Autonomy. He argues that violations of Autonomy more often reflect the interests of the state or of the supplier group than those of the patient.

## Importance of Communication

Many so called "ethical conflicts" in medical ethics are traceable back to a lack of communication. Communication breakdowns between patients and their health care team, between family members, or between members of the medical community, can all lead to disagreements and strong feelings. These breakdowns should be remedied, and many apparently insurmountable "ethics" problems can be solved with open lines of communication.

## Ethics Committees

Many times, simple communication is not enough to resolve a conflict, and a hospital ethics committee must convene to decide a complex matter. These bodies are composed primarily of health care professionals, but may also include philosophers, lay people, and clergy.

The assignment of philosophers or clergy will reflect the importance attached by the society to the basic values involved.

## Cultural Concerns

Culture differences can create difficult medical ethics problems. Some cultures have spiritual or magical theories about the origins of disease, for example, and reconciling these beliefs with the tenets of Western medicine can be difficult.

## Truth Telling

Some cultures do not place a great emphasis on informing the patient of the diagnosis, especially when cancer is the diagnosis. Even American culture did not emphasize truth-telling in a cancer case, up until the 1970s. In American medicine, the principle of informed consent takes precedence over other ethical values, and patients are usually at least asked whether they want to know the diagnosis.

## Online Business Practices

The delivery of diagnosis online leads patients to believe that doctors in some parts of the country are at the direct service of drug companies. Finding diagnosis as convenient as what drug still has patent rights on it? Physicians and drug companies are found to be competing for top ten search engine ranks to lower costs of selling these drugs with little to no patient involvement

## Conflicts of Interest

Physicians should not allow a conflict of interest to influence medical judgment. In some cases, conflicts are hard to avoid, and doctors have a responsibility to avoid entering such situations. Unfortunately, research has shown that conflicts of interests are very common among both academic physicians and physicians in practice.

### Referral

For example, doctors who receive income from referring patients for medical tests have been shown to refer more patients for medical tests. This practice is proscribed by the American College of Physicians Ethics Manual.

Fee splitting and the payments of commissions to attract referrals of patients is considered unethical and unacceptable in most parts of the world — while it is rapidly becoming routine in other countries, like India, where many urban practitioners currently pay a percentage of office-visit charges, lab tests as well as hospital care to unaccredited "quacks", or semi-accredited "practitioners of alternative medicine", who refer the patient.

### Vendor Relationships

Studies show that doctors can be influenced by drug company inducements, including gifts and food. Industry-sponsored Continuing Medical Education Programs influence prescribing patterns. Many patients surveyed in one study agreed that physician gifts from drug companies influence prescribing practices. A growing movement among physicians is attempting to diminish the influence of pharmaceutical industry marketing upon medical practice, as evidenced by Stanford University's ban on drug company-sponsored lunches and gifts. Other academic institutions that have banned pharmaceutical industry-sponsored gifts and food include the University of Pennsylvania, and Yale University.

### Treatment of Family Members

Many doctors treat their family members. Doctors who do so must be vigilant not to create conflicts of interest or treat inappropriately.

## Sexual Relationships

Sexual relationships between doctors and patients can create ethical conflicts, since sexual consent may conflict with the fiduciary responsibility of the physician. Doctors who enter into sexual relationships with patients face the threats of deregistration and prosecution. In the early 1990s it was estimated that 2-9% of doctors had violated this rule. Sexual relationships between physicians and patients' relatives may also be prohibited in some jurisdictions, although this prohibition is highly controversial.

## Futility

The concept of medical futility has been an important topic in discussions of medical ethics. What should be done if there is no chance that a patient will survive but the family members insist on advanced care? Previously, some articles defined futiliy as the patient having less than a one per cent chance of surviving. Some of these cases wind up in the courts. Advanced directives include living wills and durable powers of attorney for health care. In many cases, the "expressed wishes" of the patient are documented in these directives, and this provides a framework to guide family members and health care professionals in the decision-making process when the patient is incapacitated. Undocumented expressed wishes can also help guide decisions in the absence of advanced directives. "Substituted judgment" is the concept that a family member can give consent for treatment if the patient is unable (or unwilling) to give consent himself. The key question for the decision-making surrogate is not, "What would you like to do?", but instead, "What do you think the patient would want in this situation?"

# 13

# Clinical Ethics

Clinical ethics is defined as the field of activities that investigate what medical staff as professionals should do or how they should behave concerning a certain individual case, especially in the process of decision-making. Bioethics might also concern such issues, but not exclusively, since its main concern is general theories and not the solution of individual cases.

We need certain ethical principles for the ethical analysis of individual cases. For even if considered on a "case by case" basis, it is not as if the various cases and their analyses have nothing in common. At least the way in which we analyse and consider each case should be uniform, or else our conclusions and choices would be neither accountable, nor reasonable. This uniformity or reasonability, is acquired by basing our decisions on a set of ethical principles. There can be a viewpoint that refuses to follow such ethical principles. We are now in the field of practical case examination.

Three ethical principles in medicine:

- P1: Treat the person(s) you face as a human being(s) in medical activities!
- P2: Intend to promote the well-being of the person(s) you face through medical activities!
- P3: Maintain justice and/or equality through and in medical activities!

P1 is a deontological principle that prescribes how one should engage in one's activities, with specific reference to the process of decision-making and performing a chosen activity. P1 in detail

P2 is a teleological principle, which corresponds with the principle of beneficence and it prescribes the point of view from which an activity should be chosen. P2 in detail

P3 is a principle that takes a social point of view. It serves to check the activities of the medical staff not only by taking into account the interests of the persons they face, but also by balancing it with the interests of third parties.

## Intend to Promote the Well-being of the Person(s) You Face through Medical Activities!

With regard to P2, the term "a person's well-being" needs to be clearly defined. When we ask if a person is well or not, the question can be interpreted in two ways: if his situation is fine or if he lives his life well. The first interpretation refers to his/her given situation or circumstance. The latter one, on the other hand, refers to the person's attitude towards a particular situation, i.e. what he does or intends to do, or how he lives or intends to live in the given situation. According to both interpretations, we can derive a specialized rule under P1.

## The Bodily Situation and Quality of Living: General Assessment

First, let us examine what rule results from the first interpretation of "a person's well-being".

On the basis of the concept of Quality of Living and bodily situation, a rule results from P2:

R2-1: Intend to make the integrated sum of the Quality of Living of the person you face from the present moment until the time of death as much as possible!

Here by "Quality of Living" we primarily mean the bodily Quality of Living, but we would not restrict the term to include only the bodily aspect. Consider the example of a woman who cannot walk by herself, but can move by means of a wheelchair. In this case the weakness in her bodily Quality of Living can be compensated by another aspect of her Quality of Living i.e. her circumstance — that she can use a wheelchair. Creating such a circumstance is included in medical activities. For instance, a man with advanced cancer in his terminal stage, and in need of treatment for his bodily Quality of Living, has to be separated from his family during the course of treatment. In this case, we should estimate not only the predicted improvement in his bodily Quality of Living but also the change for the worse in his family circumstance. Thus, we should estimate not only one's bodily Quality of Living but also the other aspects of one's QOL that relate to one's bodily situation.

### The Private Attitude Towards Life: Interest Individualized

Besides R2-1, which has resulted from the second interpretation of the "person's well-being", we can arrive at another rule on the basis of its first interpretation, which explains well-being as one's attitude towards the given situation. Here P2, which directs the medical staff to "intend to promote the well-being of a person", cannot explicitly direct them to make the person live well by adopting a certain attitude towards his/her life, for this depends exclusively on the person's own ability to adopt a certain attitude. The principle, however, implicitly directs us to let the person live well, or not to prevent him/her from living well, and this is what "intend to promote one's well being" means in this respect. Thus the second specialised rule under P2 is as follows:

### Prevent the Person from Leading a Full Life!

Although P2 does not recommend that the medical staff directly help the patient lead a full life, it does recommend promoting the patient's well-being. The patient's well-being is of value insofar as it provides the patient with a chance to lead a full life, and this is what R1-we explicitly direct the medical staff to do -- improve the person's condition and attend to his/her Quality of Living or freedom from the public point of view.

On the other hand, R2-2 directs by using negative expressions. It does not direct the medical staff positively to help the patient lead a full life, as well as R2-1 doesn't, but negatively not to prevent the patient's activity. This means, they should respect the individual's own preferences and values, which besides the bodily situation and QOL, play an important role in medical decision-making. That is, the patient's overall life-plan and his/her preferences have a casting vote in many cases of decision-making. For instance, Quality of Living consists of several components: physical abilities (i.e., performance status), physical feelings (pain etc.), psychological feelings (anxiety etc.), the capacity to maintain human relationships, and so on. Thus, there can be a case where the patient considers one aspect to be more important than others in order to lead a full life. In such a case, the medics' role is to create circumstances that are conducive to the patient leading a full life. This involves taking care not to prevent him/her from leading a full life.

## Determinants of a Person's Well-being

When we ask if a person is well or not, the question can be interpreted in two ways: if he lives his life well or if his situation is fine. The first interpretation refers to the person's attitude towards a particular situation, i.e. what he does or intends to do, or how he lives or intends to live in the given situation. The latter one, on the other hand, refers to his/her given situation or circumstance. What results from the first interpretation of "a person's well-being"?

By "bodily situation", let us refer to the person's given medical situation. This situation is distinguished from other situations that the person might face, e.g. those concerning society, family, etc. "Health" and "disease", for instance, are terms that describe the bodily situation. Mental health also refers to the state of the person and, therefore, is also part of the bodily situation. The person's bodily situation is not evaluated in biomedical terms. Cancer itself, for instance, is neither good nor bad if judged only from the biological point of view. However, it is said to be bad for two reasons: first, it will result in distressing symptoms in the course of time and, second, it will shorten the patient's life. Correspondingly, the bodily situation of a person who has cancer is judged to be bad because of these predicted effects on the person, even if the person is not aware of his/her situation, or is not actually suffering from any distressing symptoms at present. Thus one's bodily situation is medically evaluated by estimating the impact that one's biological condition has on one's life as a human being, and this evaluation is based not only on one's actual present life, but also on one's predicted future life. Thus, we can define bodily situation in terms of the course of one's actual life, starting from the moment of evaluation.

In order to assess a person's life at a certain moment, we have been using the term *"quality of life"* (QOL). *QOL*, however, consists of many aspects, not all of which directly concern the bodily situation. For instance, one's quality of life is also made up of the quality of one's social and economical state, one's relationships with one's family and friends, the comfort of one's house, and other such situations that do not affect one's bodily situation, at least not directly. Therefore, the question is, which aspects of one's QOL should we consider while evaluating one's bodily situation? To answer this question, we have to clarify the general concept of QOL.

It could be observed that a person's Quality of Living is actually estimated according to the measure of his/her freedom or the actual choices that he or she has at the moment of estimation. For instance, pain and other distressing symptoms are bad because they hold the person against his will and restrict his or her chances of doing things freely. Psychological suffering (anxiety, depression, anger, etc.), physical disabilities and other factors that are negatively evaluated in the assessment of QOL are also bad for the same reason. Again, one's social circumstances might either enable one to do things freely or prevent one from doing them and, therefore, it is also involved in one's QOL. To sum up, QOL is a measure of the patient's actual freedom at the moment of estimation, and we can define the condition of one's own body and mind that concerns one's freedom as "bodily Quality of Living". On the basis of the above conception of bodily Quality of Living, we can conclude that one's bodily situation is estimated as the integrated sum of the freedom made possible by the condition of one's body and mind, from the moment of estimation until the time of death. Let "t1" be the moment of estimation and "td " be the time of death. Then, the relationship between the bodily situation and QOL can be expressed as follows:

The value of a person's bodily situation at t1 is the integrated sum of the person's bodily QOL that is and will be actualized in the course of time from t1 on until td. If you prefer a mathematical formulation, let "B(t)" be the estimated value of the bodily situation at a moment "t" and "Q(t)" be the value of the bodily quality of life at "t".

Then,

$$B(t) = \text{ç}t1_{td}\ Q(t)_{dt}$$

Thus the longer the life span and the higher the QOL at every moment, the better his present bodily situation is.

Quality of Living, i.e. the individual's freedom, at a given moment can be estimated publicly and not privately, though it is mainly estimated on the basis of the patient's self-evaluation. Also the bodily situation at a given moment is estimated in terms of the patient's freedom, though it is valued by means of medical and, therefore scientific inspection.

The rule R1-2, i.e. standing by the patient in suffering also follows from the fact that to treat someone as a human being means to maintain truthful communication with that person, which is what R1-2 prescribes. In such communication, participants can have two different positions: facing each other and facing in the same direction. When the participants face each other, they exchange words and interact with each other. When the participants face the same direction, they share the same view, feelings, ideas, intentions, etc. One position alternates with the other during communication. A patient in suffering is in great need of such communication. He needs someone who is face to face with him, takes care of him, and shares his suffering and awareness of death. The medical staff are therefore, expected to stand by the patient as humane participants in such communication.

## APPROACHES TO THE QUESTION OF DOING CLINICAL ETHICS

The question stresses that ethics consultation is a kind of action or doing and that the action is our thematic focus. Previous discussions of the broad topic of clinical ethics have failed to come to terms with the features that define it as a special type of action. Four broad approaches to the question are evident in the literature.

The first-three, namely, applied ethics, casuistry, and principlism, view clinical ethics from the perspective of ethics while the fourth approach seeks to understand clinical ethics in terms of specific techniques for addressing or resolving conflicts or disagreements. The first approach views clinical ethics, like bioethics generally, as a type of applied ethics or applied philosophy. This approach assumes that clinical ethics involves applying ethical theory and concepts to actual cases of patient care. Some have questioned the possibility and professional legitimacy of this conception of the application of normative knowledge and have pejoratively characterized applied ethics as a kind of engineering. Questions about the application of ethical knowledge, normative ethics, or ethical theory have also been mired in debates over the legitimacy of individuals claiming expertise or professional competence in ethics to testify in courts of law or serve on governmental commissions. This extensive debate, however has not addressed the question of the distinctive type of doing that makes up clinical ethics. Discussion of the application of ethical theory to cases has been conducted primarily as a theoretical or political issue, not as a fundamental issue of methodology.

A second approach views the practical functioning of clinical ethics as the dealing with concrete problems or cases. A number of authors see casuistry as the approach that can guide these activities in dealing with value conflicts and ethical dilemmas arising in medicine. Despite the advocacy for casuistry as cased-based reasoning, defenders of casuistry as a method have not really characterized how casuistry is supposed to function "on the ground," in the actual handling of clinical ethics cases. That is to say, casuistry has been promoted as an alternative to a theory-driven or principle-driven approach because it is putatively focused on the specific circumstances surrounding the problems and issues arising in individual cases. But casuists have little to say about the conditions that are presupposed such as intersubjectivity, communicative discourse, and methodology. Even though casuistry may better attend to the circumstances of cases than other approaches, casuists appear to accept these circumstances as given facts of the case. Casuistic reflection accepts the case, problem, or question as given for ethical reflection without necessarily probing beyond the giveness of the case. It does not readily address how the case came to acquire the sense or meaning that makes it an ethical problem in the first place. In the typical casuistic characterization, the function and engagement of the casuist with the case material is not an essential topic for consideration, yet in the actual doing of ethics consultation how one comports oneself, how one communicates, and how others perceive the clinical ethicist bears significantly on the construction of the meanings (ethical and otherwise) of the case and situation.

The third approach is principlism. Principlism is a broad movement that is committed to the centrality of ethical principles and theories in ethics. Despite criticism of principlism as being a "top-down approach," the best versions of principlism are not slavish to theory and do not presume that the practical process of doing ethics is something as simple as the application of principles to cases. Defenders of principlism have rightly complained that critics have vastly oversimplified what is involved in ethical theory and in the reasoning about the bearing of ethical principles on actual conduct or concrete circumstances? Principlism includes a diverse set of approaches, including Rawlsian reflective equilibrium and specified principlism. Principles are essential, in this view, because they guide the myriad complex judgments that constitute practical ethical decision-making. This point is essentially correct, even though it does not establish principlism as a viable answer to our question.

Like casuistry, principlism takes the case or problem as it is found or given for ethical analysis and reasoning. It does not seriously reflect on the actual conditions under which the ethical problems have acquired their meaning in the specific clinical setting. Furthermore, principlism tends to take theories and principles for granted just as casuistry takes for granted the paradigm cases. Apparently, neither the casuist nor principlist need be involved with the case in the flow of real time to do their work. Both approaches appear to operate comfortably from a position removed from the actual on-going circumstances or experiences of the clinical case.

The fourth approach involves advocacy for one or more specialized techniques for resolving conflicts or disagreements. Specific techniques like arbitration, conflict resolution, and mediation are recommended for effectively addressing ethical conflicts, disputes, or disagreements. Collectively, they appropriately acknowledge the engaged character of clinical ethics, but concentrate on the tasks involved in the resolution of ethical conflicts. In so doing, they overlook other actions or doings that make up clinical ethics. They focus on securing consensus or compromise with little attention given to the meaning of the ethical issue itself. Although promotion of these techniques moves in the direction of the question that we are pursuing, they do not advance us very far because they reduce clinical ethics to the task—oriented activity of resolving problems or conflicts. The utility of these techniques for clinical ethics is not in question, but rather the adequacy of a technical rather than a reflective approach for addressing the meaning of the full range of activities that make up clinical ethics.

Clinical ethics is an activity that is deeply engaged in the clinical setting. Clinical ethics consultants are involved in the cases on which they consult. They communicate with the patients, family members, physicians, nurses, and other health care professionals about the case. They are thus part of the action, on stage, as it were, and not separated from it by the proscenium. They are consultants and not just commentators on the ethical aspects of the case. They use ethical concepts and theories, reason from paradigmatic cases, derive guidance from ethical or bioethics theory for their actions and recommendations, and negotiate and arbitrate, still none of these characterizations fully captures what is distinctive about the doing of clinical ethics?

## ACTIVITIES CENTRAL TO THE FIELD OF CLINICAL ETHICS

Clinical ethics involves actions that shape the underlying structures that give meaning to the case. This involvement changes the case in ways that can be irrevocable and significant. Being involved in real time, the clinical ethicist's actions and interactions with others in the case shapes the very circumstances that give meaning to the case; clinical ethics thus becomes part of the social construction of meaning that is the clinical case. For example, ethics consultants sometimes shape not only the recommendation or interpretation of the value aspects of the case, but the very terms by which patients, families, and health professionals see and experience the situation or problem. In other words, clinical ethics regarded as an action or doing contributes to the social constitution of the meaning of the problems seen as ethical as well as to the mechanisms for their resolution or accommodation. Thus, to be adequate, an account of clinical ethics as an activity needs to make sense of this fundamental involvement of clinical ethics with and in the clinical setting. Making sense of this involvement is critical for the field because controversies about professional status or qualifications hinge on an adequate understanding of the essential nature of what it means to do clinical ethics? Stephen Toulmin claimed that medicine saved the life of ethics by giving it a relevancy that was lost as twentieth century philosophical ethics focused on the analysis of concepts and the justification of theories. This fixation on the formal, theoretical aspects of ethics eclipsed the traditional attention to practical ethical concerns. Medicine may have "saved the life of ethics" by giving it a new relevance, but it did so by drawing individual philosophers from the safe academic waters of conceptual analysis, theory construction, and justification into the more treacherous and uncharted seas of patient care. Medicine caused ethics to become re-engaged with the practical world and to address questions that impact on human well-being.

From the classrooms and lecture halls in colleges and universities, philosophers moved into professional education, where philosophical teaching in courses and seminars had to give way to isolated lectures or modules in the medical school curriculum. They had to adapt to the pedagogical innovations in medical education including the use of simulated patients and problem-based learning. Beyond these educational adaptations, philosophers found themselves serving on committees charged to protect the rights and welfare of research subjects. They were not called upon to criticize, analyze, or to elaborate theoretical distinctions, but to minimize harms or improve consent forms and the process of consent.

Drawn even further away from their home port, some philosophers found themselves in the midst of patient care – in hospitals – serving on ethics committees and providing ethics consultation services at the bedside and during ward or unit rounds. Philosophers became "strangers at the bedside" by coming into the private space of patients and the professional world of medical work, though they did so in a far less intrusive way than Rothman would have us believe. They were often called to the bedside by physicians who genuinely sought ethical advice on patient care problems or dilemmas just as they were previously invited into medical education by deans and department chairmen committed to "humanize" the next generation of physicians, who would have to face the complex questions posed by the expansion of biomedical technology and scientific findings.

Clinical ethics brought ethical reflection into the pilothouse and clinical ethicists acquired the disquieting responsibility to guide the ship of patient care safely through the shoals of ethical conflict and into the port of ethically sound clinical decision-making. This new role was filled with risk and ambiguity, especially for academics, who traditionally dealt with cases of ethical conflicts from a vantage solidly on the shore. Clinical ethics thus put these academics into positions of responsibility far beyond the calm and safe waters of the harbor and lecture hall. This role transformation and its associated anxiety that is at the heart of much of the controversy over the legitimation of clinical ethics remains stuck at the level of politics, however, because the field has not systematically faced the radical nature of this transformation and the responsibilities that it entails. A deep and understandable uncertainty about the engagement of ethics with the clinical world complicates our understanding of this transformation and the responsibilities of clinical ethics. Indeed, the claim that the philosopher or clinical ethicist can or should become so engaged has been highly controversial. The issue of expertise and professional qualifications, which has been the lightening rod of this debate, has unfortunately obscured the difficult question about the methodology of being so engaged which, in turn, has obscured the deeper and important question about the responsibilities involved in doing clinical ethics. Unfortunately, the widespread attention to and debate over the qualifications for doing clinical ethics has actually diverted attention from these questions that are so important to the field of clinical ethics..

## UNDERSTANDING ACTIVITIES OF CLINICAL ETHICS

In this context of contention and confusion, Richard M. Zaner's writings on clinical ethics are especially important for reassigning the proper priority to the question of the meaning of doing clinical ethics. Zaner has devoted a good deal of his work in clinical ethics to a consideration of the clinical nature of clinical ethics. In an early paper in the field, he provocatively asked the question: "Is 'Ethicist' Anything to Call a Philosopher?" In it, he set out the historical context of the question, but skirted the "political" concerns to address the ways in which the specific meaning of being clinical is constituted for ethics in the world of medicine.

The answer that he gives provides a solid foundation for addressing what doing clinical ethics involves? He offers the following characterization. First, clinical ethics issues arise and must be understood within the context of their occurrence, that is, within the specific clinical case and setting. Second, each case is characterized by uncertainty and ambiguity that is unique to the case. Third, the case and its issues are co-constituted by the individuals involved therein and the issues derive their fundamental ethical import from this constitution. Fourth, each case is structured by fallible assessments and decisions that have an inherent complexity that may not be readily reducible to simpler elements. Zaner offers a far more nuanced exposition of these points than can be commented upon in this paper, but three observations can provide reliable signposts on our way toward the question of the doing clinical ethics.

The first signpost is that clinical ethics is essentially and inextricably bound up with actual cases. That is, one cannot think about clinical ethics or purport to be a clinical ethicist without active engagement with actual cases of patient care. That means that academic bioethicists, who view themselves as engaged in a clinical enterprise because they think about medicine or review cases on committees are fundamentally mistaken. Clinical ethics requires an extensive and active engagement with patient care. It cannot be done from afar, but involves the clinical ethicist in the actual setting of clinical cases because the specific circumstances of the case provide the structures of ethical meaning.

The second signpost is that the meaning and interpretation of the actions in the clinical case are co-constituted by the individuals involved therein. In other words, the case as a clinical ethical reality does not exist apart from the particular individuals involved in the case. The clinical ethicist, as a participant in the case, brings skills of assessment and judgment to bear on the specific circumstances of the case. In this regard it is worth noting that Zaner's discussion of the conception of the clinical ethicist as an expert appears to be grounded in his conviction that the case, with its complex circumstances and structures of meaning, is so integral to the functioning of the clinical ethicist that a knowledge or expertise that is independent of the case will be fundamentally insufficient. That is why he sees merit in the view that the clinical ethicist is a facilitator working with others in the case? The element that is essential for Zaner, however is not the technique of facilitation as such, but the fact that the facilitation essentially involves an interpretive interaction with others in the case. This is the essential point that needs emphasis, because he does not sufficiently consider that the skills of interpretation and reflection that are so well-exemplified in his own work constitute a type of expertise – at least in the sense of discipline or skill – that are needed for effective and responsible engagement with the case in doing clinical ethics. Both elements, the possession of the skills and discipline and exercise of these capacities are essential for understanding clinical ethics.

The debate over expertise or authority in clinical ethics has unfortunately assumed the independent possession of ethical knowledge and has given little attention to the type of practical knowledge involved in doing clinical ethics. It is stressed in a discussion of the importance of the question of method for ethics consultation, the rules guiding ethics consultative activities have relevance and meaning for the practice of ethics consultation only to the extent that they are actually enacted in the particular case. Analysis of the nature of authority in ethics consultation thus leads to a consideration of the conditions under which participants in a case are able, inclined, and willing to even listen to an ethics consultant. Zaner's work helpfully makes clear that the question of the nature and scope of clinical ethics is, at bottom, a general problem of the social constitution of the meaning of clinical ethics as a practice. All individuals involved in the case thus constitute the meaning of the case as they interact, agree, and disagree. This observation highlights a corollary point, namely, that the clinical ethics essentially entails the practical function of co-constituting the ethical meanings of the case. Thus, the perspective that provides the best vantage point for accurately reflecting on the doing of clinical ethics is one that is itself engaged in the activity of clinical ethics. It is also a perspective that must accept responsibility for the involvement.

Zaner rightly characterizes this approach as a social phenomenological one, because the doing of clinical ethics is a special problem of the social constitution of the social world of the clinical ethics case. That Zaner's work stresses the clinical element in clinical ethics thus is not a conceit or an allusion to an esoteric medical knowledge, but as an essential recognition that the meaning of clinical ethics is embedded in the active social construction of meaning in the particular case.

The third signpost on the way toward the question of the meaning of the doing of clinical ethics is that the distinctively clinical character of the case is not reducible to or captured by the specific physical setting of the hospital or bedside, the interaction with patients/families or health professionals, or the possession of a specific clinical knowledge or qualification. Rather, the clinical nature of clinical ethics is bound up with being actively involved in patient care and is normatively guided by the overriding therapeutic nature of patient care. Clinical ethics is, therefore wrongly conceived as the ethics of cases or problems that happen to involve medicine and patient care; rather, it is essentially about and involved with the delivery of patient care. The therapeutic goal thus imparts a normative structure to the activities comprising clinical ethics. Since it is ultimately about therapy, clinical ethics must, quite remarkably, also incorporate and accommodate this therapeutic orientation.

These observations summarize our understanding of Zaner's complexly articulated reflections on clinical ethics. His writings are remarkably unlike those of other bioethicists, because he confronts the doing of clinical ethics from within the perspective of the activity itself. This is a difficult, even arduous, task. It requires that the one who is engaged as a clinical ethicist also must sustain a reflection on the meaning and the conditions of the activity. This undertaking, odd and difficult though it may be, is critical for the field, and Zaner's work blazes a path toward the question of what it means to do clinical ethics.

As Alfred Schu¨ tz has shown in his fundamental work on the phenomenology of the everyday social world, a social scientist can have no privileged position of observation, but is always intertwined with his subject-matter. This involvement is quite unlike the mythical distance that is supposed to exist between the natural scientist and the objects of investigation. Reflecting on clinical ethics is thus a reflection in the midst of the things themselves, namely, the active engagement in the clinical ethics enterprise itself. There is simply no substitute. There is also no special position of privilege earned by this unique undertaking. The only grounding that exists for this doing is thus to be located in the particular circumstances of the individual case as well as the assiduous adherence to methodological and evidentiar standards that are lamentably peripheral concerns for the field.

## PIVOTAL POSITION OF THE PATIENT CARE

Zaner's work moves our question of the meaning of clinical ethics forward by merging it with a broader discussion of the meaning of patient care and clinical medicine. His work shows that the term clinical ethics is ambiguous, because it includes both the activity of the person in the role of the clinical ethicist and the ethical meanings and values exhibited in the actions of all – patients, family members, physicians, and other health care professionals – who are involved in the clinical case. This broad inclusion is necessary, because the ethical meaning of the case is socially constructed, like all meanings in the everyday world of experience. From this perspective, doing clinical ethics becomes less a matter of deploying specific techniques for pre-given ethical problems than an existential and ethical encounter with the sick and their need for care.

The clinical ethicist is never just an observer or spectator, but a participant in the world of patient care that alters the meaning that makes up the real experiences underlying any narrative about the case. The presence of the clinical ethicist in the case and the reflection on the clinical situation that this presence makes possible stand in need of the most careful description. That is why before it can be explained, justified, or legitimated, the doing of the clinical ethics must be accurately described and understood.

For this reason, the clinical cases that Zaner discusses are often presented less as "ethics" cases *per se*, than as cases narrating the actual lives, feelings, and sufferings of patients, the struggles of families and health care professionals as they struggle to come to terms with illness. Even though ethical or value considerations seem to ooze from these situations and relationships, Zaner's case discussions are remarkably bereft of the typical ethical vocabulary of rights, duties, or virtues. In part this is due to his concentration on the actual clinical and scientific challenges facing physicians and other health care professionals as they diagnose and devise treatments for their patients. In an important sense, these case discussions are not presentations of ethics cases as such, but renditions of the practical experiences involved in trying to understand the structures of meaning constituted in and for the case.

The activities associated with patient care all involve a concern for relevance. Patient care is a world of work, not a realm of ideas or speculation. It is a space in which the concern for the patient primarily drives not only the therapeutic, but the analytic and intellectual functions of health professionals as well. This focus on the patient and the patient's well-being gives patient care not only an "ethical" orientation as a patient rights approach to medicine would insist, but also a distinctively practical orientation within which clinical ethics has to operate and create meaning. This practical focus sharply differentiates clinical ethics from ethics or bioethics conducted in universities where freedom of inquiry and the pursuit of knowledge for its own sake are in the main unfettered by practical demands. In the clinical setting, the purpose and vector of reflection and action is ultimately practical rather than intellectual. Problems thus emerge and are identified as "ethical" as the result of a specific interpretation of some blockage in the course of patient care. Therefore, the need for a solution is driven by a practical, not intellectual concern. This helps to explain why problems that are brought for ethics consultation are widely recognized as not strictly ethical problems, but communication problems. The accuracy of the characterization of the problem in the request for clinical ethics help is no more essential for the competent handling of the case than is the accuracy of the characterization of shortness of breath, fatigue, and nausea by a patient as "probably only a cold." The competent physician will listen to the patient's complaint and presentation of symptoms, but go further to ascertain a deeper and more relevant history of the symptoms, elicit signs of illness and, perhaps, order tests to reach a diagnosis. Similarly, although a clinical ethics case may start with the request for "ethics" help, the first activity of clinical ethics involves a probing of the structures of meaning operating in the request for assistance. Thus, it is wrong to think that clinical ethics should primarily respond with a readymade technique like mediation or conflict resolution. Instead, the first response must be the interpretive process of uncovering the actual and latent structures of ethical meaning involved in the case. Thus, to the question why one might do clinical ethics as a philosopher, Zaner gives the very reasonable answer that one cannot seriously and competently reflect on medicine and its ethics without fully engaging the concrete clinical situation.

## Case Analysis in Clinical Ethics

Clinical ethics is a practical discipline that provides a structured approach to assist physicians in identifying, analyzing and resolving ethical issues in clinical medicine. The practice of good clinical medicine requires some working knowledge about ethical issues such as informed consent, truth-telling, confidentiality, end-of-life care, pain relief, and patient rights. Medicine, even at its most technical and scientific, is an encounter between human beings, and the physician's work of diagnosing disease, offering advice, and providing treatment is embedded in a moral context. Usually, moral values such as mutual respect, honesty, trustworthiness, compassion, and a commitment to pursue shared goals, make a clinical encounter between physician and patient morally unproblematic. Occasionally, physicians and patients may disagree about values or face choices that challenge their values. It is then that ethical problems arise. Clinical ethics is both about the ethical features that are present in every clinical encounter and about the ethical problems that occasionally arise in those encounters. Clinical ethics relies upon the conviction that, even when perplexity is great and emotions run high, physicians and nurses, patients and families can work constructively to identify, analyze and resolve many of the ethical problems that arise in clinical medicine.

The authors have two purposes in writing this book: first, to offer an approach that facilitates thinking about the complexities of the problems that clinicians actually face and, second, to assemble concise representative opinions about typical ethical problems that occur in the practice of medicine. We think it is more important that clinicians develop skill at analyzing the cases they encounter rather than merely have a book in which "to look up answers." Our hope is that every clinician will acknowledge that ethics is an inherent aspect of good clinical medicine and that, ideally, every clinician will become as proficient at clinical ethics as clinical medicine. Our book is intended not only for clinicians and students who provide care to patients, but also for others whose work requires an awareness and sensitivity to the ethical issues raised in clinical care, such as hospital administrators, hospital attorneys, members of institutional ethics committees, quality reviewers and administrators of health plans. In the complex world of modern health care, all of these persons are responsible for maintain the ethics that lie at the heart of quality care.

Many books on health care ethics are organized around moral principles, such as respect for autonomy, beneficence, non-maleficence and fairness, and the cases are analyzed in the light of those principles. Our method is different. While we appreciate the importance of principles, we believe that the practitioner approaching a case needs a method that better fits the realities of the clinical setting and the reasoning of the clinician. Clinical situations are complex since they often involve a wide range of medical facts, a multitude of circumstances and a variety of values. Often decisions must be reached quickly. The authors believe that clinicians need a straightforward way to sort the facts and values of the case at hand into an orderly pattern that will facilitate the discussion and resolution of the ethical problem.

We suggest that every clinical case, when seen as an ethical problem, should be analyzed by means of four topics. These four topics are:

1. Medical Indications;
2. Patient Preferences;
3. Quality of Life,
4. Contextual Features.

That is, the social, economic, legal, and administrative context in which the case occurs. Every case can be viewed in terms of these four topics; no case can be adequately discussed without reference to them. Although the facts of each case differ, these four topics are always relevant. The topics organize the varying facts of the particular case and, at the same time, the topics call attention to the moral principles appropriate to the case. It is our intent to show readers how the topics provide a systematic way to identify, analyze and resolve the ethical problems arising in clinical medicine.

Clinicians will recall the method of case presentation that they learned at the beginning of their professional training. They were taught to "present" a patient by stating in order the patient's history, including the chief complaint, the history of the present illness, past medical history, family and social history, followed by physical findings and laboratory data. These are the topics that an experienced clinician uses to reach a diagnosis and to formulate a case management plan. While the particular details under each of these topics differ from patient to patient; the topics themselves are constant and always relevant to the task of arriving at a case management plan. Sometimes one topic, for example, the patient's family history or the physical examination, may be particularly important or, conversely, may not be relevant to the problem at hand. Still, clinicians are expected to review all topics in every case. Our four topics — (1) Medical Indications, (2) Patient Preferences, (3) Quality of Life, and (4) Contextual Features—are the ethical equivalents of these familiar clinical topics.

These topics help clinicians understand where the moral principles meet the circumstances of the clinical case. The general headings of the topics describe the major features that define the ethics of clinical medicine; each of these features takes on specific, concrete form from the circumstances of the particular case. In a given case, a patient comes to a physician, complaining of feeling ill. Medical Indications include a clinical picture of polydipsia and polyuria, nausea, fatigue and some mental confusion, with laboratory studies showing hyperglycemia, acidosis and elevated plasma ketone concentrations. A diagnosis of diabetic ketoacidosis is made. Fluids and insulin are indicated in specific doses and volumes. These particulars are the occasion for implementing the moral principle of beneficence, that is, the duty of performing actions that benefit the patient. However, in the same case, the patient may be confused and, after hearing the physician's recommendations, rejects further medical attention: these circumstances, noted under Patient Preferences, raise questions about the principle of autonomy, that is, the duty to respect the patient's wishes. As the case is described, circumstances accumulate under all four of the topics and affect the meaning and relevance of the moral principles. It is advisable to review the entire four topics in order to see how the principles and the circumstances together define the ethical problem in the case and suggest a resolution. It is rare that an ethical problem involves only one ethical principle. Every actual ethical problem is a complex collection of many circumstances. Good ethical judgment consists in appreciating how several ethical principles should be evaluated in the actual situation under consideration. We hope our method helps practitioners to do just that.

For example, the case of a Jehovah's Witness patient who refuses blood transfusion will demonstrate how the topic of Patient Preferences functions in the analysis of the ethical problem raised by a patient's refusal of an indicated medical treatment.

**Medical Indications** this topic comprises the usual content of a clinical discussion: the diagnosis and treatment of the patient's pathological condition. "Indications" refers to the relation between the pathophysiology presented by the patient and the diagnostic and therapeutic interventions that are "indicated," that is, appropriate to evaluate and treat the problem. Although this is the usual material covered in the presentation of any patient's clinical problems, the ethical discussion will not only review the medical facts, but also attend to the purposes and goals of any indicated interventions.

In Dax's case, the medical indications include the clinical facts necessary to diagnose the extent and seriousness of burns, to make a prognosis for survival or restoration of function, and the options for treatment, including the risks, benefits and probable outcomes of each treatment modality. For example, certain prognoses are associated with burns of given severity and extent. Various forms of treatment, such as fluid replacement, skin grafting and antibiotics are associated with certain probabilities of outcome and risk. After initial emergency treatment, Dax's prognosis for survival was approximately 20%. After six months of intensive care, his prognosis for survival improved to almost 100%. If his request to stop wound care and grafting during that hospitalization had been respected, he would almost certainly have died. A clear view of the possible benefits of intervention is the first step in assessing the ethical aspects of a case.

Patient preferences in all medical treatment, the preferences of the patient, based on the patient's own values and personal assessment of benefits and burdens are ethically relevant. In every clinical case, the questions must be raised: "What are the patient's goals? What does the patient want?" The systematic review of this topic requires further questions. Has the patient been provided sufficient information? Does the patient comprehend? Does the patient understand the uncertainty inherent in any medical recommendation and the range of reasonable options that exist? Is the patient consenting voluntarily? Is the patient coerced? In some cases, an answer to these questions might be "We don't know because the patient is incapable of formulating a preference or expressing one." If the patient is mentally incapacitated at the time a decision must be made, we must ask "Who has the authority to decide on behalf of this patient? What are the ethical and legal limits of that authority? What is to be done if no one can be identified as surrogate?

In Dax's case, a question about his mental capacity arose in the early days of his refusal of care. Had the physical and emotional shock of the accident undermined his ability to decide for himself? Initially it was assumed that he lacked the capacity to make his own decisions, at least about refusing life-saving therapy. The doctors accepted the consent of Dax's mother in favor of treatment, over his refusal of treatment. Later, when Dax was hospitalized in Galveston, psychiatric consultation was requested which affirmed his capacity to make decisions. Once capacity was established, the ethical implications of his desire to refuse care became central. Should his preference be respected? If not, on what grounds? Did Dax appreciate sufficiently the prospects for his rehabilitation? Are physicians obliged to pursue therapies they believe have promise over the objections of a patient? Would they be cooperating in a suicide if they assented to Dax's wishes? Any case involving the ethics of patient preferences relies on clarification of these questions.

Quality of Life. Any injury or illness threatens persons with actual or potential reduced quality of life, manifested in the signs and symptoms of their disease. The object of all medical intervention is to restore, maintain or improve quality of life. Thus, in all medical situations, the topic of quality of life must be raised. Many questions surround this topic: What does this phrase, "quality of life" mean in general? How should it be understood in particular cases? How do persons other than the patient perceive the patient's quality of life and of what ethical relevance are their perceptions? Above all, what is the relevance of quality of life to ethical judgment? This topic, which is less well worked out in the literature of medical ethics than the two previous ones, is perilous because it opens the door for bias and prejudice. Still, it must be confronted in the analysis of clinical ethical problems.

In Dax's case, we note the quality of his life prior to the accident. He was a popular, athletic young man, just discharged from the Air Force, after serving as a fighter pilot in Viet Nam. He worked in a real estate business with his father who was also injured in the explosion and died on the way to the hospital. Before his accident, Dax's quality of life was excellent. During the course of medical care, he endured excruciating pain and profound depression. After the accident, even with the best of care, he was confronted with significant physical deficits, including notable disfigurement, blindness and limitation of activity. At some stage in his illness, Dax had the capacity to determine what quality of life he wished for himself. However, in the early weeks of his hospitalization, he was probably mentally incapacitated at the time critical decisions had to be made. When he was, others would have had to make certain "quality of life" decisions on his behalf. Was the prospect for return to a normal or even acceptable life so poor that no reasonable person would choose to live? Who should make such decisions? What values should guide them? The meaning and import of such considerations must be clarified in any clinical ethical analysis.

Contextual Features Patients come to physicians because they have a problem that they hope the physician can help to correct. Physicians undertake the care of patients with the intent and the duty to make all reasonable efforts to help them. The topics of medical indications, patient preferences and quality of life bring out these essential features of the case. Yet every medical case is embedded in a larger context of persons, institutions, financial and social arrangements. Patient care is influenced, positively or negatively, by the possibilities and the constraints of that context. At the same time, the context itself is affected by the decisions made by or about the patient: these decisions have psychological, emotional, financial, legal, scientific, educational, religious impact on others. In every case, the relevance of the contextual features must be determined and assessed. These contextual features may be crucially important to the understanding and resolution of the case.

In Dax's case, several of these contextual features were significant. Dax's mother was opposed to termination of medical care for religious reasons. The legal implications of honoring Dax's demand were unclear at the time they are clearer today. The costs of sixteen months of intensive burn therapy are not insignificant although this was not emphasized in the various discussions of the case. The distress caused to medical and nursing personnel by Dax's refusal to cooperate with treatment might have influenced their attitudes toward him. These and other contextual factors must be made explicit and assessed for their relevance.

These four topics are relevant to any clinical case, whatever the actual circumstances. They serve as a useful organizing device for teaching and discussion. More important, however, is the way in which a review of these topics can help to move a discussion of an ethical problem toward a resolution. Any serious discussion of an ethical problem must go beyond merely talking about it in an orderly way: it must push through to a reasonable and practical resolution. Ethical problems, no less than medical problems, cannot be left hanging. Thus, after presenting a case, the task of seeking a resolution must begin.

The discussion of each topic raises, or presupposes, certain common ethical notions. These notions propose certain standards of behavior or attitudes that are morally appropriate to the topic. They can be called moral principles or rules: rules tend to be quite specific to particular topics, while principles are stated in broader, more general terms. For example, one version of the principle of beneficence states, "There is an obligation to assist others in the furthering of their legitimate interests." The moral rule, "physicians have a duty to treat patients, even at risk to themselves," is a specific expression of that broad principle, suited to a particular sphere of professional activity, namely, medical care. The topic of medical indications, in addition to the clinical data that must be discussed, raises the further questions, "How much can we do to help this patient?" "What risks of adverse effects can be tolerated in the attempt to treat the patient?" Answers to these questions, arising so naturally in the discussion of medical indications, can be guided by familiar moral rules applied to medical ethics such as, "Be of benefit and do no harm" or "Risks should be balanced by benefits." Rules such as these reflect in a specific way the broad principle that the philosophers have named beneficence. Similarly, the topic of patient preferences contains rules that instruct clinicians to tell patients the truth, to respect their deliberate preferences, to honor their values, etc. Rules such as these fall under the general scope of the principles of autonomy and respect for persons.

This method of analysis begins, not with the principles and rules, as do many other ethics treatises, but with the factual features of the case. We refer to relevant principles and rules as they arise in the discussion of the topics. In this way, abstract discussions of principles is avoided as is the tendency to think of only one principle, such as autonomy or beneficence, as the sole guide in the case. Moral rules and principles are best appreciated in the specific context of the actual circumstances of a case. For example, a key issue in Dax's case is the autonomy of the patient. However, the significance of autonomy in Dax's case is derived, not simply from the principle that requires we respect it, but from the confluence of considerations about preferences, medical indications for treatment, quality of life, decisional capacity, and the role of his mother, the doctors, the lawyers and the hospitals. Only when all these are seen and evaluated in relation to each other, will the meaning of the principle of autonomy be appreciated in this case.

## Sample Case Analysis

### *Case*

John, a 32 years old lawyer, had worried for several years about developing Huntington's chorea, a neurological disorder that appears in a person's 30s or 40s, bringing rapid uncontrollable twitching and contractions and progressive, irreversible dementia. It leads to death in about 10 years.

John's mother died from this disease. Huntington's is autosomal dominant and afflicts 50% of an affected parent's offspring. John had indicated to many people that he would prefer to die rather than to live and die as his mother had. He was anxious, drank heavily, and had intermittent depression, for which he saw a psychiatrist. Nevertheless, he was a productive lawyer.

John first noticed facial twitching 3 months ago, and 2 neurologists independently confirmed a diagnosis of Huntington's. He explained his situation to his psychiatrist and requested help committing suicide. When the psychiatrist refused, John reassured him that he did not plan to attempt suicide any time soon. But when he went home, he ingested all his antidepressant medicine after pinning a note to his shirt to explain his actions and to refuse any medical assistance that might be offered. His wife, who did not yet know about his diagnosis, found him unconscious and rushed him to the emergency room without removing the note.

What should the care team at the emergency room do?

## Review of Topics

### *Medical Indications*

There are 2 diagnoses/prognoses that merit consideration. The underlying chronic disease of Huntington's has no available treatment and a bleak long-term prognosis. However, there are effective treatments available for the acute diagnosis of drug overdose. How does the chronic diagnosis affect our response to the acute condition?

### *Patient Preferences*

We know from the patient's suicide note that he is refusing all medical treatment. However, what do we know about these statements of preference? Were they informed? Was the patient competent to make that decision? The answers to these questions remain unclear, but we do know that the patient does not have decision-making capacity for the present decision of whether to proceed with the gastric emptying. Is there a surrogate decision-maker available?

### *Quality of Life*

Life with Huntington's can be difficult with the onset of spasms and dementia. John was familiar with the quality of life associated with living with Huntington's as he watched his mother die of this disease. On the other hand, John does have a supportive family and continues to be able to work for the time being. How should the diminished quality of life that is anticipated in the future affect the current decision?

### *Contextual Features*

Several factors in the context of this case are significant. While the patient has a legal right to refuse treatment, he is currently unconscious and his surrogate i.e., his wife is requesting treatment. There are also certain emergency room obligations to treat emergent conditions. How should the emergency staff weigh the various competing legal and regulatory duties?

### *Case Analysis*

This is a case of treatment refusal of potentially life-sustaining treatment when the competency of the patient to decide is questionable. Also at issue is the distinction between the acute and chronic conditions of the patient.

The precedent for cases such as this one is fairly clear. When the patient's preferences are unclear, and the acute condition is easily treatable, and the harm of not treating is very great, medical teams can feel comfortable about providing the treatment for the immediate life-threatening condition, creating an opportunity to talk with the patient about his preferences regarding his chronic condition at a later time.

Notice that the facts of this particular case determine if the precedent case is applicable. If the medical team was very familiar with this patient's expressed preference to refuse any medical treatment or if the available treatment for the acute condition was considerably less certain to be effective, the case could be decided differently. The clinicians would look for a different precedent or consider whether it made a significant difference to be very clear about the patient's beliefs and certain about his competency to decide to refuse.

# Index

**Q**



**R**



**S**